WITHDRAWN

DATE DUE	
APR 0 3 1996	
MAR 0 5 1997	
JUN 1 8 1997	
~~MAY 0 2 2000~~	
MAR 0 8 2000	
MAY 0 2 2005 04/30/05	
JAN 0 3 2006	

Physical Therapy of the Shoulder
Second Edition

CLINICS IN PHYSICAL THERAPY

Other Titles Available

Cardiac Rehabilitation
Louis R. Amundsen, Ph.D., guest editor

Electrotherapy
Steven L. Wolf, Ph.D., guest editor

Rehabilitation of the Burn Patient
Vincent R. DiGregorio, M.D., guest editor

Measurement in Physical Therapy
Jules M. Rothstein, Ph.D., guest editor

Hand Rehabilitation
Christine A. Moran, M.S., R.P.T., guest editor

Sports Physical Therapy
Donna Bernhardt, M.S., R.P.T., A.T.C., guest editor

Pain
John L. Echternach, Ed.D., guest editor

Physical Therapy of the Low Back
Lance T. Twomey, Ph.D., and James R. Taylor, M.D.,
Ph.D., guest editors

Therapeutic Considerations for the Elderly
Osa Littrup Jackson, Ph.D., guest editor

Physical Therapy of the Foot and Ankle
Gary C. Hunt, M.A., P.T., guest editor

Physical Therapy Management of Arthritis
Barbara Banwell, M.A., P.T., and Victor Gall, M. Ed., P.T., guest editors

**Physical Therapy of the Cervical and
Thoracic Spine**
Ruth Grant, M.App.Sc., Grad.Dip.Adv.Man.Ther.,
guest editor

**TMJ Disorders: Management of the
Craniomandibular Complex**
Steven L. Kraus, P.T., guest editor

Physical Therapy of the Knee
Robert E. Mangine, M.Ed., P.T., A.T.C., guest editor

**Obstetric and Gynecologic Physical
Therapy**
Elaine Wilder, R.P.T., M.A.C.T., guest editor

**Physical Therapy of the Geriatric Patient,
2nd Ed.**
Osa L. Jackson, Ph.D., R.P.T., guest editor

Physical Therapy for the Cancer Patient
Charles L. McGarvey III, M.S., P.T., guest editor

Gait in Rehabilitation
Gary L. Smidt, Ph.D., guest editor

Physical Therapy of the Hip
John L. Echternach, Ed.D., P.T., guest editor

Forthcoming Volumes in the Series

**Pediatric Neurologic Physical Therapy,
2nd Ed.**
Suzann K. Campbell, Ph.D., guest editor

Pulmonary Management in Physical Therapy
Cynthia Zadai, M.S., P.T., guest editor

Physical Therapy Management of Parkinson's Disease
George I. Turnbull, M.A., P.T., guest editor

Physical Therapy of the Shoulder

Second Edition

Edited by
Robert A. Donatelli, M.A., P.T.

Instructor
School of Rehabilitation Medicine
Emory University
Co-Founder
Physical Therapy Associates of Metro Atlanta
Atlanta, Georgia

CHURCHILL LIVINGSTONE
New York, Edinburgh, London, Madrid, Milan, Melbourne, Tokyo

Library of Congress Cataloging-in-Publication Data

Physical therapy of the shoulder / edited by Robert A. Donatelli. —
  2nd ed.
       p. cm. — (Clinics in physical therapy)
    Includes bibliographical references.
    Includes index.
    ISBN 0-443-08731-8
    1. Shoulder—Wounds and injuries—Treatment. 2. Shoulder joint—
Wounds and injuries—treatment. 3. Shoulder—diseases—treatment.
4. Shoulder joint—Diseases—Treatment. 5. Physical therapy.
I. Donatelli, Robert. II. Series.
    [DNLM: 1. Physical therapy—methods. 2. Shoulder—injuries.
3. Shoulder joint—injuries. WE 810 P578]
    RD557.5.P48 1991
    617.5′ 72062—dc20
    DNLM/DLC
    for Library of Congress   90-2397
                                                CIP

Second edition© Churchill Livingstone Inc. 1991
First edition © Churchill Livingstone Inc. 1987

Distributed in the United Kingdom by Churchill Livingstone, Robert Stevenson House, 1–3
Baxter's Place, Leith Walk, Edinburgh EH1 3AF, and by associated companies, branches,
and representatives throughout the world.

Accurate indications, adverse reactions, and dosage schedules for drugs are provided in this
book, but it is possible that they may change. The reader is urged to review the package
information data of the manufacturers of the medications mentioned.

The Publishers have made every effort to trace the copyright holders for borrowed material.
If they have inadvertently overlooked any, they will be pleased to make the necessary
arrangements at the first opportunity.

Acquisitions Editor: *Kim Loretucci*
Copy Editor: *Elizabeth Bowman*
Production Designer: *Patricia McFadden*
Production Supervisor: *Jeanine Furino*

Printed in the United States of America

First published in 1991   7 6 5 4

I would like to dedicate this book to my late father, Revy Donatelli, and to my mother, Rose Donatelli. They provided the guidance, motivation, and love to help me through my college years, enabling me to pursue a career in physical therapy.

Contributors

Mark S. Albert, M.Ed., P.T., A.T.C.
Assistant Professor, Department of Physical Therapy, College of Health Sciences, Georgia State University; Assistant Athletic Trainer, Georgia Tech Athletic Association; Director and Co-owner, Private Practice, Atlanta, Georgia; Board Certified Specialist in Sports Physical Therapy, American Physical Therapy Association, 1987

Larry F. Andrews, J.D., P.T.
Supervisor, Orthopedic Physical Therapy, Emory University Hospital and Emory Clinic, Atlanta, Georgia

Edward Ayub, M.S., P.T.
Private Practice, Orthopaedic and Sports Physical Therapy, San Diego, California

Turner A. Blackburn, Jr., M.Ed., P.T., A.T.C.
Adjunct Assistant Professor, Department of Physical Therapy, Columbus College, University of Georgia; Director of Physical Therapy, Rehabilitation Services of Columbus, Inc., Columbus, Georgia

Robert Burnham, M.D., F.R.C.P.(C)
Consultant in Physical Medicine, The Glen Sather Sports Medicine Clinic, The University of Alberta Faculty of Medicine, Edmonton, and the Red Deer Regional Hospital, Red Deer, Alberta, Canada

David J. Conaway, D.O.
Clinical Associate Professor, Department of Orthopaedics, West Virginia School of Osteopathic Medicine, Lewisburg, West Virginia; Private Practice, Lilburn, Georgia

Robert A. Donatelli, M.A., P.T.
Instructor, School of Rehabilitation Medicine, Emory University; Co-Founder, Physical Therapy Associates of Metro Atlanta, Atlanta, Georgia

Martha Kaput Frame, M.S., P.T.
Instructor, Dogwood Seminars; Clinical Specialist in Orthopedics, Physical Therapy Associates of Metro Atlanta, Atlanta, Georgia

Bruce H. Greenfield, M.M.Sc., P.T.
Clinical Instructor, Graduate Program in Orthopedic Physical Therapy, Emory University School of Medicine; Private Practice, Physical Therapy Associates of Metro Atlanta, Atlanta, Georgia

Sanford E. Gruskin, D.D.S., M.S.D.
Private Practice, Jonesboro, Georgia

Carol Ann Gunnels, P.T.
Coordinator, Orthopedic Physical Therapy, Emory University Hospital and Emory Clinic, Atlanta, Georgia

Patricia Scagnelli Hartman, M.S., P.T., O.C.S.
Chief Physical Therapist, Phillips and Green, Falls Church, Virginia

Julianne Wright Howell, M.S., P.T.
Director, Hand Management Specialists, Richmond, Virginia

Kathryn Levit, M.Ed., O.T.R.
Partner, Making Progress, Alexandria, Virginia; Adjunct Clinical Faculty, Massachusets General Hospital Institute of Health Professions, Boston, Massachusetts; Coordinator/Instructor, Neurodevelopmental Treatment Association, Inc., Chicago, Illinois

Christine A. Moran, M.S., P.T.
Assistant Clinical Professor, Graduate Studies in Physical Therapy, Virginia Commonwealth University Medical College of Virginia, Richmond, Virginia; Adjunct Assistant Clinical Professor, Program in Physical Therapy, Old Dominion University, Norfolk, Virginia; Director, The Richmond Upper Extremity Center, Richmond, Virginia

Helen Owens-Burkhart, M.S., P.T.
Private Practice, Orthopedic Physical Therapy Services, Lockport, Illinois; Guest Lecturer, Northwestern University, Chicago, Illinois

David C. Reid, M.D., M.C.S.P., M.Ch.(orth), F.R.C.S.(C)
Professor of Physical Education and of Orthopaedic Surgery and Rehabilitation, University of Alberta Faculty of Medicine; Consultant in Sports Medicine, Glen Sather Sports Medicine Clinic, University of Alberta, Edmonton, Alberta, Canada

Susan Ryerson, P.T.
Partner, Making Progress, Alexandria, Virginia; Adjunct Clinical Faculty, Massachusetts General Hospital Institute of Health Professions, Boston, Massachusetts; Coordinator/Instructor, Neurodevelopmental Treatment Association, Inc., Chicago, Illinois

Linda Saboe, M.C.P.A., B.P.T.
Research Assistant, Division of Orthopaedic Surgery, University of Alberta Faculty of Medicine, Edmonton, Alberta, Canada

Sandra Richards Saunders, M.S., P.T.
Member, The American Association for Hand Surgery, Madison, Wisconsin; Orthopedic and Sports Medicine Section, American Physical Therapy Association, Washington, D.C.; Virginia Physical Therapy Association, Alexandria, Virginia

Dorie B. Syen, O.T.R./L.
Private Practice, Physical Therapy Associates of Metro Atlanta, Atlanta, Georgia; Associate Member, American Society of Hand Therapists, Phoenix, Arizona

Joseph S. Wilkes, M.D.
Associate Clinical Professor, Department of Orthopaedics, Emory University School of Medicine; Orthopedist, Orthopaedic Associates of Atlanta; Medical Director, Piedmont Hospital Sports Medicine Institute, Atlanta, Georgia; Orthopedic Consultant, United States Luge Association, Lake Placid, New York

Michael J. Wooden, M.S., P.T., O.C.S.
Instructor, Division of Physical Therapy, Emory University; Certified Specialist in Orthopaedic Physical Therapy; Partner, Physical Therapy Associates of Metro Atlanta; Co-Founder, Clinical Education Associates of Atlanta, Atlanta, Georgia

Preface

Normal function of the shoulder is critical for recreational activities, occupational performance, and activities of daily living. Given the importance of normal shoulder biomechanics, it is not surprising that changes in shoulder mechanics, altered kinematics, and anatomic deficits contribute to shoulder pathomechanics. Our role as physical therapists is to assess the intricate shoulder mechanics to determine abnormal movement patterns before we begin our treatment program.

Many rehabilitation students and clinicians are uncertain in assessing shoulder pathomechanics and in establishing treatment protocols for different shoulder pathologies. This shortcoming is due to the variety of treatment approaches to the shoulder and the complexity of the shoulder and upper quarter interrelationships.

This second edition of *Physical Therapy of the Shoulder* was written to enhance the knowledge base of musculoskeletal assessment and treatment of shoulder dysfunction. To keep pace with the ever growing knowledge base of shoulder evaluation and treatment techniques, new chapters on shoulder fractures and arthroscopic surgery have been added. In addition, five chapters — on normal mechanics and anatomy of the shoulder, evaluation, hemiplegic shoulder, shoulder isokinetics, and brachial plexus injuries — were completely revised with new concepts and ideas.

The first chapter covers the basics of shoulder mechanics needed to develop treatment protocols for mechanical dysfunction of the shoulder. Chapter 2 describes a detailed musculoskeletal evaluation of the shoulder and upper quarter. Chapters on isokinetics and postural considerations of the upper quarter complete the knowledge base in shoulder and upper quarter evaluation and interrelationships.

The chapters discussing shoulder dysfunction begin with the frozen shoulder (Chapter 5). Chapters on the hemiplegic shoulder, thoracic inlet or outlet syndrome, brachial plexus injuries, common shoulder problems in the athlete, throwing injuries to the shoulder, myofascial dysfunction, and common shoulder fractures compose the remainder of the comprehensive review of shoulder dysfunction. The authors thoroughly review the literature and discuss evaluation and treatment approaches to their specific dysfunction. The treatment of shoulder dysfunction is highlighted by the chapters on medical management of myofascial pain, mobilization of the shoulder, total shoulder replacements, and shoulder arthroscopic surgery.

Any rehabilitation professional entrusted with the care and treatment of mechanical and pathologic shoulder dysfunction will benefit from this book. We hope that its contents, like the first edition's, will meet the authors' goals— comprehensive, clinically relevant presentations that are well documented, contemporary, and personally challenging to the student and clinician alike.

Robert A. Donatelli, M.A., P.T.

Contents

1 | Anatomy and Biomechanics of the Shoulder

Martha Kaput Frame

One of the most common peripheral joints to be treated in the physical therapy clinic is the shoulder joint. The physical therapist must understand the anatomy and mechanics of this joint to evaluate and design most effectively a treatment program for patients with shoulder dysfunction. This chapter will describe the pertinent functional anatomy of the shoulder complex and relate this anatomy to mechanics of shoulder abduction, flexion, and rotation.

The shoulder joint is better termed the *shoulder complex* because a series of articulations are necessary to position the humerus in space (Fig. 1-1). Most authors, when describing the shoulder joint, discuss the acromioclavicular joint, the sternoclavicular joint, the scapulothoracic articulation, and the glenohumeral joint.[1-4] Kapanji and Kessell have expanded on this list, and also include the functional subdeltoid or subacromial joint.[5,6] Cailliet discusses the importance of considering movement at the costosternal and costovertebral joints when evaluating shoulder girdle motion.[7] Dempster relates all of these areas by using a concept of links. The integrated and harmonious roles of all the links are necessary for full normal mobility.[8]

The shoulder complex is one of the most mobile joints in the body. This wide range of mobility helps position the arm and hand for the many prehensile activities a person may perform. The shoulder can move through nearly a full arc in both the frontal and sagittal planes. This entire range is used in many athletic endeavors such as performing in the gymnastic rings or swimming the backstroke. Most activities of daily living do not require this full range of mobility. The contribution of the shoulder to upper extremity function may be

1

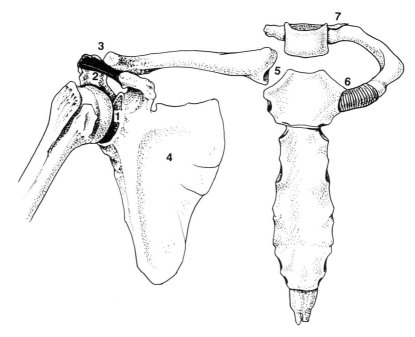

Fig. 1-1. The components of the shoulder joint complex: (*1*) glenohumeral joint; (*2*) subdeltoid joint; (*3*) acromioclavicular joint; (*4*) scapulothoracic joint; (*5*) sternoclavicular joint; (*6*) first costosternal joint; (*7*) first costovertebral joint.

small if the person can compensate with motion at the cervical spine and distal upper extremity joints. This contrast may explain the presence of shoulder dysfunction at both ends of the mobility spectrum—hypermobility associated with shoulder dislocations and hypomobility seen with adhesive capsulitis. Shoulder motion differs between individuals. Some of this variability is due to anatomic considerations.[9,10]

ANATOMY

Glenohumeral Joint

Osteology

The glenohumeral joint contributes the greatest amount of motion to the shoulder complex. This joint has been described as a ball and socket joint. Saha confirmed this description in 70 percent of the specimens he studied. In the other 30 percent, the radius of curvature of the humeral head was greater than the radius of curvature of the glenoid. Thus, the joint was not a true enarthrosis.[10] Saha further described the joint surfaces, especially on the head

A

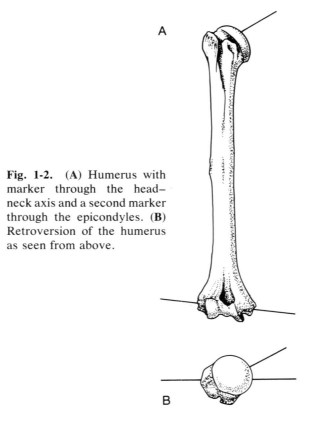

Fig. 1-2. (A) Humerus with marker through the head–neck axis and a second marker through the epicondyles. (B) Retroversion of the humerus as seen from above.

B

of the humerus, as very irregular and having a great amount of individual variation.[10]

The head of the humerus is a hemispherical, convex, articular surface that faces superiorly, medially, and posteriorly. The articular surface is inclined 130° to 150° to the shaft of the humerus and is retroverted 20° to 30° (Fig. 1-2).[3] This retroversion of the head of the humerus corresponds to the forward inclination of the scapula so that free pendulum movements of the arm do not occur in a straight sagittal plane, but at an angle of 30° across the body.[6] This corresponds to the natural arm swing evident in ambulation. This is also one reason why functional movements of the shoulder occur in diagonal patterns. This retroversion also gives rise to the radial groove.[10]

The head of the humerus is large in relation to the glenoid fossa; therefore, only one-third to one-half of the humeral head can contact the glenoid fossa at a given time.[1,6] The glenoid fossa is a shallow structure deepened by the glenoid labrum. The labrum is wedge shaped when the glenohumeral joint is in the resting position and changes shape with various movements. The functional significance of the labrum is questionable. *Gray's Anatomy* lists the labrum's functions as deepening the articular concavity, protecting the edges of the joint and aiding in joint lubrication, similar to a meniscus.[11] Peat states that the labrum may serve as an attachment for the glenohumeral ligaments.[12] Most investigators agree that the labrum is a weak supporting structure, especially in the young.[13,14] Moseley and Övergaard considered the labrum a redundant fold of the capsule composed of dense fibrous connective tissue but generally devoid of cartilage except in a small zone near its osseous attachment.[13]

The glenoid fossa faces laterally. There is some discrepancy regarding the superior or inferior tilt of the glenoid. Freedman and Munro found that the glenoid faced downward in 80.8 percent of the shoulders they studied with radiographs.[15] Basmajian and Bazant described a superior tilt, and hypothesized that it aided in stability of the joint.[16] Another factor lending stability to this joint is a backward-facing glenoid. Saha found a 7.4° retrotilt of the glenoid in 73.5 percent of his normal subjects.[17] Both the humeral and glenoid articular surfaces are lined with articular cartilage. The cartilage is thickest at the periphery on the glenoid fossa and at the center of the humeral head.[11]

Periarticular Structures

The capsule and ligaments reinforce the glenohumeral joint. The capsule is a relatively large structure that has twice the surface area of the humeral head. The capsule attaches around the glenoid rim and forms a sleeve around the head of the humerus, attaching on the anatomic neck except medially, where the capsule is reflected downward one-half inch. The fibrous capsule encompasses the long head of the biceps tendon and is lined with a synovial membrane.[11] The capsule is a lax structure; the head of the humerus can be distracted one-half inch when the shoulder is in a relaxed position.[11] To aid in stability, the capsule is reinforced anteriorly and posteriorly by ligaments and muscles. There is no additional support inferiorly, which causes weakness of this portion of the capsule. This inferior portion of the capsule lies in folds when the arm is adducted. This redundant portion of the capsule adheres to itself and limits motion in adhesive capsulitis.[6]

The anterior capsule is reinforced by the glenohumeral ligaments. The support these ligaments lend to the capsule is insignificant, and the ligaments are not consistently present in each individual.[18] Turkel et al. described the inferior glenohumeral ligament as the thickest and most consistent structure.[19] Moseley and Övergaard found the inferior as well as the superior ligaments to be consistent in their cadaver population.[13] Reeves determined the anterior capsule and ligaments to be especially weak in the elderly population. These structures were stronger in the younger cadavers.[20]

The coracohumeral ligaments are the strongest supporting ligaments of the glenohumeral joint. They are also thickenings of the capsule. These ligaments arise from the coracoid process and extend to the greater and lesser tuberosity. They blend with the supraspinatus muscle and help maintain the normal resting position of the glenohumeral joint.[11]

In addition to ligamentous reinforcement, the capsule is also reinforced by muscles. The tendon of the subscapularis muscle is an important reinforcer against the clinically common anterior dislocation. The strength of this tendon diminishes with age secondary to heterotopic calcifications.[20] Other muscle tendon units that reinforce the capsule are the supraspinatus, which reinforces superiorly, and the infraspinatus and teres minor, which lend support posteriorly. These rotator cuff muscles have been termed the *musculotendinous glenoid*, which describes their important role in stabilizing the glenohumeral joint.[21]

Between the supporting ligaments and muscles lie synovial bursa or recesses. They are located between adjacent moving structures to allow for free gliding. Anteriorly, there are three distinct recesses. The superior recess is the subscapular bursa. This important bursa lies between the neck of the scapula and the subscapularis tendon and protects the tendon as its passes over the scapula. Separated from the subscapular bursa by the width of the subscapularis tendon is the axillary pouch or recess. The middle synovial recess lies posterior to the subscapularis tendon.[22,23]

Myology

The major muscles that act on the glenohumeral joint are the scapulohumeral and axiohumeral muscles. The muscles of the scapulohumeral group originate on the scapula and insert on the humerus. The rotator cuff muscles insert on the tuberosities and along the upper two-thirds of the anatomic neck.[11] The subscapularis has the largest amount of muscle mass of the four rotator cuff muscles.[4]

The deltoid comprises 41 percent of the scapulohumeral muscle mass.[4] This muscle, in addition to its proximal attachment on the acromion process and the spine of the scapula, also arises from the clavicle. The distal insertion is on the shaft of the humerus at the deltoid tubercle. The mechanical advantage of the deltoid is enhanced by the distal insertion and the evolution of a larger acromion process.[4] The deltoid is a multipennate and fatigue-resistant muscle. This may explain the rare involvement of the deltoid in shoulder pathology.[24]

The next muscle group is the axiohumeral muscles. The pectoralis major, pectoralis minor, and latissimus dorsi form this group. Besides being prime movers of the arm, they can act on a fixed arm to move the trunk upward and forward, as in climbing.[11]

Sternoclavicular Joint

The sternoclavicular joint is the only articulation that binds the shoulder girdle to the axial skeleton. This is a synovial sellar joint; the sternal articulating surface is greater than the clavicular surface, providing stability to the joint.[5] The joint is also stabilized by its articulating disc, joint capsule, ligaments, and reinforcing muscles.[8,25] The articular disc attaches superiorly to the clavicle

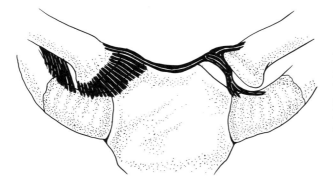

Fig. 1-3. Diagram showing the upper and lower attachments of the meniscus and the upper and lower ligaments of the sternoclavicular joint.

and inferiorly to the first costocartilage and rib.[8,11,25] (Fig. 1-3). The disc binds the joint together and divides the joint into two cavities. This anatomic arrangement permits the disc and its attachments to function as a hinge, increasing the range of motion (ROM) at the joint while allowing for stability of the joint.[12] Without this disc attachment, forces transmitted from the shoulder to the axial skeleton would tend to dislocate the clavicle over the sternum. Clinically, this is rarely seen; a more common scenario is a clavicular fracture.

The capsule surrounds the joint and is thickest on the anterior and posterior aspects. The section of the capsule from the disc to the clavicle is more lax, allowing more mobility in this area than between the disc, sternum, and first rib.[11] The interclavicular ligament reinforces the capsule anteriorly and superiorly. The rhomboid-shaped costoclavicular ligament connects the clavicle to the first rib.[11] This strong supporting ligament limits elevation of the medial aspect of the clavicle. Muscles, especially the sternocleidomastoid, sternohyoid, and sternothyroid, provide further support.[25] One important function of the clavicle is to provide attachment sites for six muscles.[6] The clavicle itself forms a double curve that is convex medially and concave laterally.[4] The double curve allows the clavicle to act as a crankshaft. Clavicular rotation and elevation occur simultaneously at the acromioclavicular joint. The combined movement of rotation and elevation is referred to as the *crankshaft effect*.[4]

Acromioclavicular Joint

At the other end of the clavicle is the acromioclavicular joint. This plane synovial articulation is characterized by variability in size and shape of the clavicular facets and the presence of an intra-articular meniscus.[25] The acromioclavicular joint allows the scapula to glide forward and back and to rotate on the clavicle. This helps to maintain the congruency between the glenoid fossa and the humeral head.[11] This joint's capsule is more lax than that of the sternoclavicular joint; thus, more motion occurs at the acromioclavicular joint and it is more prone to dislocations.[8] There are three major supporting ligaments. The conoid and trapezoid ligaments are collectively called the *cora-*

coclavicular ligament. It is through this ligament that scapular motion is translated to the clavicle.[8] The trapezoid ligament prevents the clavicle from overriding the acromion in the event of a fall on the outstretched arm.[11] The acromioclavicular ligament, along with the intertwined tendinous attachment of the trapezoid and deltoid muscles, strengthens the superior aspect of the joint.[25]

Scapulothoracic Joint

The scapulothoracic joint is not an anatomic joint but an important physiologic joint that adds considerably to the motion of the shoulder girdle. The scapula is concave, articulating with a convex thorax.[1] The scapula is without bony or ligamentous connections to the thorax, except from its attachments at the acromioclavicular joint and coracoclavicular ligament. The scapula is primarily stabilized by muscles. The axioscapula muscles include the trapezius, rhomboid major and minor, serratus anterior, and levator scapula. The tone in the upper trapezius is the chief mechanism for suspension of the entire shoulder girdle.[4]

Subacromial Joint

The functional subacromial joint is formed by the acromioclavicular joint and ligament and the coracoacromial ligament from above and the tuberosities and head of the humerus from below.[5,6,26] There is an intervening subacromial bursa acting as a joint capsule. This bursa separates the deltoid muscle from the rotator cuff muscles. The bursa is attached to the acromion process from above and the rotator cuff tendons and greater tuberosity from below. The bursa has no attachments laterally; its lateral walls are free to move during elevation, allowing gliding to occur.[6]

The normal space in the subacromial joint is 7 to 14 mm. Narrowing of this interval is associated with a rotator cuff tear.[27] Clinically, a painful arc of movement between 60° to 120° of abduction indicates a disorder of the subacromial region.[26]

BIOMECHANICS

Anatomic structures both promote and limit movement. The shoulder joint complex is designed for movement. Three important movements for function are shoulder abduction, flexion, and rotation. During each of these movements, synchronous motion is occurring at the five major component joints of the shoulder complex.

Abduction

Shoulder abduction is the most extensively studied shoulder motion.[4,7,9,15,28–32] Traditionally, abduction is movement in the coronal plane.[4,7,32] This movement of the humerus in relation to the trunk actually places the glenohumeral joint in an extended position.[6] Recent reports in the literature describe abduction utilizing the plane of the scapula. In this plane, the mechanical axis of the humerus approximates the mechanical axis of the scapula[28,30,33] (Fig. 1-4). This is not a fixed plane. The plane of the scapula is approximately 30° to 45° anterior to the coronal plane.[29,31] Movement in this plane is more natural and functional. Anatomically, movement in this plane prevents twisting of the inferior fibers of the capsule and allows the fibers of the surrounding muscles to maintain a parallel and optimal length-tension relationship.[28]

Arthrokinematics

The amount of shoulder abduction varies between individuals with an average of 148° to 182° of osteokinematic motion.[15,34] Approximately 104° to 135° of this motion occurs at the glenohumeral joint.[4,10,34] The motion occurring at the joint surfaces is arthrokinematic motion, of which there are three types: rolling, gliding, and rotation (Fig. 1-5). Rolling occurs when various points on a moving surface contact various points on a stationary surface. Gliding occurs when one point on a moving surface contacts multiple points on a stationary surface. When rolling or gliding occurs, there is a significant change in the contact area between the two joint surfaces. The third type of arthrokinematic movement is rotation, which occurs when one or more points on a moving

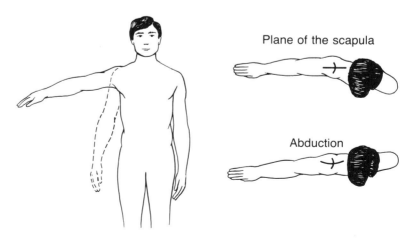

Plane of the scapula

Abduction

Fig. 1-4.   Abduction in the plane of the scapula.

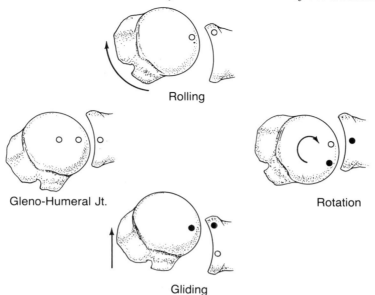

Rolling

Gleno-Humeral Jt.

Rotation

Gliding

Fig. 1-5.   Arthrokinematic motion occurring at the glenohumeral joint: rolling, rotation, and gliding.

surface contact one point on a stationary surface. There is little displacement between the two joint surfaces in rotation.

All three arthrokinematic movements can occur at the glenohumeral joint, but they do not occur in equal proportions. These motions are necessary for the large humeral head to take advantage of the small glenoid articulating surface.[10] Saha investigated the contact area between the head of the humerus and the glenoid with abduction in the plane of the scapula[10] and found that the contact area on the head of the humerus shifted up and forward while the contact area on the glenoid remained relatively constant, indicating a rotation movement. Poppen and Walker measured the instant centers of rotation for the same movement.[30] They found that in the first 30°, and often between 30° and 60°, the head of the humerus moved superiorly in the glenoid by 3 mm, indicating rolling or gliding. At more than 60°, there was minimal movement of the humerus, indicating almost pure rotation.[30]

Concomitant external rotation of the humerus is necessary for abduction in the coronal plane.[4,10,11,28,32] Some investigators have postulated that this motion is necessary for the greater tuberosity to clear the acromion and the coracoacromial ligament.[1,2,32] Although a decrease in the distance between the humeral head and the coracoacromial ligament has been associated with rotator cuff dysfunction,[27] there is sufficient room to prevent bone impingement.[10] External rotation also remains necessary for full coronal abduction even after the acromion and the coracoacromial ligament are surgically removed. Saha has reasoned that external rotation is necessary to prevent the humeral head from impinging on the glenoid rim.[10]

External rotation of the humerus is not necessary for full abduction in the plane of the scapula.[28] Poppen and Walker found that the humerus and scapula moved synchronously into external rotation at 90° of abduction so there was little relative rotation of the humerus on the glenoid with abduction in the plane of the scapula.[30]

Forces

A significant amount of force is generated at the glenohumeral joint during abduction through muscle contractions. Since most of the muscles acting on the glenohumeral joint have a line of pull that is oblique to the plane of the glenoid fossa, a combination of shearing and compressive forces are produced.[4,29] In the early stages of abduction, the loading vector is beyond the upper edge of the glenoid.[17] During this stage of abduction, the pull of the deltoid produces an upward shear of the humeral head.[35] This shearing force peaks at 60° of abduction and is counteracted by the transverse compressive forces of the rotator cuff muscles[29] (Fig. 1-6). At 90° of abduction, the loading vector is still eccentrically placed in the upper glenoid; however, at this range, the compressive forces are maximum, resulting in compressive stability.[35] Poppen and Walker estimated this compressive force to be 0.89 times body weight.[29] Inman et al. also describe a maximum compressive force at 90°, which is slightly less than Poppen and Walker's calculations.[4] At the end ranges of abduction, the loading vector is directed into the central axis of the glenoid, and the forces are equalized through all portions of the glenoid.[35]

Scapulohumeral Rhythm

Along with movement at the glenohumeral joint, a synchronous movement also occurs at the adjacent articulations. Inman et al. investigated scapulohumeral rhythm in subjects abducting their shoulders in the coronal plane.[4] In

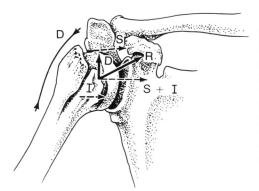

Fig. 1-6.   In the early stages of glenohumeral abduction, the deltoid reactive force (D) is located outside the glenoid fossa. This force is counteracted by the transverse compressive forces of the supraspinatus (S) and infraspinatus (I) muscles. The resultant reactive force (R) is therefore more favorably placed within the glenoid fossa for joint stability.

their often referenced study, they found that after the first 30° of motion a fairly constant ratio of 2° humeral motion to every degree of scapular motion was present. More recent studies investigating scapulohumeral rhythm in the plane of the scapula reveal much more complex relationships. These relationships are also not static but dynamic, changing through the various portions of the range. Bagg and Forrest evaluated 20 subjects and found three distinctive patterns of scapulohumeral rhythm.[34] Each pattern had three phases with varying ratios of humeral to scapular movement. The most common pattern had 3.29° of humeral motion for every degree of scapular motion in the 20.8° to 81.8° ROM. The humeral component then decreased to 0.71° for abduction between 81.8° to 139.1°. During end ranges of abduction between 139.1° and 170° the humeral contribution to movement again increased to 3.49°. Doody et al. found a similar pattern of movement with a ratio of 7.24° to 1 early in the range and less than 1 to 1 later in the range.[9] Freedman and Munro also found a varying ratio of glenohumeral motion to scapular rotation throughout the ROM.[15] They found the glenohumeral contribution to be greatest at end ranges of abduction. Doody et al., along with Freedman and Munro, have attributed this increase in scapular rotation at midranges of abduction to the relative strength of the scapula rotators over the deltoid and supraspinatus muscles.[9,15] When Doody et al. added weight to the arm the scapula moved sooner but contributed less to the overall range.[9]

Eight of Bagg and Forrest's 20 subjects had scapulohumeral patterns different from those listed above.[34] One group demonstrated a scapular contribution to arm abduction greater than the glenohumeral contribution until the arm reached 130° of abduction. Glenohumeral contribution then increased to 6.51° for every degree of scapular motion. In the third group, there was a relatively constant 2 to 1 ratio through most of the ROM. Bagg and Forrest speculated that the variance in patterns may be secondary to anatomic considerations, especially the weight of the arm and relative muscle imbalances between the scapula rotators and the deltoid. A person with a heavier arm or with weak deltoids would have an increased need for scapular rotation earlier in the range of abduction.[34] In most of the literature, there are reports of common trends along with considerable variation. Therefore, when possible, the clinician should compare the scapulohumeral rhythm bilaterally on an individual patient. The comparison will reveal more useful information than comparing a patient's rhythm to a set norm.

Movement of the scapula is permitted by movement in the acromioclavicular and sternoclavicular joints. The relative contribution of these two joints changes throughout the ROM depending on where the instant center of rotation (ICR) lies.[34] Initially, the ICR lies near the root of the scapular spine. As the arm is abducted past 60° to 90°, the ICR shifts laterally, reaching the acromioclavicular joint between 120° to 150° of abduction.[34] This suggests that clavicular elevation occurs at the sternoclavicular joint during the first 120° to 150° of abduction and that rotation of the scapula around the acromioclavicular joint starts at 60° to 90° of abduction and continues to near end range.[34] Inman et al. found different results, with sternoclavicular motion occurring between

0° to 90° of abduction and acromioclavicular motion occurring before 30° and after 135°.[4] One reason for the difference may be that these investigators looked at two different motions. Bagg and Forrest investigated abduction in the plane of the scapula whereas Inman et al. investigated in the coronal plane.

Muscle Activity

Muscles are active in moving the shoulder into abduction. Saha describes the rotator cuff muscles, active throughout the range of abduction, as steerers, because they are responsible for positioning the humeral head in the glenoid.[17,33] During abduction, the force vectors of the infraspinatus, teres minor, and subscapularis pass very close to the ICR. Therefore, these muscles cannot contribute significantly to abduction of the upper limb.[36]

The role of the supraspinatus and deltoid in shoulder abduction is controversial. Earlier literature indicated that the supraspinatus initiated abduction and the deltoid carried out the motion. Electromyograph (EMG) studies demonstrate that both muscles are active throughout the ROM.[4,37] However, there is an earlier rise in tension in the supraspinatus. This muscle activity helps to fixate the humeral head so that the deltoid works at an improved mechanical advantage.[2,4,18,37] With paralysis of either the supraspinatus or deltoid, the arm can be elevated, but with a loss of power. Impairment of the supraspinatus results in a more significant loss of power.[38]

The axioscapular muscles fixate the scapula, allowing the scapulohumeral muscles to raise the arm.[4] The major muscles that act as a force couple to rotate the scapula on the thoracic wall are the upper, middle, and lower trapezius and the serratus anterior. During abduction in the plane of the scapula, EMG activity in these muscles increases as the angle of abduction increases.[39] The EMG pattern of each muscle is also characterized by a plateau phase in midrange. Bagg and Forrest speculate that this plateau phase may be related to the changing mechanical advantage of the various muscles as the ICR migrates from the root of the spine of the scapula to the acromioclavicular joint.[39] Of these muscles, the serratus anterior is functionally the most significant. Paralysis of this muscle limits elevation of the arm to 90°.[40]

Flexion

The movement of flexion has been less thoroughly investigated. Flexion is movement in the sagittal plane. Full flexion to 162° to 180° is possible only with synchronous motion in the glenohumeral, acromioclavicular, sternoclavicular, and scapulothoracic joints.[29] The movement is similar to that of abduction.

Arthrokinematics

Saha has shown that the contact area on the head of the humerus shifts anteriorly and superiorly as the shoulder moves through flexion. The contact area on the glenoid remains fairly stationary.[10] This indicates that the major arthrokinematic motion is rotation. To enhance muscle power, scapular and clavicular movements occur earlier in flexion than in abduction.[4,10]

For full flexion in the sagittal plane, concomitant internal rotation is necessary.[41,42] Blakely and Palmer analyzed internal rotation with flexion and found that 94.9° plus or minus 13.5° internal rotation accompanied full flexion. When the glenohumeral joint was held in full external rotation, flexion was limited to 30.2° plus or minus 6.5°.[41]

Muscle Activity

Similar muscle activity is present in the rotator cuff muscles during flexion and abduction.[4] However, the subscapularis is active earlier in the range from 30° to 120°. The anterior fibers of the deltoid and the clavicular portion of the pectoralis major are the most significant shoulder flexors.[18] These same muscles are also internal rotators; therefore, the motions of flexion and internal rotation are coupled together.[41]

Rotation

As described previously, rotation occurs concomitantly with both flexion in the sagittal plane and abduction in the coronal plane. Internal and external rotation can also occur in isolation. The amount of rotation depends on the position of the arm.[6,10,37,43] Most studies report a decrease in the amount of rotation present at the shoulder as the arm is abducted. Bechtol, without citing a source, reports a 180° rotation occurring with the arm adducted. This amount of rotation decreased to 90° with the arm abducted to 90°. In full abduction, little rotation is available.[38] Bechtol speculated that the ROM may decrease with increased abduction because of capsular tightness and winding of the rotator cuff muscles.[38] A study by Clarke et al. measured only 67° of external rotation with the arm adducted, while the total of internal and external rotation increased to 159° with the arm abducted to 90°.[43]

Arthrokinematics

Saha described posterior gliding of the humeral head with internal rotation and anterior gliding with external rotation.[10] More recent work by Howell et al. using radiographs has documented a posterior placement of the humeral head when the shoulder was externally rotated and extended.[44] Mobilization techniques of posterior glides to restore internal rotation and anterior glides to restore external rotation have been used by manual therapists; therefore, the manual techniques may be successful because they are stretching the opposing soft tissue rather than restoring the normal gliding of the humeral head on the glenoid. This is confirmed by Kummel, who demonstrated that the anterior capsule must be extensible for external rotation to occur.[22] Scapular movement is also important for full mobility into rotation. Scapular adduction is associated with external rotation, and scapular abduction is associated with internal rotation.[5]

Muscle Activity

Generally, more muscle force can be generated in internal rotation than in external rotation.[5] Scheving and Pauly describe the latissimus dorsi as the most important internal rotator.[45] Harms-Ringdahl et al. investigated EMG activity of the internal rotators during resistive activity and found that the sternoclavicular portion of the pectoralis major was the most activated muscle.[46] The infraspinatus and teres minor muscles are the chief external rotators.[11]

Glenohumeral Stability

No single structure is responsible for glenohumeral stability as the shoulder is moved through its full ROM. Osseous, periarticular structures, and muscles are stabilizing structures.[10,16,18,19,21] Generally, the supporting structures are more superior when the shoulder is adducted and shift to more inferior structures as the shoulder is abducted.

Osteology

The position and size of the glenoid fossa and humeral head will help determine stability of the glenohumeral joint. Saha found that if the ratio of the diameter of the glenoid to the diameter of the humeral head was less than 0.75 in the vertical direction and less than 0.57 in the transverse direction, the joint was inherently less stable.[17] He also found that a posterior tilting fossa and humeral head enhanced the stability of the joint.[17]

Periarticular Structures

Various periarticular structures support the glenohumeral joint as the shoulder moves through different ranges of motion. Dempster showed that with various movements, the capsule and ligaments become taut, binding the joint

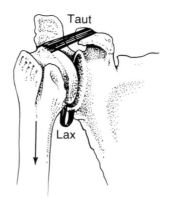

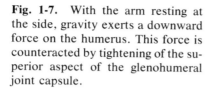

Fig. 1-7. With the arm resting at the side, gravity exerts a downward force on the humerus. This force is counteracted by tightening of the superior aspect of the glenohumeral joint capsule.

together and limiting further movement.[8] The structures opposite the side of movement become the tightest (Fig. 1-7). For example, the superior aspect of the capsule and its coracohumeral ligamentous reinforcements prevents inferior movement of the humeral head when the arm is resting at the side.[16] Structures in the anterior aspect of the glenohumeral joint provide stability when the arm is moved into abduction and external rotation.[2] The supporting structures shift from superior to inferior as the angle of abduction increases. At 45° of abduction, the middle glenohumeral ligament and the anterior superior fibers of the inferior glenohumeral ligament stabilize against anterior dislocations of the humeral head. At 90° of motion, the inferior glenohumeral ligament prevents dislocation; this structure is an especially important stabilizer at end ranges of abduction.[19] Kaltsas showed the anterior inferior portion to be the capsule's weakest part.[47] This corresponds to the number of anterior dislocations seen clinically. The labrum may also provide a limited anterior buttressing effect.[48]

Muscles

The supraspinatus, deltoid, and subscapularis muscles are active stabilizers of the glenohumeral joint. When the arm rests at the side, the supraspinatus acts with the superior aspect of the joint capsule to support the joint.[16] If a load is carried in the hand, there is increased EMG activity in the supraspinatus and in the posterior fibers of the deltoid.[16] During abduction, the subscapularis tendon reinforces the anterior ligamentous stability.[19] This muscle and tendon is strongest up to the third decade of life and is a primary stabilizer in the young.[14] The subscapularis is most active up to 130° of abduction; therefore, this muscle provides the most support during the early and middle ranges of abduction.[4,19]

SUMMARY

Patients with shoulder dysfunction are routinely treated in the physical therapy clinic. An understanding of the anatomy and biomechanics of this joint can help provide the physical therapist with a rationale for evaluation and treatment. Most studies involving shoulder anatomy and biomechanics reveal a common pattern along with a wide variation among subjects. The physical therapist should keep this variation in mind when treating an individual patient.

Treatment may be directed toward restoring mobility, providing stability, or a combination of the two. The shoulder is an inherently mobile complex, with various joint surfaces adding to the freedom of movement. The shallow glenoid with its flexible labrum and large humeral head provides mobility. At times, this vast mobility occurs at the expense of stability. The shoulder relies on various stabilizing mechanisms, including shapes of joint surfaces, ligaments, and muscles to prevent excessive motion. Nearly 20 muscles act on this joint complex in some manner and at various times can be both prime movers and stabilizers. Harmonious actions of these muscles are necessary for the full function of this joint.

REFERENCES

1. Kent BE: Functional anatomy of the shoulder complex. A review. Phys Ther 51:867, 1971
2. Lucas D: Biomechanics of the shoulder joint. Arch Surg 107:425, 1973
3. Sarrafian SK: Gross and functional anatomy of the shoulder. Clin Orthop Rel Res 173:11, 1983
4. Inman VT, Saunders M, Abbott LC: Observations on the function of the shoulder joint. J Bone Joint Surg 26A:1, 1944
5. Kapanji IA: The Physiology of the Joints—Upper Limb, Vol. 1. Churchill Livingstone, New York, 1970
6. Kessell L: Clinical Disorders of the Shoulder. 2nd Ed. Churchill Livingstone, Edinburgh, 1986
7. Cailliet R: Shoulder Pain. FA Davis, Philadelphia, 1966
8. Dempster WT: Mechanism of shoulder movement. Arch Phys Med Rehabil 46A:49, 1965
9. Doody SG, Freedman L, Waterland JC: Shoulder movements during abduction in the scapular plane. Arch Phys Med Rehabil 51:595, 1970
10. Saha AK: Theory of Shoulder Mechanism: Descriptive and Applied. Charles C Thomas, Springfield, IL, 1961
11. Warwick R, Williams P (eds): Gray's Anatomy. 35th British Ed. WB Saunders, Philadelphia, 1973
12. Peat M: Functional anatomy of the shoulder complex. Phys Ther 66:1855, 1986
13. Moseley HP, Övergaard B: The anterior capsular mechanism in recurrent anterior dislocations of the shoulder: morphological and clinical studies with special reference to the glenoid labrum and glenohumeral ligaments. J Bone Joint Surg 44B:913, 1962

14. Reeves B: Experiments in the tensile strength of the anterior capsular structures of the shoulder in man. J Bone Joint Surg 50B:858, 1968
15. Freedman L, Munro RR: Abduction of the arm in the scapular plane: scapular and glenohumeral movements. A roentgenographic study. J Bone Joint Surg 48A:1503, 1966
16. Basmajian JV, Bazant FJ: Factors preventing downward dislocation of the adducted shoulder joint: an electromyographic and morphological study. J Bone Joint Surg 41A:1182, 1959
17. Saha AK: Dynamic stability of the glenohumeral joint. Acta Orthop Scand 42:491, 1971
18. Basmajian J: The surgical anatomy and function of the arm-trunk mechanism. Surg Clin North Am 43:1475, 1963
19. Turkel SJ, Panio MW, Marshall JL, Girgis FG: Stabilizing mechanisms preventing anterior dislocation of the glenohumeral joint. J Bone Joint Surg 63A:1208, 1981
20. Reeves B: Experiments in the tensile strength of the anterior capsular structures of the shoulder in man. J Bone Joint Surg 50B:858, 1968
21. Himeno S, Tsumura H: The role of the rotator cuff as a stabilizing mechanism of the shoulder. p. 17. In Bateman S, Welsh P (eds): Surgery of the Shoulder. CV Mosby, St. Louis, 1984
22. Kummel BM: Spectrum of lesions of the anterior capsular mechanism of the shoulder. Am J Sports Med 7:111, 1979
23. Moore KL: Clinically Orientated Anatomy. Williams & Wilkins, Baltimore, 1980
24. Hagberg M: Electromyographic signs of shoulder muscular fatigue in two elevated arm positions. Am J Phys Med 60:111, 1981
25. Moseley HF: The clavicle: its anatomy and function. Clin Orthop Rel Res 58:17, 1968
26. Kessel L, Watson M: The painful arc syndrome. J Bone Joint Surg 59B:166, 1977
27. Weiner DS: Superior migration of the humeral head: a radiological aid in the diagnosis of tears of the rotator cuff. J Bone Joint Surg 52B:524, 1970
28. Johnston TB: Movements of the shoulder joint—plea for use of "plane of the scapula" as plane of reference for movements occurring at humero-scapula joint. Br J Surg 25:252, 1937
29. Poppen NK, Walker PS: Forces at the glenohumeral joint in abduction. Clin Orthop Rel Res 135:165, 1978
30. Poppen NK, Walker PS: Normal and abnormal motion of the shoulder. J Bone Joint Surg 58A:195, 1976
31. Saha AK: Mechanism of shoulder movements and a plea for the recognition of "zero position" of glenohumeral joint. Clin Orthop Rel Res 173:3, 1983
32. Codman EA: The Shoulder. Thomas Dodd, Boston, 1934
33. Saha AK: Mechanics of elevation of glenohumeral joint. Acta Orthop Scand 44:668, 1973
34. Bagg, Forrest WJ: A biomechanical analysis of scapular rotation during arm abduction in the scapular plane. Am J Phys Med Rehabil 67:238, 1988
35. Elfman H: Biomechanics of muscle with particular application to studies of gait. J Bone Joint Surg 48A:368, 1966
36. De Duca CS, Forrest WJ: Force analysis of individual muscles acting simultaneously on the shoulder joint during isometric abduction. J Biomech 6:385, 1973
37. Perry J: Biomechanics of the shoulder. p. 21. In Rowe CR (ed): The Shoulder. Churchill Livingstone, New York, 1988
38. Bechtol C: Biomechanics of the shoulder. Clin Orthop Rel Res 146:37, 1980

39. Bagg DS, Forrest WJ: Electromyographic study of the scapular rotators during arm abduction in the scapular plane. Am J Phys Med 65:111, 1986
40. Brunstrom S: Muscle testing around the shoulder girdle. J Bone Joint Surg 23A:263, 1941
41. Blakely RL, Palmer ML: Analysis of rotation accompanying shoulder flexion. Phys Ther 64:1214, 1984
42. Steindler A: Kinesiology of the Human Body. Charles C Thomas, Springfield, IL, 1966
43. Clarke GR, Willis LA, Fish WW, Nichols PJR: Assessment of movement at the glenohumeral joint. Orthopaedics 7:55, 1974
44. Howell SM, Galinat BJ, Renzi AJ, Marone PJ: Normal and abnormal mechanics of the glenohumeral joint in the horizontal plane. J Bone Joint Surg 70A:227, 1988
45. Scheving L, Pauly J: An electromyographic study of some muscles acting on the upper extremity of man. Anat Rec 135:239, 1959
46. Harms-Ringdahl K, Ekholm J, Arborelius UP, et al: Load moment, muscle strength and level of muscular activity during internal rotation training of the shoulder. Scand J Rehabil Med, suppl., 9:125, 1983
47. Kaltsas DS: Comparative study of the properties of the shoulder joint capsule with those of other joint capsules. Clin Orthop Rel Res 173:20, 1983
48. Townley C: The capsular mechanism in recurrent dislocations of the shoulder. J Bone Joint Surg 32A:370, 1950

2 | Evaluation of the Shoulder: A Sequential Approach

Christine A. Moran
Sandra Richards Saunders

The shoulder patient can be regarded either as a challenge or a drudgery. The evaluation of such a patient is often clouded by the multiple joints and muscles involved. Frequently, the therapist becomes frustrated. The final degree of motion achieved by the patient is usually less than satisfactory.

The sequential approach to shoulder girdle evaluation described in this chapter is designed to clarify the picture. Each step of the evaluation, as outlined in Figure 2-1, aids the patient. It may be necessary to bypass one or more steps, but, at the completion of this sequential evaluation, the therapist will have much more information than is provided by traditional evaluation and will be able to establish a more specific treatment program. All limiting factors relating to the specific diagnosis as well as to associated problems are identified. As has been observed clinically, the associated problems often frustrate the therapist, frequently causing a less than complete result from treatment.

HISTORY TAKING

The initial step in evaluation is history taking (Fig. 2-1). Detailed, specific questions regarding such factors as injury, surgery, and pain are asked. By taking time for a detailed history, the therapist determines the direction of the remaining evaluation. The initial diagnosis should not limit the fact-finding

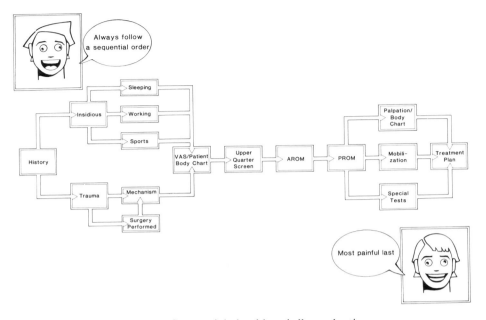

Fig. 2-1. Sequential shoulder girdle evaluation.

nature of the history. If the patient describes pain and limited motion before a recent surgical procedure, the therapist should be alerted to examine more carefully the areas of pain, soft tissue limitation through range of motion (ROM), joint play assessment, and abnormal posturing. The subsequent evaluation sequence is then determined from the history information.

First, the patient must be questioned as to the onset of symptoms. Was the onset of the problem traumatic or insidious? This question is not as clearcut as it may seem. Many injuries may be of a traumatic onset, yet a period of time may elapse between injury and treatment and/or surgery. In situations of repetitive use, a significant period of time could have elapsed before the shoulder problem or shoulder surgery. In these cases, information must be obtained regarding not only the mechanism of injury and surgery performed, but also how the problem is affected by sleeping, working, and sport postures, activities, and self-observed motion limitations.

Examination of the patient with shoulder pathology requires a knowledge of microtrauma versus macrotrauma. As discussed by Jobe and Moynes, macrotrauma can be easily identified as some sort of frank trauma, such as a rotator cuff rupture or humeral neck fracture.[1] Microtrauma, on the other hand, is the persistent irritation of periarticular tissues that provokes local inflammatory response. Insidious pain can develop from sleep, work, and sports postures. Continued irritation can cause scarring, tendinitis, muscular trigger points, and progressive shoulder limitation. This form of trauma develops over periods of weeks and months, and the patient often describes the pain and limitation as "coming on gradually."

INSIDIOUS ONSET

Travell and Simons define idiopathic frozen shoulder as the activation of trigger points in the subscapularis muscle (Fig. 2-2), with subsequent sensitization of surrounding shoulder girdle muscles and progressive motion restrictions.[2] Evaluation of insidious shoulder pain from this perspective requires knowledge of referred pain and trigger points. Studies by Kellgren[3] and Inman and Saunders[4] identified specific reproducible patterns of pain activated when selective connective tissue and muscle structures were irritated[3,4] (Figs. 2-2 and 2-3) Travell and Simons[2] compiled common referral patterns from muscles of the upper extremity. Figures 2-4 to 2-6 are referral patterns of three muscles in the shoulder that commonly develop trigger points.

The key factors in the identification of trigger points are (1) constant locus of referred pain and (2) the ability to reproduce the pain consistently.[2-7] Knowledge of referral patterns from specific muscles aid the therapist in discovering the source of pain and restriction. This is addressed in detail in Chapter 12. Sola and Kuitert examined 100 patients with complaints of loss of motion, pain, and stiffness of the shoulder and neck.[7] Most patients had been unsuccessfully treated for bursitis, neuritis, or myositis. Of the 80 patients with complaints of shoulder pain, 61 patients had trigger points in the infraspinatus muscle; 41 patients had trigger points in the levator scapulae muscle; and 9, 4, 3, and 2 patients exhibited trigger points in the teres minor, supraspinatus, rhomboid major, and trapezius muscles, respectively. Very often, these muscles not only have become sensitized and developed trigger points, but also have shortened adaptively owing to lack of motion. Using only the limited available motion, the patient provokes further irritation to the shortened muscles, ligament, and capsule. The glenohumeral joint capsule also demonstrates a specific referral pattern to the area about the deltoid insertion. Again, the key factors in identification are consistent reproduction of the patient's pain and a characteristic pattern of presentation.

Finally, the evaluator should consider the possibility that the patient is compensating for local trauma. Such compensation can lead to altered biomechanics; this in turn can lead to trigger point activation, which refers pain that mimics the primary pathology. The compensating movement of the upper extremity may produce muscle microtrauma in the infraspinatus muscle, which then develops into a trigger point. The infraspinatus muscle can refer pain to the anterior shoulder; this may be confused with a local pathology. Palpation performed during evaluation of the patient will help distinguish between a local and a referred problem.

Trigger points can also occur secondarily from the altered biomechanics of the postsurgical recovery period. Comparison of preinjury and postsurgery pain diagrams can shed light on this subject. The pain may be the same or

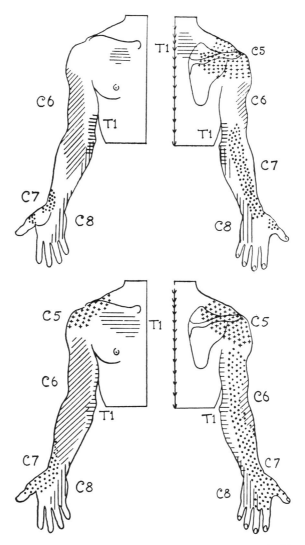

Fig. 2-2. Mappings of referred pain from local irritation of rhomboids (crosses), flexor carpiradialis (oblique hatching), abductor pollicis longus (stippling), third dorsal interosseous (vertical hatching), and first intercostal space (horizontal hatching). (From Kellgren,[3] with permission.)

different. More often, it is not exactly the same, implying a different source of pain than the site of surgery.

A more traditional interpretation of insidious shoulder pain is use of the term *frozen shoulder*. This term appears to identify the patient's lack of function rather than provide information regarding precipitating factors. Although this

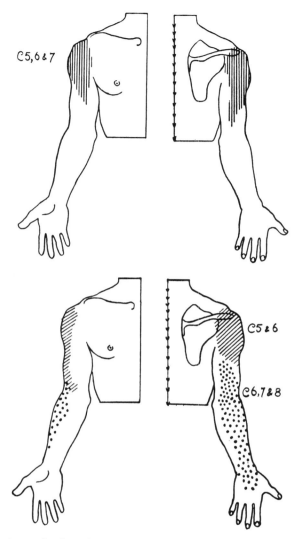

Fig. 2-3. Mappings of referred pain from local irritation of serratus anterior (vertical hatching) and latissimus dorsi (stippling). (From Kellgren,[3] with permission.)

term has been used interchangeably with the term *adhesive capsulitis* and other diagnostic descriptors, investigators are encouraging a distinction between these two frequently used terms.[8–10] Reeves described an arthrographic difference between patients with frozen shoulders and patients with post-traumatic stiff shoulders.[8] In patients with frozen shoulders, he arthrographically observed a failure to fill the subscapularis bursa, bicipital tendon sheath, and axillary pouch; the stiff shoulder patients demonstrated loss of the inferior

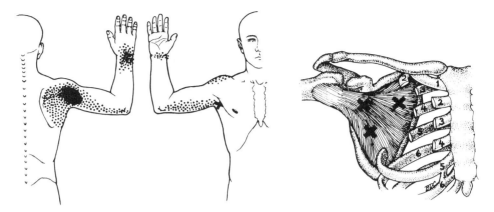

Fig. 2-4. Location of trigger points and areas of referred pain for the subscapularis muscle. (From Travell and Simons,[2] with permission.)

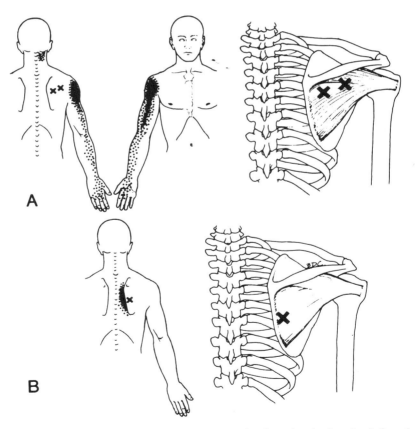

Fig. 2-5. Location of trigger points and areas of referred pain for the infraspinatus muscle.

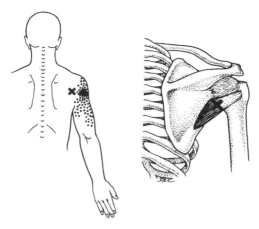

Fig. 2-6. Location of trigger points and corresponding referred pain area of the teres minor muscle. (From Travell and Simons,[2] with permission.)

pouch while the subscapular bursa becomes full. Continuing his arthrographic observations, in 1975 Reeves noted that patients with frozen shoulders displayed spontaneous onset of shoulder pain with movement restriction in every direction and loss of capsular volume.[9]

Over the course of many years, Neviaser has discussed frozen shoulder pathology and adhesive capsulitis pathology; however, two more recent articles provide a clear update.[10,11] In attempting to distinguish these shoulder pathologies, Neviaser and Neviaser observed that stiff, painful shoulders were caused by any condition causing pain, but no true capsule contracture could be detected.[10] The onset of pain may be more acute and possibly related to overhead activity or repetitive use. Arthrographs revealed normal volumetric capacity of the joint capsule.

Adhesive capsulitis, however, was noted to have a distinct inflammatory reaction within the capsule and synovium.[10] A preadhesive stage is detectable in stage I via arthroscopic visualization, while stage II demonstrates acute synovitis with adhesion formation. Loss of the axillary fold occurs during stage III, with mature adhesions and marked joint restrictions identified in stage IV. Patients with adhesive capsulitis were characterized as women, 40 to 60 years of age who describe gradual onset of stiffness and pain. The loss of motion is usually described as the result of immobilization secondary to another problem (i.e., hand injury).

The following case study describes a patient with insidious shoulder pain, who described her pain as one of gradual onset that began as an inability to sleep comfortably through the night. Finally, the patient was referred with a diagnosis of thoracic outlet syndrome; later, the diagnosis was changed to frozen shoulder.

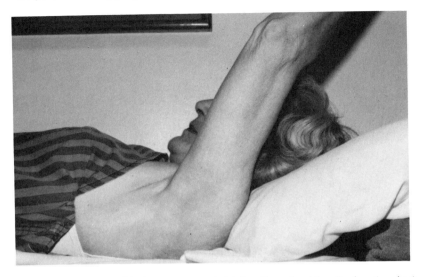

Fig. 2-7.   Patient (L.S.) demonstrates initial active shoulder flexion (supine).

Case Study 1

A 52-year-old, right-dominant woman noticed a gradual onset of left shoulder pain during the summer of 1984. She could not associate any particular event or posture with her shoulder complaint. In November 1984, the pain was severe enough to cause her to seek medical attention, and she was referred for physical therapy with a diagnosis of thoracic outlet syndrome. Initial findings indicated that she was unable to sleep supine or on her left shoulder, had pain during the day with constant use, and was unable to dress or comb her hair. Active range of motion (AROM) was limited except in forward flexion (Figs. 2-7 to 2-10), and passive range of motion (PROM) was limited and painful in all shoulder motions.

Pain diagram: Figure 2-10
Upper quarter screen: Limited cervical rotation, but non-painful.

AROM:		Supine	Sitting
Flexion		135°	115°
Extension		90°	50°
Abduction		90°	80°
Internal rotation at	45° abduction	45°	45°
External rotation at	0° abduction	25°	—
	45° abduction	—	—
	90° abduction	—	—

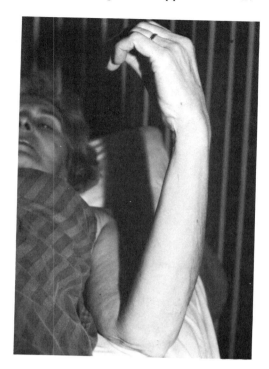

Fig. 2-8. Patient (L.S.) demonstrates initial external rotation.

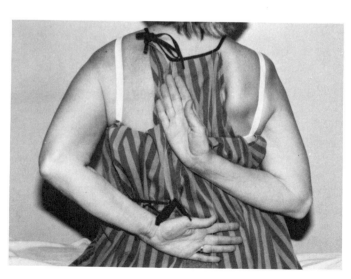

Fig. 2-9. Patient (L.S.) demonstrates initial active internal rotation; note lack of scapular mobility.

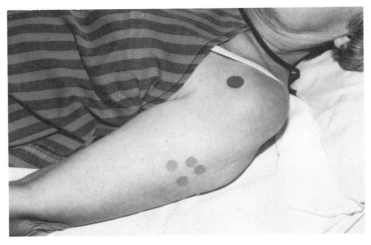

Fig. 2-10.   Patient (L.S.) reproduces referred pain (small dots) from the anterior capsule (large dot).

PROM:	Not tested.
Mobilization:	Anterior glide—limited and extremely painful; posterior glide—mildly painful; distraction—painful.
Special tests:	Supraclavicular Tinel's sign—negative; costoclavicular maneuver—negative.
Palpation:	Trigger point in infraspinatus.
Initial thoughts:	As revealed by the initial evaluation, the patient's chief complaint is that of a painful shoulder, not thoracic outlet symptoms. The cervical restriction was longstanding and did not affect her activities. The most painful area elicited in the examination was the anterior capsule, identified in the active/passive motion testing of external rotation and anterior glide mobilization testing. This information was confirmed in the history by her description of functional level and sleeping postures. Treatment was directed toward relieving the anterior capsule pain and the secondary trigger point in the infraspinatus muscle. All stretching and mobilization was then directed toward the capsule. The patient was discharged with pain-free, full shoulder mobility.

Trigger points can also occur secondarily from the altered biomechanics of the postsurgical recovery period. Comparison of pre-injury and postsurgery pain diagrams can shed light on this subject. The pain may be the same or different. More often, it is not exactly the same, implying a different source of pain than the site of surgery. The following case study is an example of a

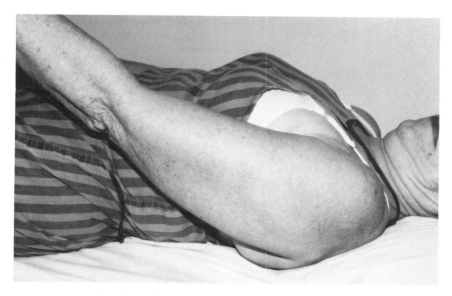

Fig. 2-11. Patient's (A.B.) initial supine flexion.

postsurgical patient with trigger points. Were the trigger points preexisting or secondary to immobilization?

Case Study 2

A. B., an avid golfer, complained of persistent left shoulder pain of 2 years' duration that occurred between 60° and 120° of shoulder elevation and at night. She underwent an arthrogram, which revealed no significant rotator cuff tear. On November 20, 1984, she underwent an acromioplasty that included a release of the coracoacromial ligament. She was seen in our clinic on December 11, 1984, with complaints of decreased shoulder motion (Fig. 2-11) and severe shoulder pain.

Visual analogue scale: 3
Pain diagram: Pain over incision, deltoid insertion, and anterior shoulder.
Upper quarter screen: Normal.

AROM:	Supine	Sitting
Flexion	20°	45°
Extension	68°	60°
Internal rotation	30°	50°
External rotation	45°	30°
Abduction	Not tested	45°
Elevation	Not tested	35°

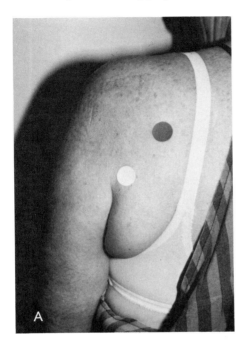 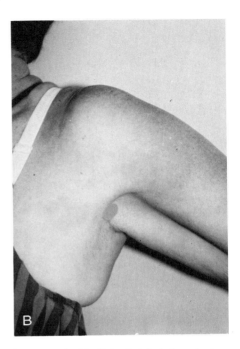

Fig. 2-12.   Latent trigger points in the teres minor muscle (A, light dots), infraspinatus muscle (A, dark dots), and subscapularis muscle (B) (patient A.B.).

PROM:

Flexion	50°
Extension	60°
Internal rotation at 30° abduction	55°
External rotation at 0° abduction	45°
45° abduction	35°
90° abduction	Not tested

Mobilization: Limited inferior glide, external rotation, distraction, anterior glide, scapular distraction.

Special tests: Not applicable.

Palpation: Trigger points in the infraspinatus, subscapularis, and teres minor muscles (Fig. 2-12).

Initial thoughts: Initially, we thought the patient had a dual problem: the acromioplasty and trigger points that limited motion and caused her pain. Her inability to sleep at night preoperatively was thought to be caused by the trigger points, probably preexisting and brought on by the repetitive motion of golf. We therefore chose to treat her soft tissue pain first by use of soft tissue stretching techniques, pain-relieving modalities over the trigger points, and grade I and II mobilization techniques. Her pain was under con-

	trol after the first week, at which time more vigorous mobilization techniques were used. The patient led a very active life prior to her injury, and we felt that she could tolerate such vigorous treatment. The trigger points were reevaluated throughout treatment.
Results:	Full ROM, no pain while playing golf (18 holes) at least three times a week.

Rotator cuff injuries are the most common example of insidious injury to tendons. Neer and Welsh described impingement of the suprasupine tendon and, to a lesser extent, the infraspinatus and long head of biceps tendon on the anterior edge of the coracoacromial ligament and the anterior one-third of the acromion.[12] They described three stages: (1) edema and hemorrhage, (2) thickening and fibrosis, and (3) tearing of the rotator cuff and biceps tendon. The first stages have been recognized in athletes but also occur in non-athletic individuals and in workers. The patient initially reports anterior shoulder pain after use, then during use; by stage 3, the patient reports almost constant pain.[11] In stages 1 and 2, conservative measures geared toward protecting the involved structures and decreasing inflammation are effective. By stage 3, surgery is recommended.[13]

During history taking, information should be obtained to enable the therapist to determine if the pain is primarily after use (stage 1), during use (stage 2), or almost constant (stage 3). Even if a single incident is reported as the reason for the patient to seek medical care, a history of recurrent pain should alert the therapist to microtrauma and resultant weakened tissue.

Special tests and palpation will direct the therapist to the injured tissue. Watson and Kessel classify painful arc syndrome into three forms: the anterior form, the superior form, and the posterior form.[13,14] The three forms are distinguished by palpation. The anterior form involves tenderness over the lesser tuberosity (subscapularis tendon) and is associated with pain with active abduction and external rotation. The superior form involves tenderness to palpation in and around the greater tuberosity (supraspinatus, infraspinatus). It is necessary to sometimes adduct the shoulder to palpate the entire insertion of the supraspinatus. The posterior form involves the insertion of the infraspinatus and, to a lesser degree, the teres minor. The pain is precipitated by internal rotation and abduction.

Watson and Kessel believe that the anterior and posterior forms can be treated conservatively, but the superior form can worsen. This is due to the relative avascularity of the supraspinatus tendon insert (watershed area or critical zone) impeding the natural healing process. Meticulous identification of the irritated and/or damaged structures guides the therapist toward selection of resting postures and/or exercises. Sports medicine literature will aid the therapist in selecting proper activity to stress different structures. In treating the non-athlete, it is also important that the therapist learn what kind of life the patient leads. A sedentary patient will not have the same tensile strength in the injured structure and surrounding tissue as an active or athletic person.

SHOULDER PROBLEMS IN ATHLETES

In addition to what has been described regarding rotator cuff pathology, the onset of shoulder pain in athletes is well documented.[12-20] Repetitive overuse of the shoulder in swimmers and baseball players demonstrates the cumulative effect of microtrauma but is often overlooked in the athlete who plays only occasionally. Intensive weekend play or improper shoulder postures can contribute to muscular, tendinous, and capsular complaints. Pain is typically associated with the pull-through or follow-through phase of the arm movement pattern. Characteristically, such patients display the same referred pain pattern shown by the insidious shoulder pain patient. Examination of the athlete must include a careful evaluation of the sports movement. How is the shoulder held? What is the relationship of the arm and hand during the movement? This topic is discussed further in Chapters 9 and 10.

OVERUSE PROBLEMS IN WORKERS

Attention has been directed to the shoulder area as a potential region of overuse or ergonomically related problems. Overuse or cumulative trauma disorders are the result of repeated exertions and movements and, as observed by Armstrong, may be higher than studies indicate through Workers' Compensation reports.[21] Herberts et al. observed that arm elevation and hand load had the greatest effect on muscle involvement and strain in the shoulder.[22] Specifically, they observed that the infraspinatus muscle showed the greatest dependence on hand load and was strained in an arm position of forward flexion; the supraspinatus muscle was more often involved when the arm was abducted. They also identified an earlier onset of supraspinatus tendinitis in workers who performed static work and a later onset in workers who performed dynamic work.

A study by Delacerda outlined the development of myofascial shoulder girdle syndrome in assembly line workers[23] who developed trigger points in the muscles stabilizing the scapula. Westgaard and Bjorklund[24] observed in their small series that muscular tension varies in the trapezius and rhomboid muscles during hand assembly movements, but these muscles exhibit tension despite the low variability of load. In a 1981 study of six females performing maximum voluntary isometric shoulder elevations against a strain gauge, Hagberg[25] observed significant correlations between muscle electrical activity and shoulder torque. In particular, the work load on the shoulder directly related to the electrical output of the trapezius muscle. He felt that this was due to the trapezius muscle's function, which is to prevent downward scapular rotation during elevation. In conjunction with other reports, Hagberg also observed that fatigue developed in the trapezius muscle after repetitive shoulder tasks. These findings did not correlate with any significant deltoid involvement. Chaffin[26] observed that when the elevated arm is supported, the work load on the shoulder girdle musculature is reduced.

In a longitudinal study of shipyard workers, Berg et al.[27] observed that despite retirement, musculoskeletal symptoms continued during reevaluation 3 years later. They suggested that "normal aging" symptoms had taken over from the physical load symptoms. In those workers still active at the shipyard, they also observed a statistically significant ($P < .01$) decrease in shoulder symptoms. Aaras et al.[28] recently suggested the implementation of postural angle assessment of the shoulder and neck region as a better predictor of overuse among workers. In their series, female workers adopting a shoulder flexion position of less than 15° and a shoulder abduction position of less than 10° had lower sick leave incidence than those workers who used higher shoulder positions.

SHOULDER PAIN AND SLEEPING POSTURES

Characteristically, the patient with shoulder pain caused by abnormal sleeping postures describes morning pain or being awakened during the night by pain. Much information can be gathered by having the patient demonstrate his or her usual sleeping positions.[1] If the patient sleeps on one side with the shoulder joint protracted, the pain may be caused by an overstretched infraspinatus muscle and an adaptive shortened subscapularis muscle, pectoralis major muscle, or anterior shoulder capsule secondary to the posture. A patient who sleeps with an arm under the head may describe impingement-like pain because this sleeping posture forces the humeral head against the acromion, impinging the supraspinatus tendon and subdeltoid bursa. These patients should be asked how many pillows they use when sleeping. Although this question seems more appropriate in the case of a patient with neck pain, overstretching of the levator scapulae muscle through improper head and neck alignment can provoke shoulder problems. A sensitized levator scapulae muscle causes a downward tilt of the glenoid fossa. Because the glenoid fossa is normally positioned in an upward tilt, such rotational shifting of the scapula subsequently alters elevation. When a patient with a painful shoulder sleeps supine, the glenohumeral joint is unsupported. During the patient's sleep, the shoulder slowly falls toward the bed, stressing painful and/or adaptively shortened anterior structures. This is especially true of postsurgical patients who complain of pain during the night. The following case study describes a patient with insidious shoulder pain, who described her pain as one of gradual onset that began as an inability to sleep comfortably through the night. The patient was referred with a diagnosis of thoracic outlet syndrome; later, the diagnosis was changed to frozen shoulder.

This third case study identifies the role that postures can play in causing shoulder pain.

Case Study 3

A 51-year-old, third-grade schoolteacher presented with a 1-year history of bilateral shoulder pain. She had undergone a left arthroscopic decompression 3 weeks before her initial appointment. Her chief complaints were lateral arm pain and limitation of motion. The pain was always present but was worse at night. She could recall no trauma but did report many years of leaning forward over schoolchildren's desks. She also reported that her family continually reminded her of her poor posture. Three weeks post-operatively, she complained of the same pain.

Visual analogue scale: 7
Pain diagram: Lateral arm to elbow.
Upper quarter screen: Limited cervical motion all directions—painful.

AROM:	Supine	Sitting
Flexion	100°	100°
Extension	—	50°
Abduction	80°	63°
Internal rotation at 45° abduction	60°	
90° abduction	Not tested	
External rotation at 0° abduction	25°	
45° abduction	50°	
90° abduction	Not tested	

PROM:	Supine
Flexion	130°
Abduction	95°
Internal rotation at 45° abduction	60°
90° abduction	50°
External rotation at 0° abduction	35°
45° abduction	50°
90° abduction	30°

Mobilization:	Inferior and anterior glides limited, and anterior capsule very painful.
Special tests:	Not applicable.
Palpation:	Local trigger points in infraspinatus, pectoralis major, levator scapulae, and teres major muscles. Subacromial area and anterior capsule are tender to palpation.
Posture:	Kyphosis (Figure 2-13), forward head, elevated scapula (Fig. 2-14), anteriorly positioned humerus (Fig. 2-15), and left sloping shoulder (Fig. 2-16).
Initial thoughts:	The patient's posture is most likely the predisposing factor. The trigger points are probably secondary to her capsular pain. Her night pain could be that her sleeping pos-

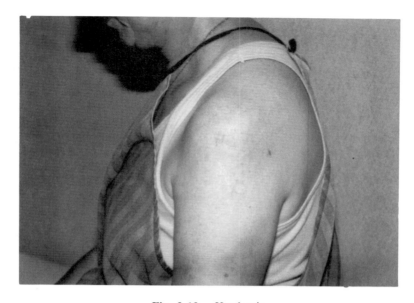

Fig. 2-13.   Kyphosis.

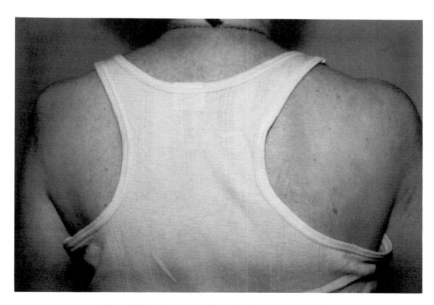

Fig. 2-14.   Forward head, elevated scapula.

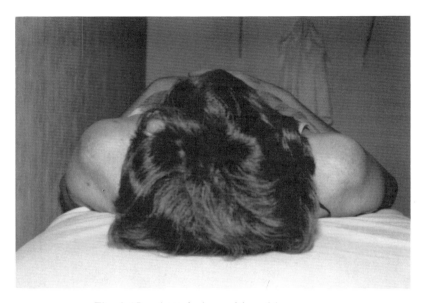

Fig. 2-15.   Anteriorly positioned humerus.

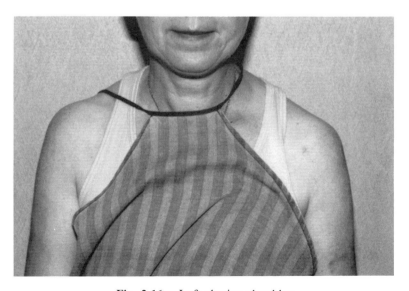

Fig. 2-16.   Left sloping shoulder.

ture stresses the anterior capsule as well as maintains her muscles containing trigger points in an elongated position. During the day, the muscles containing the trigger points are at a biomechanical disadvantage owing to her anterior shoulder posture. To control her pain, sleeping posture stresses, improper biomechanics, and capsular restrictions must all be addressed. Mobilization must release anterior capsule stress by increasing inferior glide. Pain modalities must be directed at the anterior capsule. At the same time, the thoracic kyphosis and scapular position must be addressed to relieve the biomechanics imbalance. The local trigger points must be continually monitored and treated since the postural changes may activate the trigger points to refer pain into the arm. After 1 month, the patient was pain free and had functional range of motion such that the contralateral side could be arthroscoped. In Figure 2-17, note the improved anterior/inferior capsule mobility in the testing position of 90° abduction/external rotation. In Figure 2-18, the left sloping is less obvious and continued to change as therapy was pursued on the left shoulder for an additional month.

Insidious onset of shoulder pain can be the result of a variety of circumstances and/or tissue irritations. The patients develop shoulder pain from microtrauma injury to tendon, ligament, muscle, or capsule owing to athletic

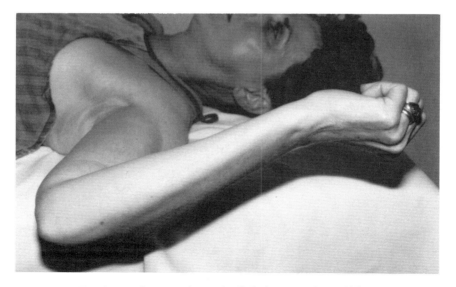

Fig. 2-17. Improved anterior/inferior capsule mobility.

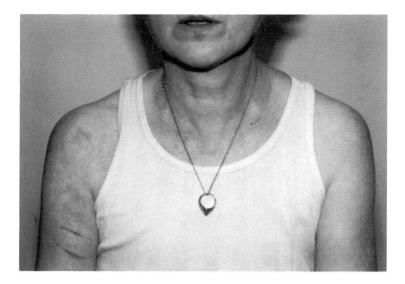

Fig. 2-18.   Left sloping is less obvious.

endeavors, work postures, sleeping postures, or the classic onset without a particular cause.

TRAUMATIC ONSET OF SHOULDER PAIN

Traumatic onset of shoulder pain and instability can range from a simple contusion to a fracture or dislocation. Although the latter is a surgical challenge for the physician, the physical therapist must manage the persistent soft tissue pain which may result from the contusion. Four concepts must be considered: secondary soft tissue damage, preinjury lifestyle, a series of microtrauma or macrotrauma events, and altered biomechanics leading to secondary and primary trigger points. Even if the mechanism and pathology seem very straightforward, these concepts should be addressed, as should specific questions that indicate specific pathology. Here, for clarification, we review a case study.

Case Study 4

S. P., a 34-year-old man, sustained a clavicular fracture and acromioclavicular separation on January 9, 1984. Treatment consisted of immobilization with velcro straps for 6 to 7 weeks. The patient reported much discoloration and edema in the area of the teres major, subscapularis, and infraspinatus muscles. He was allowed to exercise independently for 1 week and was then referred to a physical therapist. At that time, active flexion was approximately

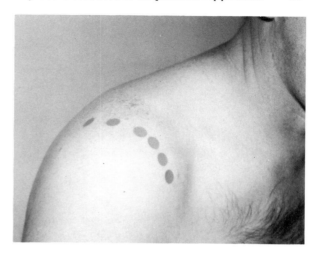

Fig. 2-19. Pain produced with active elevation (patient S.P.).

60°. The treatment consisted of heat, joint mobilization, and exercise. No soft tissue mobilization was reported. The patient obtained functional ROM after 1 month, but continued to experience pain. He received cortisone injections two or three times, but obtained no permanent pain relief. In February 1985, he was given a 10 percent disability settlement and was discharged from the attending physician's care. The patient refused settlement and sought care from another physician, who performed arthroscopic surgery after noting a necrotic spot on the humeral head and scar tissue that was limiting the patient's motion. Surgical release of the scar tissue adhesions afforded the patient increased ROM, especially into horizontal adduction. The patient was sent to our clinic for the goals of increasing ROM, decreasing pain, and increasing strength. His functional complaint, apart from pain, was an inability to throw a ball. Initial evaluation revealed the following:

Visual analogue scale: 7
Pain diagram: Figures 2-19 to 2-21
Upper quarter screen: Normal.

		Supine	Sitting
AROM:			
Flexion		150°	140°
Internal rotation at	90° abduction	60°	—
External rotation at	0° abduction	85°	—
	45° abduction	85°	—
	90° abduction	85°	—
Abduction		160°	132°

Mobilization: Inferior glide—painful and limited; scapular distraction—limited; posterior glide—painful.
Special tests: Negative.

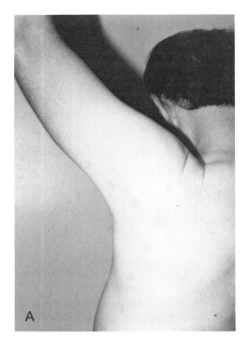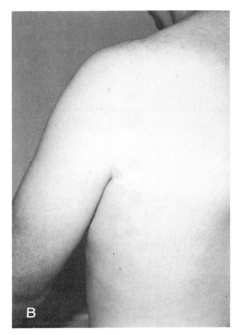

Fig. 2-20.   Pain produced when patient (S.P.) abducts (A) and extends elbow (B).

Palpation:	Local tenderness—pectoralis major muscle, teres minor muscle, long head triceps tendon insertion, and subscapularis muscle.
Initial thoughts:	This was a patient whose history revealed soft tissue injury (discoloration and edema in the area of the teres major, subscapularis, and infraspinatus muscles) as well as a clavicular fracture and acromioclavicular separation. Initially, the fracture was treated. The resulting frozen shoulder was then treated, but the original soft tissue damage was never addressed; thus, the patient had continuing pain from his teres minor, long tendon of the triceps, and subscapularis muscles. We believe that if the secondary soft tissue damage had been addressed initially, the rehabilitation period would have been shortened. His inability to throw a ball was the result of an abnormal scapulohumeral rhythm demonstrated in active and passive flexion (scapula protrusion); that is, the scapula was excessively protracted and upwardly rotated during flexion, a movement that places the rotator cuff muscles at a mechanical disadvantage. Continued attempts to throw would lead only to compensation by other muscles, development of secondary trigger points, and further pain. Prior to injury, the patient had led an

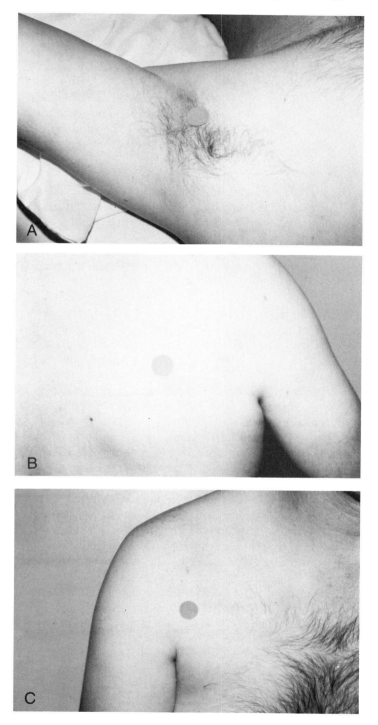

Fig. 2-21. Latent trigger points of patient (S.P.) in the subscapularis muscle (A), infraspinatus muscle (B), and pectoralis major muscle (C).

	active life. Further questioning revealed no previous recurrent shoulder pain during or after activities, which allowed the evaluator to assume that the patient had no preexisting microtrauma and that treatment can be vigorous.
Treatment plan:	The patient's treatment consisted of soft tissue mobilization treatment of trigger point with transcutaneous electrical nerve stimulation, phonophoresis, scapular isometrics, and resistive exercise/stretching with scapular stabilization.

The history should elucidate the four concepts mentioned above: secondary soft tissue damage, preexisting lifestyle, previous microtrauma, and altered biomechanisms leading to secondary and primary trigger points.

PATIENT PAIN DIAGRAM AND VISUAL ANALOGUE SCALE

Pain mapping, a way to localize the patient's pain, is the next step in the evaluation sequence. Figure 2-22 is an example of the body diagram used in our clinic. The patient places marks on the body diagram exactly where the pain is located. When the diagram is complete, the therapist reviews it with the patient, making sure that nothing has been overlooked and that it contains information regarding the quality of the patient's pain. Is the pain constant or intermittent? Often, the patient will first claim that the pain is constant, but questioning by the therapist may reveal that it is intermittent. If pain occurs while the patient assumes stationary positions, the therapist should seek a muscular component. Constant pain is less common and occurs with serious pathology that is beyond the scope of physical therapy treatment or is caused by a complex soft tissue problem with severely altered biomechanics that do not allow structures to rest. Is the pain sharp or diffuse? A sharp pain on movement may indicate an instability or abutment of structures in which the diffuse pain is the result of either a chronic situation of multiple trigger points, cervical involvement, or thoracic outlet syndrome. Such answers allow the therapist insight into the patient's problems, but are not diagnostic.

The therapist should note any skin changes (as identified in case study 4), scars, surgical procedures, and edema. The progression of pain with respect to microtrauma and macrotrauma should also be noted. It may be enlightening for the therapist if surgical patients fill out two pain diagrams—one representing the pain that existed before surgery and the second representing postsurgical pain. This can help the therapist determine whether there is an irritated surgical area, whether preexisting trigger points are still producing pain, or whether new pain is being produced by immobilization or surgery.

When all information regarding location, quality, and precipitating factors has been collected, the quantitative aspect of the patient's pain must be as-

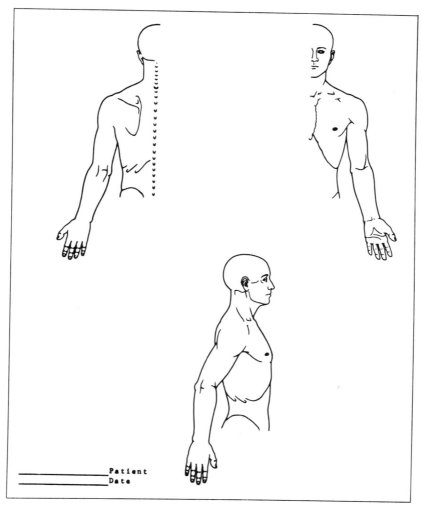

Patient
Date

Fig. 2-22. Body diagram used for patient's and therapist's identification of local and referred pain.

sessed. The use of a visual analogue scale (VAS) serves this purpose (Fig. 2-23). The VAS, as described by Price et al.,[29] is a 15-cm line. One end is designated as "the most intense sensation imaginable"; the other end is designated "no sensation." It is important for the purpose of validity that these exact words be used because this analogue scale has been proven experimentally using ratio data.

Unpleasantness of pain can also be assessed with the VAS. The ends of the 15-cm line are then designated respectively as "the most intense bad feeling for me" and "not bad at all." This second aspect represents the degree of

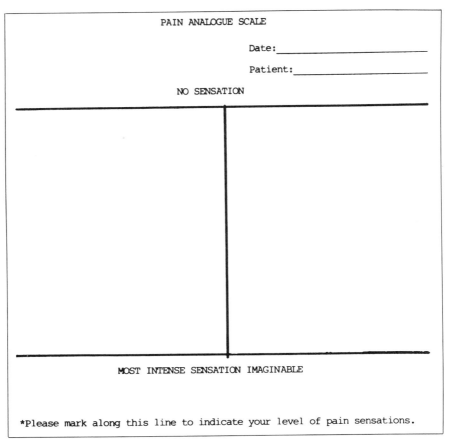

PAIN ANALOGUE SCALE

Date:_____

Patient:_____

NO SENSATION

MOST INTENSE SENSATION IMAGINABLE

*Please mark along this line to indicate your level of pain sensations.

Fig. 2-23.   The pain analogue scale is used to quantify the patient's complaint of pain. The patient marks on the line the level of painful sensation that is experienced. The scale is a 15-cm line. The "X" on the scale corresponds to a numerical value.

disturbance the pain causes the patient. In evaluating the chronic pain patient, both of these scales are helpful. We have encountered patients who say they are still hurting but are improving functionally. By using both scales—pain intensity and unpleasantness—both aspects of pain are evaluated. Other professionals have used similar VASs to rate function, anxiety, etc. These scales are acceptable for the therapist's own knowledge, but have not yet been deemed valid.

The body diagram and VAS produce a clear picture of the patient's complaints and relevant history. Much information has been obtained before a hand has been placed on the patient. At this point, and with this information, the therapist determines irritability, limitations, and precautions that determine which manual tests should be included. Progression of evaluation should always proceed from the most benign tests to the most provoking so that the picture of the pain and mechanics is not clouded. Certain evaluation steps may be postponed until an appropriate time.

UPPER QUARTER SCREEN

In keeping with the philosophy of evaluating the most benign condition first and ruling out concomitant pathology, an upper quarter evaluation is completed next. This is particularly important in light of direct access in many states, and is a systematic way of evaluating all structures that could contribute to or be the sole cause of the patient's chief complaint. It is designed to be quick yet comprehensive. The upper quarter screen was developed by W. J. Personius at the Medical College of Virginia (Fig. 2-24).

It is advisable to evaluate even postoperative patients with a modified screen, the obvious rationale being a search for secondary limitations due to immobilization. Less obvious conditions may be discovered—subtle irritations or abnormalities that either add to the present problem or that may be aggravated during the rehabilitation of the primary problem. If such conditions are not treated initially, the patient's recovery is hampered.

The first three steps are self-explanatory and require only a few seconds. Step four requires a short description of the position in which the arm is held and used. With regard to the patient's posture, the therapist should look for scapular position (protraction/retraction/elevation) and head position, all of which may signal abnormal biomechanics. Under functional tests, the cervical region is examined first by the active cervical motion of forward bend, back bend, left rotation, right rotation, left side bend, right side bend, axial compression (Fig. 2-25), and axial distraction (Fig. 2-26). The latter two are manually administered. Both the mechanics (degree and quality of motion) and pain location and severity are recorded. After each active motion, overpressure is applied while pain is located and severity is assessed. Many therapists refuse to apply overpressure if pain is present on active motion. The decision is made by the therapist with regard to the particular patient. The cervical motion and mechanics evaluation is made to identify or exclude pathology originating in the cervical region. The neurologic examination is a quick manual muscle test that checks for weakness. The therapist stands behind the patient (Fig. 2-27) and gives resistance bilaterally to the following movements, evaluating motor functions at that level:

C2	Axial flexion
C3–C4	Shoulder shrug
C5	Shoulder abduction at 90°
C6	Elbow flexion
C7	Elbow extension
C8	Wrist extension
T1	Finger abduction

Patient _____
Date _____

Observation and Inspection
1. Body build: endo _____ , ecto _____ , meso _____ ; ht _____ ; wt _____
    Unusual features _____
2. Assistive devices _____
3. Skin _____
4. Upper Quarter Functions
    Position _____
    Use _____
5. Posture
    Lateral _____
    Posterior _____
    Anterior _____

Function Tests

1. Cx ROM   active   OP
        FB   ___ M ___ ;   ___ P _____   ___ P _____
        BB   ___ M ___ ;   ___ P _____   ___ P _____
        LRot   ___ M ___ ;   ___ P _____   ___ P _____
        RRot   ___ M ___ ;   ___ P _____   ___ P _____
        LSB   ___ M ___ ;   ___ P _____   ___ P _____
        RSB   ___ M ___ ;   ___ P _____   ___ P _____
        Comp   ___ M ___   ___ P _____
        Trac   ___ M ___   ___ P _____

2. Neuro
    Motor
            C1   ___
            C2,3   ___
            C3,4   ___
            C5   R ___   =   L ___
            C6   ___   =   ___
            C7   ___   =   ___
            C8   ___   =   ___
            T1   ___   =   ___

    Sensory
            Dizziness: ☐ yes   ☐ no
            Tinnitus: ☐ yes   ☐ no
            Light Touch & Pinprick   R   LT   L   R   PP   L
                    C4   ___   =   ___   ___   =   ___
                    C5   ___   =   ___   ___   =   ___
                    C6   ___   =   ___   ___   =   ___
                    C7   ___   =   ___   ___   =   ___
                    C8   ___   =   ___   ___   =   ___
                    T1   ___   =   ___   ___   =   ___

    Reflex   R   L
            C5,6   ___   =   ___
            C7   ___   =   ___

3. Vascular
    Radial Pulse
    Thoracic Outlet

4. Peripheral Joints
    Shoulder
            UE Elevation   ___ M ___ ;   ___ P _____   (OP) _____
            Locking Position   ___ M ___ ;   ___ P _____
            Quadrant Position ___ M ___ ;   ___ P _____
    Elbow   (OP)
            Flex RL   ___ M ___ ;   ___ P _____   ___ P _____
            Ext   ___ M ___ ;   ___ P _____   ___ P _____
    Forearm
            Sup   ___ M ___ ;   ___ P _____   ___ P _____
            Pro   ___ M ___ ;   ___ P _____   ___ P _____
    Wrist
            Flex   ___ M ___ ;   ___ P _____   ___ P _____
            Ext   ___ M ___ ;   ___ P _____   ___ P _____
            RD   ___ M ___ ;   ___ P _____   ___ P _____
            UD   ___ M ___ ;   ___ P _____   ___ P _____

Fig. 2-24. Upper quarter scanning examination. (Developed by Walter J. Personius, Ph.D., P.T., Fall 1980, Medical College of Virginia Department of Physical Therapy.)

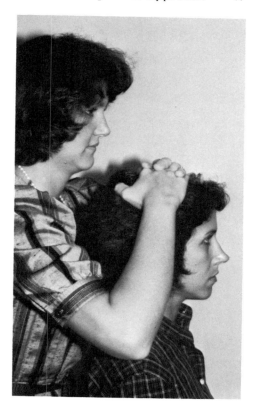

Fig. 2-25. Axial compression maneuver as part of upper quarter screen.

The sensory component involves looking for and asking about dizziness and tinnitus to rule out vascular problems. The therapist tests sensation by running the fingers and a pin over all dermatome areas of the patient bilaterally, looking for differences in sensation in the patient's right side compared with the left. The dermatomes are represented as follows:

C4	Top of the shoulder
C5	Deltoid area
C6	Lateral arm to thumb
C7	Middle finger
C8	Ulnar aspect of hand
T1	Medial upper arm

The reflexes of the biceps (C5, C6) and triceps (C7), which are two-level innervated, are tested with a reflex hammer. Results are compared right to left. The radial pulse is palpated in the resting and elevated positions to determine strength and regularity.

Finally, each peripheral joint is examined for mechanics and pain. Overpressure is applied, where appropriate, to discover pain. The locking position

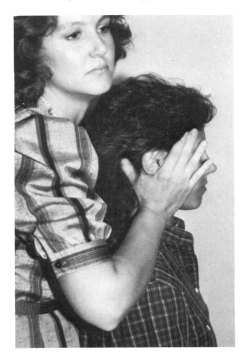

Fig. 2-26.   Cervical distraction as part of upper quarter screen.

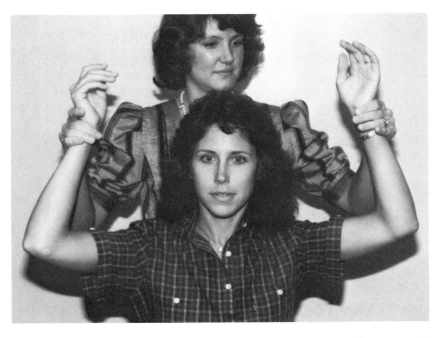

Fig. 2-27.   Therapist stands behind the patient, giving bilateral resistance to elbow extension as part of upper quarter screen.

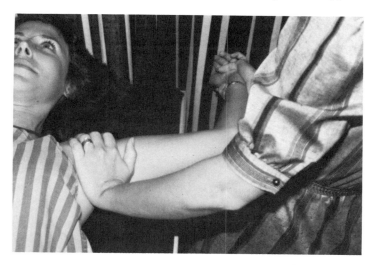

Fig. 2-28. Quadrant position maneuver performed as part of upper quarter screen; patient's arm is placed in abduction and external rotation.

and quadrant position are evaluated with the patient supine. The shoulder is abducted to 90°, then externally rotated (quadrant position) (Fig. 2-28); it is then internally rotated and placed in abduction (locking position) (Fig. 2-29).

It is obvious that for most postsurgical patients tests such as the quadrant position, locking position, and thoracic outlet (radial pulse in elevation) cannot be performed. They should be omitted initially and be evaluated at the appro-

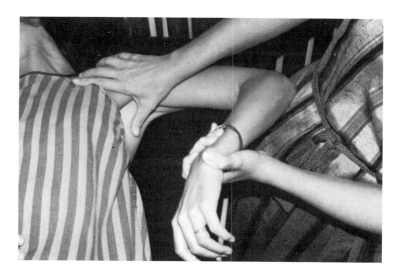

Fig. 2-29. Locking position maneuver performed as part of upper quarter screen.

priate time. In other patients, it may be that only at these extreme positions—where the capsule is taut and maximal stress is placed on the ligaments—that pain will be reproduced or abnormal mechanics observed.

The screening examination is just that, a scan of the total upper quadrant to rule out problems and note areas that need more specific testing. For example, a thoracic outlet test that shows diminished radial pulse in elevation is a red flag to the therapist to pursue this area in more detail and with more reliable tests. The whole procedure should take no more than 5 minutes, producing a volume of information.

ACTIVE RANGE OF MOTION

Active range of motion demonstrates to the therapist the patient's ability to utilize muscular strength and coordinated action about a particular joint.[30–33] If AROM limitation exists, then muscular weakness or some tissue irritation is inhibiting the movement pattern. Measurements are typically taken supine and sitting to observe for painful arcs, substitution patterns, and specific muscular weakness. Besides yielding goniometric measurements, AROM should demonstrate the coordinate movements of the rotator cuff muscles and the kinesiologic patterns of the entire shoulder girdle complex. As the patient performs shoulder motions, the therapist can key in on these points for later muscle testing or passive joint assessment. For example, when the patient is asked to abduct the shoulder, is scapular protraction noted? Or, does the patient perform the movement in the frontal rather than saggital plane?

Laumann[34] and Moseley[35] have published reports on kinesiologic movements, which are expansions of earlier works, particularly of Inman et al.[36] Laumann suggested that during elevation, four essential muscles must function throughout the AROM and that loss of any of these muscles would cause significant limitation.[34] These muscles are the deltoid, trapezius, supraspinatus, and serratus anterior muscles. Moseley,[35] on the other hand, ascertains that muscular force couples guide the shoulder girdle through elevation. These muscular force couples are (1) levatorscapulae/lower trapezius, (2) upper trapezius/pectoralis minor, and (3) middle trapezius/serratus anterior.

In applying these studies to evaluation of the clinical shoulder patient, the therapist is encouraged to observe and test these specific muscles as well as to assess them later for passive extensibility and/or potential trigger points.

In the literature, several investigators have identified shoulder elevation (abduction) in the plane of the scapula.[37–39] This plane is 30° to 45° anterior the frontal plane, corresponding to the anterior positioning of the glenoid fossa and the retroverted position of the humeral head. In this position, shoulder elevation is truly measured without the extra external rotation needed for abduction or the component of internal rotation needed for flexion.[40]

Several other observations may also be included during active motion assessment. First, scapular rotation monitoring might be helpful in identifying any restriction during active motion.[41] It has been noted that scapular rotation is greatest during 80° to 140° of abduction and when total rotation is 60° in

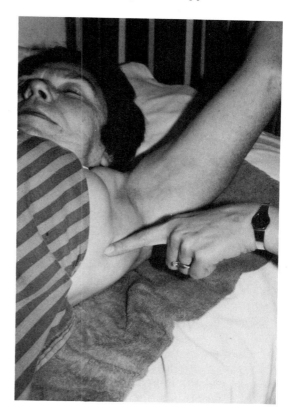

Fig. 2-30. In active elevation, the scapula "wings" or glides laterally, indicating shortening of the posterior shoulder girdle muscles.

addition to a medial tilt of 40° and a downward tilt arc of 24°.[42] Second, in observing scapular protraction, or the "winging" of the scapula that occurs during AROM, retraction/stabilization of the scapula on the chest wall can be performed, and decreased active motion be observed (Figs. 2-30 and 2-31). Since the rotator cuff muscles may have adaptively shortened following trauma or immobilization, the scapula will move laterally off the chest rather than rotating to accommodate the inferior movement of the humeral head.

Third, to determine if restrictions of elevation are due to tight musculature, two overpressure techniques can yield information. In supine elevation, overpressure can provide information about pectoralis major muscle tightness. If this muscle is tight, with overpressure, the inferior thoracic cage will raise. In the sitting position, a tight triceps (long head) may restrict elevation. The patient is asked to place his or her involved extremity hand over the C7 spinous process, then passive elevation overpressure at the elbow is applied.

Finally, as shown in Figure 2-32, selective stressing of muscle and non-contractile structures can be performed in three testing positions of external rotation. In each position tested and measured actively and passively, information can be obtained about restrictive structures. This testing sequence will be described in the passive motion section.

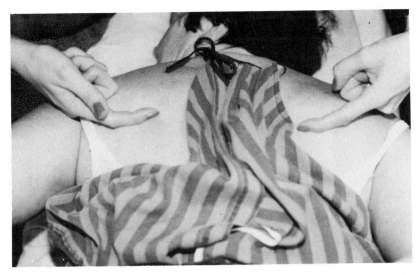

Fig. 2-31. Examination of the heights of inferior scapular angles to assess levator scapulae muscle irritation, which provokes elevation and downward rotation of the scapula.

Throughout the active motion assessment, notations are made on the body diagram of limitations, local versus referred pain, and scapular protraction as the patient performs the movement patterns.

PASSIVE RANGE OF MOTION

Passive motion and joint play assessment permit a further evaluation of contractile versus non-contractile structure restriction.[43-45] Notations can again be made on the body diagrams regarding pain and specific restrictions. Cyriax's capsular patterns can be observed at this time, as can the unique capsular pattern of the diabetic shoulder pattern.[6,46]

Joint play techniques performed on all joints of the shoulder girdle, glenohumeral joint, acromioclavicular joint, sternoclavicular joint, and scapulothoracic joint yield specific information regarding the specific joint arthrokinematics and the status of surrounding tissues.[43-45] These specific maneuvers are listed in Chapter 11 as treatment techniques but also can be used for assessment.

Interest in the stabilizing structures of the shoulder girdle has yielded three recent studies that sequentially identified stabilizing structures via cadaver studies. In 1981, Turkel and associates sequentially analyzed the stabilizing influences of the structures about the shoulder girdle in 36 cadaver shoulders.[47] The analysis was conducted in the positions of 0°, 45°, and 90° external rotation.

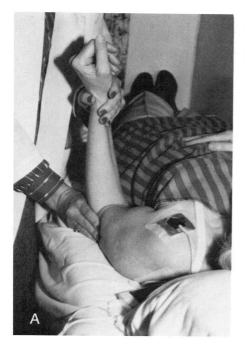

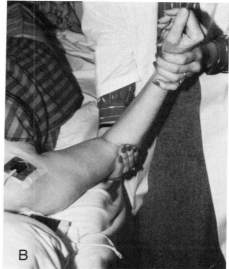

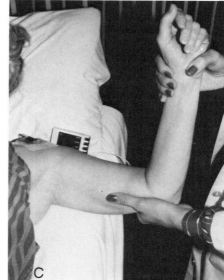

Fig. 2-32. Identification of external rotation/elevation limitation by test position: (A) 0° abduction—subscapularis, (B) 45° abduction—middle, anterior-superior glenohumeral ligament, subscapularis, and (C) 90° abduction—inferior glenohumeral ligament.

They reported that in the 0° position, the subscapularis muscles, the middle glenohumeral ligament (MGHL), and the superior and inferior portions of the inferior glenohumeral ligament (IGHL) stabilized the joint; in the 45° position, the subscapularis muscle, the MGHL, and the inferior portion of the IGHL stabilized and in the 90° position, the inferior and posterior portions of the IGHL stabilized.

In 1987, Schwartz et al. observed in posterior instability patterns, like anterior instability patterns, that when the capsule was cut interiorly, the humeral head began to sublux.[48] However, when the entire inferior capsule was incised, posterior subluxation occurred.

Therefore, using the external rotation testing positions passively, the following was observed: the 0° position tests the extensibility of the superior/anterior capsule, superior band IGHL, subscapularis muscle, and MGHL; the 45° position tests the extensibility of the subscapularis muscle, superior portion of the IGHL, and the MGHL; and the 90° position tests the extensibility of the posterior and inferior bands of the IGHL and the axillary pouch (lower anterior capsule).

In 1985, Ovesen et al.[49] studied serial sections of 10 cadaver shoulders. They observed that the most stabilizing structure was the subscapularis muscles, and that the lower portion of the anterior capsule stabilized during increasing abduction.

Although all of these investigators pursued their studies in different ways, their data are similarly conclusive in terms of the area of passive stability offered about the glenohumeral joint.

To summarize all of the information discussed above, with the exception of special tests and tissue palpation, some general guidelines follow:

1. Anatomically, the patient must be able to achieve true scapular elevation. Excessive humeral protraction or collapsed humeral head fracture would alter the 45° angle relationship of humeral head to glenoid fossa.[39]

2. Anterior structure extensibility can determine the potential for abduction, extension, elevation, external rotation, and medial rotation (combined extension and internal rotation).

3. Inferior structure extensibility can determine the potential for flexion, elevation, and abduction.

4. Posterior structure extensibility can determine the potential for horizontal adduction, internal rotation, and shoulder elevation/elbow extension.

5. Scapular mobility provides information regarding the extensibility of levator scapulae, rhomboid, posterior rotator cuff, trapezius, and serratus anterior muscles.

There is one report regarding a clinical functional assessment for the shoulder. In 1987, Constant and Murley[50] reported the compilation of pain, activities of daily living, ROM (goniometry), and power (Cybex, Ronkonkoma, NY) to determine functional outcome in 100 patients. Using three different observers, the error average was 3 percent.

SPECIAL TESTS

Various special tests described in this chapter have been developed to test specific lesions in the shoulder girdle. The therapist must remember that these are called special tests because they test special conditions, not because they are particularly reliable. Much controversy exists as to the value of certain tests. The therapist must acknowledge that each test is only a small piece of the total picture and not predictive in itself.

Impingement Syndromes

Impingement syndrome tests have been described by Neviaser and Neviaser,[10] Neer and Welsh,[12] and Hawkins and Kennedy.[13] The tests are similar, but each investigator believes his or her variation has a better predictive value. Neer and Welsh produce impingement pain by forceful elevation (flexion) of the humerus, which forces the abutment of the rotator cuff tissues into the anterior third of the acromion.[12] If pain is eliminated during this procedure by injection of 10 mL of 1 percent Xylocaine (lidocaine) into the subacromial space, the test is positive. Hawkins and Kennedy believe that the pain is better reproduced by 90° of humeral flexion with forceful internal rotation, which drives the rotator cuff tissue under the coracoacromial ligament.[13]

Neviaser and Neviaser describe the impingement test and the palm-down abduction test as being helpful for both acute and chronic rotator cuff tears,[51] and the "drop arm" test to be more often positive in acute tears.[10]

If complete rupture of the supraspinatus tendon exists, the therapist should perform a drop arm test. That is, if the arm is placed in 90° of abduction, the patient is unable to lower the arm slowly and smoothly. This is not to be confused with "dead arm syndrome," which was recently described in the sports literature and is probably related to neurovascular compromise.[52]

Bicipital Tendinitis

Another condition with symptoms similar to those of rotator cuff pathology is tendinitis of the biceps long head. Many investigators have described test variations for this condition. Yergason's test, based on one case study in 1931, is still widely used, but its reliability is being questioned.[53] The test is performed by having the patient supinate actively against the examiner's resistance with the patient's elbow flexed 90° and forearm pronated. The patient will experience pain in the anterior, inner aspect of the shoulder. Lippman's test, on the other hand, relies on palpation of the tendon. Unfortunately, the tendon is difficult to palpate in the muscular shoulder of an athlete. In this test, the examiner displaces the patient's tendon from the side, producing a sharp pain.[54] The reverse of Lippman's test was described by deAnquin: in this test, the examiner rotates the patient's shoulder internally and externally while palpating the anterior portion of the shoulder.[30] The test is positive if the most tender spot occurs as the biceps tendon passes under the examiner's fingers. In Ludington's test, a patient grasps the top of his or her head, and then actively flexes the affected elbow, producing sharp pain.[55] Hawkins and Kennedy elicit pain by having the patient resist humeral flexion with an extended elbow; thus, their test is called the straight arm test.[13]

Transverse Humeral Ligament Rupture

To test for rupture of the transverse humeral ligament, the therapist positions the patient's arm in shoulder abduction and external rotation. The arm should be internally rotated while the examiner palpates over the bicipital groove. If the transverse ligament holding the tendon of the biceps long head is ruptured, the tendon can be felt snapping in and out of the groove.[30]

Anterior/Posterior Shoulder Instability

In trying to identify shoulder instability beyond the "apprehension test"[32] and before arthroscopy,[56] recent papers have suggested additional clinical observation. O'Brien et al.[57] describe the sulcrus sign, in which multidirectional instability is identified. The clinical picture is a prominent depression anteriorly on the patient's shoulder below the acromion while traction is placed on the wrist inferiorly. Schwartz et al.[48] identified the need to identify more clearly posterior instability as it is typically missed 60 to 80 percent of the time during the first examination. The physical examination of the painful shoulder should reveal a prominent coracoid process, the glenoid fossa emptying anteriorly and bulging posteriorly. Specifically, Schwartz et al. noted that the patient cannot supinate the involved forearm while flexing simultaneously. Finally, they observed two clinical differences between those patients with anterior instability and those with posterior instability: the apprehension test is positive in the anterior instability group, and pain rather than instability is the primary problem of the posterior instability group.

Thoracic Outlet Syndrome

Although numerous thoracic outlet syndrome tests exist, their relationship to the pathology is questionable. Most tests rely on the vascular component of the entrapment, which is discussed in more detail in Chapter 7. However, the pathology does not have a vascular component.[58] Adson's sign, most commonly used, consists of palpating for the loss of the radial pulse while the patient extends the affected arm, rotates the head to the opposite side, and simultaneously takes a deep breath.[59] Wright's test adds abduction of the shoulder to 90° and full external rotation to Adson's test manuever.[58] In the costoclavicular compression maneuver, both neurologic (tingling) or vascular (decreased radial pulse) components are evaluated. While the patient allows shoulder slumping, traction is added inferiorly to the arm. The 3-minute abduction stress test and the supraclavicular Tinel's sign test use neurologic indicators and are reported to be positive in 80 percent of cases.[60] The patient's arms are in 90° of abduction and external rotation while the patient flexes and extends the fingers for 3 minutes. The examiner elicits a positive supraclavicular Tinel sign by tapping on the patient's brachial plexus in the supraclavicular area. The special tests listed are indicated by the upper quarter examination, history, and general shoulder evaluation. However, more recent reports suggest that double crush syndrome may also occur in conjunction with thoracic outlet syndrome. This would require additional sensory testing distally.[61]

PALPATION

Because palpation is a strong stimulus for pain, it must be performed at the end of the evaluation. If palpation is performed early in the evaluation, it may produce persistent pain, clouding the remainder of the evaluation and rendering further information useless. The examiner must choose, based on the information from the evaluation sequence, the least painful area to examine first (local versus referred pain). If the patient reports a history of a "snap" in the shoulder and now complains of anterior shoulder pain, palpation of the tendon of the long head of the biceps should be done last. Remote trigger points should be evaluated first. Last, it is important to make sure that the pain produced by palpation is the patient's chief complaint and not a new pain produced by the examiner. By pressing hard enough, the examiner can produce pain in many structures of the shoulder. In the shoulders of many persons who are not muscularly overdeveloped, the rotator cuff tendons, biceps tendon (long head), transverse humeral ligament, acromioclavicular joint, and sternoclavicular joint can be palpated.

The rotator cuff and biceps tendon are best palpated with the patient seated and the examiner standing behind the patient. As the examiner's finger drops off the patient's acromion anteriorly, it should palpate the bicipital groove. This can be confirmed by having the subject rotate the shoulder internally and externally. The examiner feels for elevation on each side of the depression or groove, which contains the tendon of the long head of the biceps. Medial to the groove is the lesser tuberosity with the insertion of the subscapularis. Lateral to the groove (greater tuberosity) is the tendinous insert of the supraspinatus, the most commonly afflicted tendon. If the subject's shoulder is internally rotated and adducted behind the patient's back, the cuff insertions of the supraspinatus, infraspinatus, and teres minor muscles become more anterior. They can be palpated from the anterior to posterior as the supraspinatus, infraspinatus, and teres minor muscles. In persons who are less muscular, a firm roundness can be felt at the supraspinatus and infraspinatus tendons. These tendons should be palpated for pain, but the edema, increased temperature, or crepitus should also be sought by using palpation in the same manner. The examiner palpates from the prominent anterior curve of the clavicle laterally to find the acromioclavicular joint. The clavicle sits superiorly to the acromion and can be distinguished from the flat acromion by its roundness. Bilateral symmetry, crepitus with flexion and extension of the shoulder, and local pain should be noted. The sternoclavicular joint is found at the medial end of the clavicle, immediately lateral to the sternal notch. Again, symmetry, crepitus, and pain should be noted.

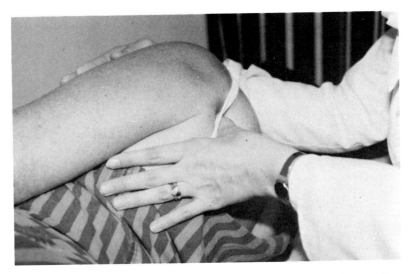

Fig. 2-33. Palpation of infraspinatus muscle/tendon to identify a trigger point and referred pain.

All muscles innervated by the same segmental level as the area of chief complaint (dermatome) must be evaluated by palpation. If the patient reports pain on palpation, the examiner must ask if it is the original pain or a new pain. Designation must be made between active and latent trigger points. The trigger point should be marked by an "X" on the pain diagram, and the area of referral pain should be designated by dots or slashes. For referral patterns, those of Travell and Simons,[2] Kellgren,[3] and Inman and Saunders[4] are suggested. Although these investigators differ on the segmental relationship between trigger point and referral area, the clinical importance of the two symptoms is clear. If the patient complains of anterior shoulder pain and the history suggests referred pain, the palpation examination should first rule out a local problem and then proceed to the more pain-producing trigger point palpation. Because the anterior shoulder is C5 dermatome, all muscles innervated by C5 should be evaluated. These include the subscapularis, infraspinatus, teres minor, teres major, supraspinatus, serratus, anterior, latissimus dorsi, pectoralis major, pectoralis minor, deltoid, and biceps muscles. We have found that the infraspinatus muscle most commonly refers pain to the anterior shoulder area (Fig. 2-33). This clinical finding concurs with the findings of Sola and Kuitert regarding trigger point incidence in shoulder patients.[7]

SUMMARY

Evaluation of the shoulder girdle complex requires examination of all soft tissue structures and involved synovial joints that comprise this mobile unit. Traditionally, goniometric measurements, muscle testing, and special tests were performed. However, as we learn more about the effects of connective tissue immobilization and the synovial joint biomechanics needed for functional movement, these traditional means of assessment do not provide a complete picture. As a consequence, our results are not optimal, and both patient and therapist are dissatisfied. Use of new evaluation techniques as well as resurrection of older techniques yields more specific information that better directs our treatment efforts. Our treatment goals become more specific. New parameters of the shoulder girdle evaluation will permit specific identification of symptoms and limitations that will help direct a more exact course of treatment.

REFERENCES

1. Jobe FW, Moynes RD: Delineation of diagnostic criteria and a rehabilitation program for rotator cuff injuries. Am J Sports Med 10:336, 1982
2. Travell JG, Simons DG: Myofascial Pain and Dysfunction. The Trigger Point Manual. Williams & Wilkins, Baltimore, 1983
3. Kellgren J: Observations of referred pain arising from muscle. Clin Sci 3:175, 1938
4. Inman VT, Saunders JB: Referred pain from skeletal structures. J Nerve Ment Dis 99:660, 1944
5. Forester O: The dermatome in man. Brain 56:1, 1938
6. Cyriax J: Textbook of Orthopaedic Medicine. Vol. I: Diagnosis of Soft Tissue Lesions. 2nd Ed. Williams & Wilkins, Baltimore, 1975
7. Sola AE, Kuitert JH: Myofascial trigger point pain in the neck and shoulder girdle. Northwest Med 54:980, 1955
8. Reeves B: Arthrographic changes in frozen and post-traumatic shoulders. Proc R Soc Med 59:827, 1966
9. Reeves B: The natural history of frozen shoulder syndrome. Scand J Rheumatol 4:193, 1975
10. Neviaser R, Neviaser T: The frozen shoulder: diagnosis and management. Clin Orthop 223:59, 1987
11. Neviaser T: Adhesive capsulitis. Clin Orthop North Am 18:439, 1987
12. Neer CS, Welsh RP: The shoulder in sports. Orthop Clin North Am 8:583, 1977
13. Watson M: The impingement syndrome in sportsmen. In Bayley I, Kessel L (eds): Shoulder Surgery. Springer-Verlag, Berlin, 1982
14. Kessel L, Watson M: The painful arc syndrome: clinical classification as a guide to management. J Bone Joint Surg 59:166, 1977
15. Hawkins RJ, Kennedy JC: Impingement syndromes in athletes. Am J Sports Med 8:151, 1980
16. Collins RH, Wilde AH: Shoulder instability in athletics. Orthop Clin North Am 4:759, 1973
17. Jobe FW, Jobe CM: Painful athletic injuries of the shoulder. Clin Orthop 173:124, 1983
18. Cofield RH, Simonet WT: The shoulder in sports. Symposium on sports medicine: part 2. Mayo Clin Proc 59:157, 1984
19. Penny JN, Welsh RP: Shoulder impingement syndromes in athletes and their surgical management. Am J Sports Med 9:11, 1981
20. Ciollo JV, Stevens GG: The prevention and treatment of injuries to the shoulder in swimming. Sports Med 7:182, 1989

21. Armstrong TJ: Ergonomics and cumulative trauma disorders. Hand Clinic 2:553, 1986
22. Herberts P, et al: Shoulder pain and heavy manual labor. Clin Orthop Rel Res 191:166, 1984
23. Delacerda F: A comparative study of three methods of treatment for shoulder girdle myofascial syndrome. J Orthop Sports Phys Ther 4:51, 1982
24. Westgaard RH, Bjorklund R: The generation of muscle tension additional to body posture. Ergonomics 30:911, 1987
25. Hagberg M: Work load and fatigue in repetitive arm elevations. Ergonomics 24:543, 1981
26. Chaffin DB: Localized muscle fatigue. J Occup Med 15:346, 1973
27. Berg M, Sanden A, Torell G, Jarvholm B: Persistence of musculoskeletal symptoms: a longitudinal study. Ergonomics 31:1281, 1988
28. Aaras A, Westgaard RH, Stranden E: Postural angles as an indicator of postural load and muscular injury in occupational work situations. Ergonomics 31:915, 1988
29. Price DD, McGrath PA, Rafi A, Buckingham B: The validation of visual analogue scales as ratio scale measures for chronic and experimental pain. Pain 17:45, 1983
30. Booth RE, Marvel JP: Differential diagnosis of shoulder pain. Orthop Clin North Am 6:353, 1975
31. Moore M: Clinical assessment of joint motion. p. 192. In Basmajian J (ed): Therapeutic Exercises. 4th Ed. Williams & Wilkins, Baltimore, 1984
32. Mosley HF: Examination of the shoulder. In Mosley HF (ed): Shoulder Lesions. Williams & Wilkins, Baltimore, 1969
33. Neviaser RJ: Anatomic considerations and examination of the shoulder. Orthop Clin North Am 11:187, 1980
34. Laumann U: Kinesiology of the shoulder. p. 23. In Kolbel, Helbig, Blouth (eds): Shoulder Replacement. Springer-Verlag, Berlin, 1981
35. Moseley HF: The clavicle: its anatomy and function. Clin Orthop 58:17, 1968
36. Inman VT, Saunders JB, Abbott LC: Observation on the function of the shoulder joint. J Bone Joint Surg 26A:1, 1944
37. Poppen N, Walker P: Normal and abnormal motion of the shoulder. J Bone Joint Surg 58A:195, 1976
38. Saha AK: Dynamic stability of the glenohumeral joint. Acta Orthop Scand 42:491, 1971
39. Kapandji I: Upper Limbs. Vol. I. in: Physiology of the Joints. Churchill Livingstone, New York, 1983
40. Blakely RL, Palmer ML: Analysis of rotation accompanying shoulder flexion. Phys Ther 64:1214, 1984
41. Bagg SD, Forrest WJ: A biomechanical analysis of scapular rotation during arm abduction in the scapular plane. Am J Phys Med Rehabil 67:238, 1988
42. Kondo M, Tazoe S, Yamada M: Changes of the tilting angle of the scapula following elevation of the arm. p. 12. In Bateman JE, Welsh RP (eds): Surgery of the Shoulder. BC Decker, Philadelphia, 1984
43. Brodin H: Principles of examination and treatment in manual medicine. Scand J Rehabil Med 11:181, 1979
44. Moritz U: Evaluation of manipulation and other manual therapy. Scand J Rehabil Med 11:173, 1979
45. Nicholson G: The effects of passive joint mobilization on pain and hypermobility associated with adhesive capsulitis of the shoulder. J Orthop Sports Phys Ther 6:238, 1985

46. Friedman NA, LaBan MM: Periarthrosis of the shoulder associated with diabetes mellitus. Am J Phys Med Rehabil 68:12, 1989
47. Turkel S, Panio M, Marshall J, Gagis F: Stabilizing mechanisms preventing anterior dislocation of the glenohumeral joint. J Bone Joint Surg 63A:1208, 1981
48. Schwartz E, Warren R, O'Brien S, Fronek J: Posterior shoulder instability. Orthop Clin North Am 18:409, 1987
49. Ovesen J, Nielsen S: Stability of the shoulder joint. Acta Orthop Scand 56:149, 1985
50. Constant CR, Murley AHG: A clinical method of functional assessment of the shoulder. Clin Orthop 214:160, 1987
51. Neivaser R: Rupture of the rotator cuff. Orthop Clin North Am 18:387, 1987
52. Leffert RD, Gumley G: The relationship between dead arm syndrome and thoracic outlet syndrome. Clin Orthop 223:20, 1987
53. Yergason RM: Supination sign. J Bone Joint Surg 13:160, 1931
54. Lippman RK: Frozen shoulder: periarthritis, bicipital tenosynovitis. Arch Surg 47:283, 1943
55. Ludington NA: Rupture of the long head of the biceps tendon cubiti muscle. Ann Surg 77:358, 1923
56. Caspari R, Savoic F: Shoulder arthroscopy: present status of a promising technique. J Musculoskel Med 39, 1989
57. O'Brien SJ, Warren RF, Schwartz E: Anterior shoulder instability. Orthop Clin North Am 18:395, 1987
58. Wright JS: The neurovascular syndrome produced by hyperabduction of the arm. Am Heart J 29:1, 1945
59. Adson AW, Coffey JR: Cervical rib: a method of anterior approach for relief of symptoms by division of the scalenus anticus. Ann Surg 85:839, 1927
60. Jaeger SH, Read R, Smullens SN, Breme P: Thoracic outlet syndrome: diagnosis and treatment. p. 378. In Hunter J, Mackin E, Bell J, Callahan A (eds): Rehabilitation of the Hand. CV Mosby, St Louis, 1984
61. Wood V, Twilo R, Verska J: Thoracic outlet syndrome. Orthop Clin North Am 19:131, 1988

3 | Isokinetic Evaluation and Treatment of the Shoulder

Mark S. Albert
Michael J. Wooden

Isokinetic exercise has become a popular form of resistive exercise in the physical therapy clinic. Since the late 1960s, the literature has consisted primarily of research data and clinical information relating to the knee. However, recent advances in equipment have made it possible to use positioning to apply isokinetics effectively to most other extremity joints, including the shoulder complex. The purposes of this chapter are to list some advantages of isokinetics in shoulder evaluation and treatment, to describe the adaptability of several dynamometers to shoulder diagonal patterns, to discuss principles of isokinetic testing and training with emphasis on shoulder positioning, and to describe considerations of test data interpretation.

PRACTICAL ADVANTAGES OF ISOKINETICS

Isokinetic exercise, unlike isotonic exercise, offers totally accommodating resistance to a muscular contraction.[1-3] Because the speed of movement is constant, resistance to the movement varies according to the amount of force applied to the resistance arm. Therefore, in a maximum-effort isokinetic contraction, the muscle is loaded maximally at each point in the range of motion (ROM).[1-3]

With isotonic equipment or free weights, because the speed of movement is not preset, resistance to muscle contraction will vary owing to gravity, positioning, lever arm lengths (in the equipment and in the patient's limbs), and cam sizes.[3] If, owing to these factors, effective resistance occurs only at a certain point in the range, it is possible that the muscle is being strengthened only at that point.

The primary advantage to isokinetic exercise, then, is the ability to load a muscle effectively throughout its ROM by fixing the speed of movement.

Isokinetics offers several other clinical advantages, such as the capacity for a wide range of speeds, both for testing muscle function and for rehabilitation or strength training.[4] This allows the clinician to determine at what velocities muscle torque deficits occur: at low speeds (so-called "strength" deficits), or high speeds ("power" and "endurance" deficits).[2] Testing and training at higher speed attempts to simulate normal activities in which angular velocities (as in walking, running, swimming, throwing, and other activities) are far in excess of most isotonic speeds.[3] Even the highest speeds of the MERAC (Universal Corp., Cedar Rapids, IA), at 500°/s, are not fast enough to match many activities, especially sports activities. However, exercising at different speeds may cause quantitative and qualitative recruitment of different muscle fiber types; therefore, most or all of the muscle can be loaded.[5–8]

Studies have shown that an increase in speed of isokinetic contraction decreases both torque output and electromyographic activity of the muscle.[1,5–8] Therefore, compressive reaction forces at the joint should also decrease. In joints that exhibit an inflamed or painful response to exercise, increasing the speed may temporarily "spare the joint" by reducing joint reaction forces. Whether training solely at high speeds contributes to an increase of strength at low speeds is controversial, however.[4,5] Nevertheless, the use of higher speeds is an important safety factor in reactive joint conditions.

Whether at fast or slow speeds, isokinetic resistance will accommodate to pain levels, further ensuring safety, because if the patient needs to decrease or stop the contraction suddenly because of pain, the resistance will decrease immediately, since resistance will never exceed the amount of force applied.[3] Unlike in isotonic exercise, little momentum factor is involved. In cases of pain or suspected joint reaction problems, another safe means of isokinetic exercise is submaximal effort, whereby the patient is instructed to reduce the contractile effort purposely. Decreasing the force used in isokinetic resistance exercise will, in turn, decrease joint reaction forces as produced in submaximal effort. Additional advantages of submaximal training include modification of pain, selective recruitment of muscle fiber type (slow twitch or type I), and improved joint lubrication.

In addition to the advantages already discussed, Davies[3] cites many other physiologic and clinical advantages of isokinetics. Also listed are a few disadvantages, some of which should be mentioned here.

A major physiologic limitation of the Cybex II (Cybex Inc., Ronkonkoma, NY) is its inability to exercise muscle eccentrically. Because muscle generates the most amount of tension eccentrically[9] and because much of functional movement requires eccentric contraction, rehabilitation and testing of the glenohumeral joint in an eccentric mode have important applications and have received increasing emphasis from clinicians and investigators.[10-13] Isotonic exercise incorporates eccentric muscle loading; however, for reasons previously stated, it does not fully accommodate for length–tension changes. With the advent of recent technology in dynamometry, instruments such as the Kincom (Chattanooga Corp., Chattanooga, TN), Biodex (Biodex, Shirley, NY), and Lido (Loredan Biomedical, Inc., Davis, CA) have the capability of applying eccentric isokinetic loading with the inherent length–tension accommodation. Controversy exists as to the safety of robotic instruments when applied to human subjects, and continued research is needed to clarify this issue. A key concept to robotic testing and training involves thorough understanding of the alterations in the force–velocity curve that are produced by robotics.

Another consideration is that the resistance mechanism, at least on Cybex equipment, is uniaxial. Extremity joints, of course, are multiaxial, as their instantaneous centers of rotation change constantly through movement.[10-14]

Some practical disadvantages of isokinetics in the clinic include the high cost of equipment, the amount of floor space required, and the time required to change positions and attachments to test the different movements. The latter is a particular problem with shoulder evaluation, because so many positions and motions are recommended. Testing of diagonal patterns reduces the time required for multiple dynamometer position changes, while assessing multiple muscle groups.

The testing and training protocols implemented before readiness for diagonal patterns require decisions about the positioning of the glenohumeral joint. To protect injured tissues while maintaining effective strengthening techniques, several important biomechanical principles warrant consideration. The 90° abducted position (90° AP) as described in the Cybex manual[4] can produce optimal external rotation torque and work values.[12,15] In addition, the proximity of the position may risk glenohumeral joint impingement.[15-18] The 90° AP also involves long-lever arm forces that are contraindicated in cases of joint instability and significant rotator cuff weakness.[19] The 90° AP is deleterious when restricted internal rotation ROM is present,[20] as torsion forces are transmitted from the scapula through the coracoclavicular ligaments into the acromioclavicular joint.

In contrast, the neutral position (elbow adducted close to the patient's chest wall) produces the optimal internal rotation torque values as well as high external rotation values. Two negative considerations of this position are the microvascular wringing out effect,[3,21] which deprives the active supraspinatus of necessary blood flow, and stress on the anterior capsular mechanism with forced stretching of the often inflexible subscapularis muscle.

Both Hinton[12] and Soderberg and Blaschak[15] suggest the need for multiple positions for testing and training and, not surprisingly, that no single patient or glenohumeral position is optimal for all clinical purposes. However, a compromise position that is safe from both vascular and biomechanical perspectives is the intermediate, or 45°, abducted position. Although Hageman et al.[22] found high concentric and eccentric torque values for both external and internal rotation at 45° AP, appropriate protection for both the anterior and posterior capsular and labral mechanisms also was found to exist. Interestingly, the 45° AP closely simulates the modified base position advocated by Davies[3] and can be readily adapted to conform to the plane of the scapula, which creates low capsular stress and produces peak isokinetic rotator cuff torque.[23,24] The 45° AP is also simply applied to all dynamometer setup capacities.

EVALUATION OF SHOULDER DIAGONALS

The Cybex II manual contains detailed information on testing all the cardinal plane movements of the shoulder.[4] Photographs and descriptions of positioning and machine settings allow for isolated testing of abduction, adduction, flexion, extension, and internal and external rotation. These procedures provide excellent information on specific muscles or muscle groups and are indicated for certain pathologies. The process of testing all of these movements as part of a comprehensive shoulder evaluation is quite time-consuming, however, and can be clinically unmanageable. The time management problem can be solved by evaluating overall muscle function with two diagonal movements, thus eliminating several lengthy steps.

In addition to its practical benefits, diagonal movement testing may also be more functional than cardinal plane movements, which fail to isolate and measure motion of the acromioclavicular, sternoclavicular, and scapulothoracic joints.[4] Of course, movement of these joints occurs throughout the range of glenohumeral motion. Resisted diagonal movement will load muscles which effect movement at all joints in the shoulder girdle. Knott and Voss,[25] pioneers in proprioceptive neuromuscular facilitation (PNF), first described "mass movement patterns" as being inherently diagonal in nature. These diagonals are dictated by anatomy—shapes of joints, lines of muscle pull, and soft tissue restrictions—and are those movements observed to be most used in everyday activities.[25] The movements to be described in this chapter are similar to the classic upper extremity PNF patterns.

TESTING PROCEDURE

The first diagonal movement described is the combination of extension, abduction, internal rotation (Ext/Abd/IR) and flexion, adduction, external rotation (Flex/Add/ER). Figure 3-1A shows the initiation of the Ext/Abd/IR movement, and Figure 3-1B shows the end of that same diagonal, blocked manually to prevent hyperextension. Figure 3-1C illustrates the end positions for the Flex/Add/ER movement.

For both movements, the patient is instructed to try to keep the elbow straight and to rotate the arm internally or externally, depending on which movement is being performed. To allow for rotation, a swivel handle is used. It should be pointed out, however, that the rotational component cannot be

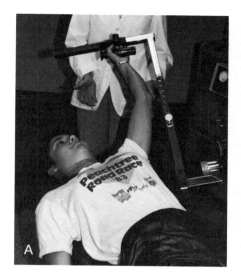
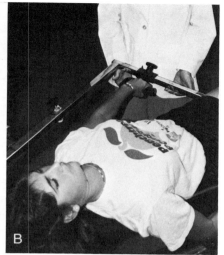
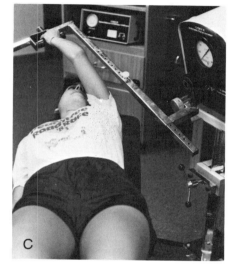

Fig. 3-1. (A) Initiation of the diagonal movement Ext/Abd/IR. (B) End of diagonal movement Ext/Abd/IR. (C) End of diagonal movement Flex/Add/ER.

resisted by the apparatus, as would be the case if manual resistance were used in PNF.[25] The dynamometer is tipped forward 15° to account for trunk movement and the forward-inclined plane of the scapula.[23,26]

Figure 3-2A is the normal torque curve for the diagonal Ext/Abd/IR and Flex/Add/ER in a post-anterior dislocation patient who has recovered most of her ROM. The shoulder is tested at 60°/s (low speed) and 180°/s (high speed), the speeds recommended by Cybex for flexion and extension.[4] An athlete or unusually strong person can also be tested at higher speeds as long as measurable torque is being produced. Figure 3-2B represents the torque curve for the injured side in the same patient. The lower foot-pound readings for the

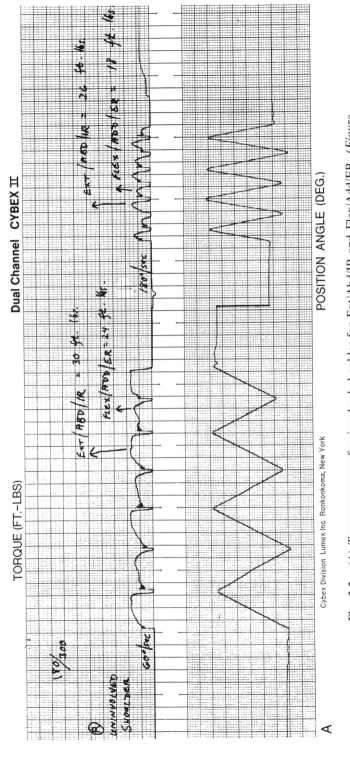

Cybex Division Lumex Inc Ronkonkoma, New York

Fig. 3-2. (A) Torque curves of uninvolved shoulder for Ext/Abd/IR and Flex/Add/ER. (*Figure continues.*)

68

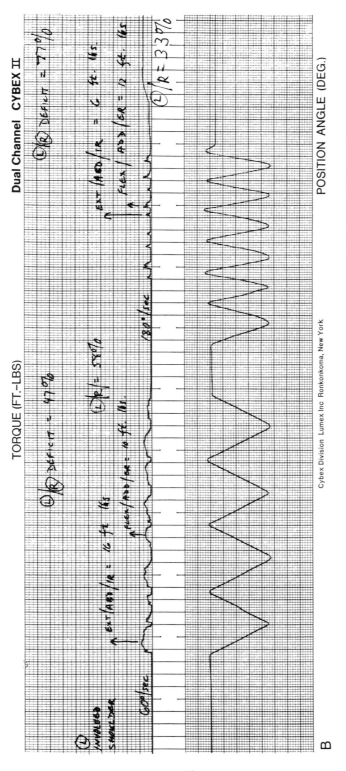

Dual Channel **CYBEX** II

TORQUE (FT.-LBS)

POSITION ANGLE (DEG.)

B

Cybex Division Lumex Inc Ronkonkoma, New York

Fig. 3-2 (*Continued*). (**B**) Torque curves of involved shoulder for Ext/Abd/IR and Flex/Add/ER.

69

Table 3-1. Summary of Peak Torque Deficits

Diagonal	Speed	Right Uninvolved (ft-lb)	Left Uninvolved (ft-lb)	Deficit (%)
Ext/Abd/IR	60°/s	30	16	47
	180°/s	26	6	77
Flex/Add/ER	60°/s	24	10	58
	180°/s	18	12	33

(Data from Figure 3-2.)

"left involved shoulder" indicate strength deficits, at low and high speeds, ranging from 33 to 77 percent. Table 3-1 is a summary of the torque measurements taken from Figure 3-2.

Not only can strength deficits be computed, but the shapes of the torque curves in Figure 3-2 can also be compared. The low-speed curves (60°/s) for the involved shoulder show a slower "rate of rise" than for the normal side. That is, the weaker side took longer to reach its peak torque. In addition, the duration of each Ext/Abd/IR and Flex/Add/ER contraction at low and high speed is shorter, as compared with the opposite side, indicating the inability to sustain tension. These variations in curve shape are further indications of muscle weakness that should improve after appropriate isokinetic training. Last, a comparison of the lower "position angle" scale indicates limitations at the extremes of ROM, although in this case the differences are slight.

This evaluation procedure can also be done for a second diagonal, the combination of Ext/Add/IR and Flex/Abd/ER. The sequence of these movements is illustrated in Figure 3-3. The start and finish positions for Ext/Add/IR are shown in Figure 3-3A and B, and Figure 3-4A&B, and initiation of Flex/Abd/ER is shown in Figure 3-3C. In this diagonal, the extreme of the flexion movement was blocked either manually or, as shown, using UBXT (Cybex Inc., Ronkonkoma, NY) attachments. Torque deficit computation and shape of curve comparisons were done as previously described.

INTERPRETATION OF ISOKINETIC TEST PARAMETERS

Traditional clinical practice with isokinetics has focused on the knee, with consideration of a specific agonist to antagonist torque ratio (hamstring to quadriceps) as a key clinical parameter. Similarly, the glenohumeral joint presents a key clinical parameter with external rotation to internal rotation (ER/IR) ratio expressed as a percentage. Two studies[27,28] have reported ER/IR ratios of 80 percent or greater; however, most studies[3,12,13,15,18,29,33] have consistently demonstrated normative ratios of 60 to 70 percent (Table 3-2). Consequently, the ER/IR ratio of 60 to 70 percent provides a basis for clinical description of normal force couple synergy and muscular tension capacity. The parameters of total work and endurance should also be examined as they provide an ad-

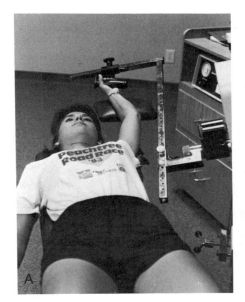

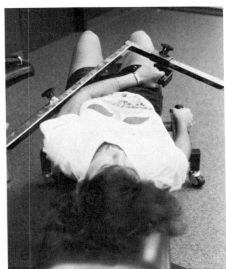

Fig. 3-3.   (A) Initiation of diagonal movement Ext/Add/IR. (B) End of diagonal movement Ext/Add/IR. (C) Initiation of diagonal movement Flex/Abd/ER.

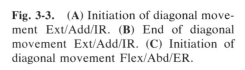

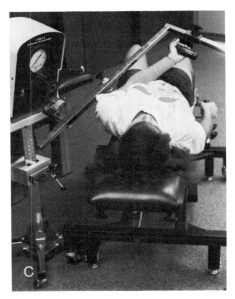

ditional perspective for clinical decision making and discharge status, and perhaps have greater functional significance than peak torque values.[19]

Because the upper extremity muscles are smaller in cross-sectional area than most lower extremity muscles, they tend to demonstrate smaller normative peak torque to body weight (PT/BW) relationships. The strongest muscle groups of the upper extremity also produce the highest PT/BW ratios: 45 to 56 percent for adductors and 25 to 26 percent for abductors, as consistently re-

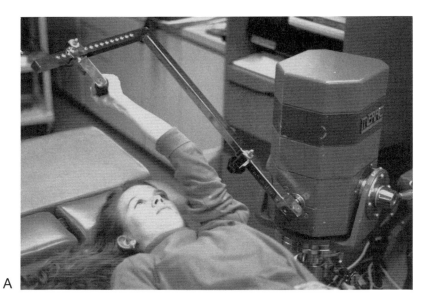

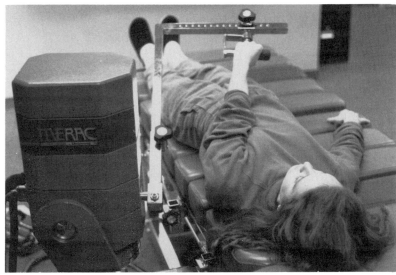

Fig. 3-4. MERAC isokinetic diagonal patterns. (**A**) Initiation of diagonal movement Ext/Add/IR. (**B**) End of diagonal movement Ext/Add/IR.

Table 3-2. Comparisons of Upper Extremity Muscle Torque

Study	Subjects	Speeds	Flexion/Extension	Abductors/Adductors	External Rotation/Internal Rotation
Cook et al.[28]	Male pitchers and non-pitchers	180°/s	70–81% 76–99%	NA	70–81% 81%[a]
Soderberg and Blaschak[15]	Males, nonathletes	60°, 180°, 300°/s	NA	NA	57–69%
Davies[3] (Ch. 12)	20 Males and females	60° and 300°/s	60% Males, 48% females	66% Males, 52% females	64%[a]
Ivey et al.[27]	31 Normals, mixed activity	60° and 180°/s	66% Males, 73% females	61% Males, 57% females	67%[a]
Alderink and Kuck[13]	24 Males, high school and college pitchers	90°, 120°, 180°, and 300°/s	48–55%	50–57%	66–76%[a]
Hinton[12]	26 Pitchers, high school	90° and 240°/s	NA	NA	56–62%[a]
Connelly-Maddux et al.[18]	21 Males, 20 females	60°/s	NA	NA	63% Males, 71% females

NA, not available.
[a] Data from 90° shoulder abducted position.

ported by Davies[3] and Alderink and Kuck.[13] No consensus regarding external rotation and internal rotation PT/BW ratios has been reported, with external rotation values ranging from 8 to 16 percent and internal rotation values ranging from 13 to 22 percent.[3,13,18]

The limited number of studies regarding shoulder isokinetic parameters and normative data have been performed with a variety of patient populations (mostly small numbers), differing test speeds and dynamometers, inconsistent methodology, and varied patient positions. Consequently, applying the normative data to a given population or to predicting functional progress or discharge status must be done with caution. However, useful and consistent concepts have emerged from available isokinetic normative shoulder studies that provide general guidelines for clinical decision making.

Bilateral comparison testing, in which peak torque at the injured joint is expressed as a percentage of deficit compared with the uninvolved ("normal") side, is one method of interpretation of isokinetic test data commonly used in the clinical setting. Unfortunately, this method fails to account for differences in strength that may arise from hand dominance, sports activity, occupational demands, and pre-existing injury. Common disagreements on whether strength differences occur between the dominant and non-dominant sides provide a dilemma for clinical consideration. Ivey et al.,[29] Connelly-Maddux et al.,[18] and Reid et al.[28] found no statistical difference between dominant and non-dominant sides, while Alderinck and Kuck[13] concurred with the exception of shoulder adductors and extensors. In contrast, Cook et al.[27] and Coleman[30] described strength differences between sides in baseball throwers, and Davies[3] determined 10 to 25 percent differences between non-dominant and dominant extremities. Perhaps, then, a small strength difference should be expected in a patient with vigorous and repetitive occupational or sports use of the dominant arm, but normal use in activities of daily living (ADLs) does not produce an expectation for greater peak torque of the dominant side.

When possible, industrial or sports prescreening with isokinetic testing provides an ideal situation to establish "normal" values for a given individual that are useful if injury or dysfunction occurs.

TREATMENT PROTOCOLS

In general, isokinetic rehabilitation of the shoulder can be initiated when the joint complex has progressed to tolerance of resisted exercise through a given ROM. Fractures, dislocations, muscle tears, and other soft tissue injuries should be well healed, stable, and past the acute stage. Although full active ROM is not required, it should be painless at its extremes. In postsurgical cases, knowledge of the surgical procedure (review of the dictated surgical report is extremely helpful) is essential in determining direction of resisted movement. Table 3-3 reviews resistive exercise progressions that are effective preparatory stages for isokinetics and indicates the appropriate timing of isokinetic resistance modes.

Table 3-3. Exercise Progression Based on the Time/Healing
Stages (Earliest to Latest)

Multiple angle isometrics (submaximal effort)
Multiple angle isometrics (maximal), inertial
Short-arc concentric isokinetics (submaximal), inertial
Short-arc isotonics
Short-arc concentric isokinetics (maximal)
Full ROM concentric isokinetics (submaximal)
Full ROM isotonics
Full ROM concentric isokinetics (maximal)

(Adapted from Davies,[3] with permission.)

Isokinetic training should be applied after consideration of patient position, dynamometer position, and attachments. In addition, the patient's scapular control, parameters of repetition, rest periods, speeds, allowable ROM for the particular pathology, and stage of healing should be considered.

Despite careful clinical planning with isokinetics, some patients will respond negatively with varied inflammatory responses of the tendon, capsule, and synovium, requiring immediate treatment. The use of cryotherapy post-isokinetics is useful to prevent such symptomatic responses. Our clinical experience, in agreement with Engle and Canner,[19] indicates that each isokinetic training session should be followed by continual reassessment of program tolerance and results, and progression to more challenging training should be preceded by two or three trial sessions of fixed intensity.

In all cases of painful arc, joint restriction, and instability, appropriate use of stops to block movement is necessary, especially when using faster speeds in excess of 180°/s. Blocking may be produced manually or as a function of the dynamometer with mechanical or electronic technology. Each patient problem dictates individualized blocking; however, anterior glenohumeral instability problems require restriction of external rotation with abduction, while posterior instability requires restriction of internal rotation with flexion.

In choosing which speed to use in isokinetic rehabilitation, several criteria are used. The most simple determination is based on the evaluation. For the most part, low-speed torque deficits require low-speed training, whereas faster speeds are used for high-speed deficits. Often, however, deficits occur at both testing speeds, as the curves in Figure 3-2 indicate. In this case, a helpful guideline is the "25 percent rule." That is, if the strength deficit at the 60°/s testing speed is greater than 25 percent, rehabilitation at that speed is indicated. If the deficit is less than 25 percent at the lower testing speed, training should be at 180°/s or faster.

There are several exceptions to this rule. As mentioned previously, the need to reduce joint reaction forces may necessitate high-speed training even though major deficits at the low testing speed are found. The same is true for a painful joint when the patient will not tolerate movement at the indicated speed. Contractile pain is usually less at faster speeds, although occasionally slow-speed exercise is tolerated better. Other ways of lessening pain include submaximum effort and short-arc contraction, which avoids pain localized to

Table 3-4. Guidelines for Isokinetic Speed and Protocol Selection in Shoulder Rehabilitation

Isokinetic Speed	Protocol
60°/s	1. Strength deficit >25% 2. Patient too weak to generate torque at higher speeds 3. High-speed movement too painful
180°/s	1. Strength deficit <25 2. Low-speed contraction too painful 3. Decrease joint reaction forces
Velocity spectrum protocol	Train at several speeds; simulate speeds used in normal activities
Short-arc contraction	To avoid painful ranges; possible instability at end range
Submaximum effort contraction	1. Not ready for maximum effort at any speed due to pain, inflammation, incomplete healing, etc. 2. Poor tolerance to initial test done at maximum effort

a portion of the ROM. Some general guidelines for selecting speeds and pain-reducing protocols are listed in Table 3-4. Submaximum effort training is some-times done for a few treatment sessions prior to actual testing of a patient who is not yet ready for the maximum effort contractions that are necessary for bilateral strength comparisons.

GENERAL TEST AND WARM-UP CONSIDERATIONS

Before maximal effort isokinetic testing, it is important to provide a warm-up stimulus to increase intra-articular temperature and influence the visco-elastic properties of collagenous tissues to reduce strain potential. Warm-up sessions can consist of upper extremity repetitive, low-load isotonics and/or sub-maximal aerobics for up to 5 minutes' duration, avoiding muscular fatigue. Apparatuses such as the Schwinn AirDyne (Schwinn Bicycle Co., Chicago, IL), UBE (Cybex Inc., Ronkonkoma, NY), or the pulley mechanism of the Nordic Trak (Chaska, MN) can all provide the aerobic component. Warm-up repetitions are then provided on the dynamometer with 5 to 10 graduated efforts at 120°/s and five warm-ups at each test speed.

As a general rule, test speeds will vary from 60° to 300°/s.[27] Based on clinical experience, 60°/s is excessively slow for initial training and test speeds because of the production of large shear forces that are contraindicated in cases of acute injury, capsular sprains, and joint instability. Davies[3] and Soderberg and Blaschak[15] support early clinical training with intermediate speeds (120° to 180°/s) and gradual change to velocity spectrum rehabilitation protocol (VSRP) with increased velocities up to 300°/s and, finally, incorporating slow speeds (60° to 90°/s) during late-stage rehabilitation. As described by Wallace et al.[31] 120°/s is easily controlled and tolerated by most individuals and provides the basis for our preferred initial warm-up speed.

Maximal effort testing of the glenohumeral joint after most traumatic in-

Table 3-5. Velocity Spectrum Rehabilitation Protocol

Repetitions per Speed	Velocities in Degrees per Second
10	60–90–120–150–180–210–180–150–120–90–60

(Adapted from Davies,[2] with permission.)

juries, arthroscopy, rotator cuff pathology, or arthrotomy should not be instituted until good tolerance of submaximal work has been demonstrated, at least 1 month after the procedure. Retest sessions should be scheduled at 1-month intervals to avoid negative reinforcement to the patient, owing to the predicted gradual changes in muscle physiology and force development that may manifest only 5 percent increases per week.[32]

Questions regarding numbers of repetitions and frequency of training sessions are difficult to answer since there is great variability among patients and the conditions requiring rehabilitation. A recommended starting protocol for low-speed diagonal training is 100 repetitions (e.g., 10 sets of 10 repetitions) at 60°/s. To avoid overuse, patients work out no more than three times a week at regular intervals, with repetitions added depending on tolerance, until several hundred are performed. Patients are routinely retested after each six sessions to determine when workouts can be advanced to higher speeds.

High-speed training can be progressed in a similar way at 180°/s, although Davies[3] recommends the use of several speeds at each session, using the VSRP.[3] Again, patients build up to hundreds of repetitions that are divided among many speeds of movement. Table 3-5 is an example of VSRP.

In general, when retesting shows strength deficits to be reduced to ≤10 percent, isokinetic training is discontinued. It is important to emphasize functional activities and ongoing home exercises at this stage to promote full recovery.

SUMMARY

A method of evaluating and treating shoulder girdle muscle weakness and joint dysfunction has been described. Diagonal movements relate closely to normal activity and provide time-saving and practical means of applying isokinetics to the shoulder. For specific weakness of a muscle or small muscle group (e.g., in rotator cuff tears), the isolated movements described in the isokinetic manual may be more helpful. Similarly, certain injuries or surgical repairs may necessitate isolation of movement to a cardinal plane with blocked motion as appropriate.

Both isokinetic testing and training sessions should be preceded by warm-up techniques. Clinical decisions with isokinetics include timing of application, number of repetitions, amount of patient effort, and, importantly, the patient and glenohumeral positioning used. While both the neutral and 90° AP have specific advantages, it appears that the 45° position offers the optimal compromise of physiologic, safety, and strengthening goals for clinical training.

Normative data for the shoulder indicate a strength/torque hierarchy as follows: adductors and extensors followed by flexors and abductors and, finally, the internal and external rotators. Side to side torque differences tend to be minimal unless specific vigorous preferred activities, such as baseball pitching, are involved. Peak torque to body weight ratios range from 45 to 46 percent for the strongest adductor group to a variable 8 to 22 percent for the external and internal rotators, respectively. A clinically important value for normal shoulder function and synergism is the ER/IR ratio, which should be 60 to 70 percent for most test positions.

Although clinically useful normative data exist, this new area of isokinetic practice needs continued research. Similarly, existing clinical protocols and positions require additional research investigation, with the goal of improved patient care and potentially new uses for isokinetic technology as applied to the dynamic stabilizer system that is so critical to functional capacity of the human upper extremity.

REFERENCES

1. Moffroid M, Whipple R, Hofkosh J, et al: A study of isokinetic exercise. Phys Ther 49:735, 1969
2. Laird C, Rozier C: Toward understanding the terminology of exercise mechanics. Phys Ther 59:287, 1979
3. Davies G: A Compendium of Isokinetics in Clinical Usage: Workshop and Clinical Notes. S & S Publishers, LaCrosse, WI, 1984
4. Cybex: Isolated Joint Testing and Exercise: A Handbook for Using Cybex II and the UBXT. Cybex, Ronkokoma, NY, 1983
5. Moffroid M, Whipple R: Specificity of speed of exercise. Phys Ther 50:1693, 1970
6. Barnes WS: The relationship of motor unit activation to isokinetic muscular contraction at different contractile velocities. Phys Ther 60:1152, 1980
7. Thorstensson A, Grimby G, Karlsson J: Force velocity relations and fiber composition in human knee extension muscles. J Appl Physiol 40:12, 1976
8. Smith M, Melton P: Isokinetic versus isotonic variable resistance training. Am J Sports Med 9:275, 1981
9. Rasch P, Burke R: Kinesiology and Applied Anatomy. 3rd Ed. Lea & Febiger, Philadelphia, 1967
10. Jobe FW, Tibone JE, Perry J, Moynes D: EMG analysis of the shoulder in pitching. A preliminary report. Am J Sports Med 11:3, 1983
11. Ellenbecker TS, Davies GJ, Rowinski MJ: Concentric versus eccentric isokinetic strengthening of the rotator cuff: objective data versus functional test. Am J Sports Med 16:64, 1989
12. Hinton RY: Isokinetic evaluation of shoulder rotational strength in high school baseball pitchers. Am J Sports Med 16:274, 1988
13. Alderink GJ, Kuck DJ: Isokinetic shoulder strength of high school and college age baseball pitchers. J Orthop Sports Phys Ther 7:163, 1986

14. Williams P, Warwick R: Gray's Anatomy. 3rd Ed. WB Saunders, Philadelphia, 1980

15. Soderberg GJ, Blaschak MJ: Shoulder internal and external rotation peak torque production through a velocity spectrum in differing positions. J Orthop Sports Phys Ther 8:518, 1987

16. Elsner RC, Pedegrana LR, Lang J: Protocol for strength testing and rehabilitation of the upper extremity. J Orthop Sports Phys 4:229, 1983

17. Einhorn AR, Jackson DW: Rehabilitation of the shoulder. p. 103. In Jackson DW (ed): Shoulder Surgery in the Athlete. Techniques in Orthopedics. Aspen Publications, Rockville, MD, 1985

18. Connelly-Maddux RE, Kibler WB, Uhl T: Isokinetic peak torque and work values for the shoulder. J Orthop Sports Phys Ther 1:264, 1989

19. Engle RP, Canner GC: Posterior shoulder instability: approach to rehabilitation. J Orthop Sports Phys Ther 10:488, 1989

20. Kibler WB, Chandler TJ: Functional scapular instability in throwing athletes. Unpublished study, Lexington, KY, 1988

21. Rathbun JB, McNab I: The micro-vasculature pattern of the rotator cuff. J Bone Joint Surg 52:540, 1970

22. Hageman PA, Mason DK, Rylund KW, et al: Effects of position and speed on eccentric and concentric isokinetic testing of the shoulder rotators. J Orthop Sports Phys Ther 11:64, 1989

23. Johnston T: The movements of the shoulder joint. A plea for the plane of the scapula as the plane of reference for movement occurring at the humero-scapular joint. Br J Surg 2:252, 1952

24. Greenfield B, Donatelli R, Wooden M, Wilkes J: Comparison of isokinetic shoulder rotation strength in plane of scapula vs. frontal plane. Am J Sports Med 18(2):124, 1990

25. Knott M, Voss D: Proprioceptive Neuro-muscular Facilitation: Patterns and Techniques. 2nd Ed. Harper & Row, New York, 1968

26. Gardner E, Gray D, O'Rahilly R: Anatomy: A Regional Study of Human Structure. 2nd Ed. WB Saunders, New York, 1963

27. Cook EE, Gray VL, Savinar-Nogue E, Medeiros J: Shoulder antagonist strength ratios: a comparison between college-level baseball pitchers and nonpitchers. J Orthop Sports Phys Ther 8:451, 1987

28. Reid DC, Salboe L, Burnham R: Current Research of Selected Shoulder Problems. In Donatelli R (ed): Physical Therapy of the Shoulder. Churchill Livingstone, New York, 1987

29. Ivey FM, Calhoun JH, Rusche K, et al: Isokinetic testing of shoulder strength: normal values. Arch Phys Med Rehabil 66:384, 1985

30. Coleman AE: Physiological characteristics of major league baseball players. Phys Sports Med 10:51, 1982

31. Wallace WA, Barton MJ, Murray WA: The power available during movement of the shoulder. In Bateman, Welsh (eds): Surgery of the Shoulder. BC Decker, Philadelphia, 1984

32. Cote C, Simoneau JA, LaGasse P, et al: Isokinetic strength training protocols: do they induce skeletal muscle fiber hypertrophy? Arch Phys Med Rehabil 69:281, 1988

33. Loredan Co: Lido isokinetic normative values for shoulders. Unpublished clinical study, Davis, CA, 1987

4 | Posture and the Upper Quarter

Edward Ayub

The upper quarter consists of the occiput, the cervical spine, and the upper extremities, including the clavicles and scapulas. Through an interdependent process, positions of the component parts are related so that a change in the position of one structure may influence the position of related structures. An immediate relationship is perceived when one realizes that the occiput is connected to the cervical spine which, through muscular attachments, is connected to the shoulder girdle.

A disturbance in upper quarter muscle balance may lead to observable deviations in structural position and become evident as a postural deviation. Muscles that become tight tend to pull body segments to which they attach, causing deviations in alignment. The antagonistic muscles may become weak and allow deviation of body parts owing to their lack of support.[1] The muscle tone will change via afferent impulses from the joint structures such as capsule, synovial membrane, ligaments, and tendons.[2] These impulses reflexively influence the tone of muscles.[2] Although the function of a joint is movement, a disturbance in mobility may lead to pathology.[2] A joint may have a restriction in movement or an abnormal range of movement that results in shortening or lengthening of the muscles acting on it. These changes may result in impaired movement patterns that in turn result in pain or disability in the upper quarter. The most frequent clinically observed postural deviation of the upper quarter involves abnormal positioning of the head and cervical spine. However, the evaluation of faulty positional mechanics necessitates an understanding of normal posture to judge the degree of deviation.

POSTURE

By definition, good posture is that state of muscular and skeletal balance that protects the supporting structures of the body against injury or progressive deformity, irrespective of the attitudes (erect, lying, sitting, squatting, stooping) in which the structures are working or resting.[3] Although posture is described as a matter of alignment, observable changes in body contours may translate to some degree of variation in skeletal alignment. The spinal curve must transect a plumb line to remain in balance with gravity, such that an increase in any one curve may be compensated by a proportionate increase or decrease in the other curves. Around this line, the body is hypothetically in a position of equilibrium, which implies a balanced distribution of weight as well as a stable position of each joint. Balance is efficient with less expenditure of energy if the body remains in line with the vertical axis. Body deviation from this efficient positioning may be significant in understanding how posture may influence the upper quarter.

Faulty posture may cause prolonged mechanical deformation of a tissue and a structural change in inherent form. This prolonged deformation may produce a pain felt distally if pressure on pain-sensitive tissue is acute, whereas loss of function is more likely to occur if pressure is prolonged and continuous.[4] Maintenance of erect upright posture and performance of voluntary movements are highly integrated coordinated functions of groups of skeletal muscles. Inhibition of select postural muscles may be reflected in abnormal upper quarter postural deviations.

Of importance in the evaluation of the upper quarter is the position of the head, which is significant in the determination of overall body posture, as well as limb control.[5] Abnormal positioning of the head on the cervical spine is increasingly significant when one considers the importance of the upper cervical spine (occiput on atlas and atlas on axis) on the regulation of body posture. The essential afferent impulses for the static and dynamic regulation of body posture, as well as the ability to produce reflex changes in the motor unit activity of all four limb muscles, arise from the receptor systems located in the connective tissue structures and muscles within the upper vertebral synovial joints.[5] One may view the balancing of the head on the cervical column as a lever system whose fulcrum lies at the level of the occipital condyles, whereas the center of gravity of the head is near the sella turcica. The apex of the cervical lordosis is located at the posterior–inferior border of C4.[6]

Therefore, the center of gravity lies anterior to the fulcrum. It becomes apparent that motionless, erect posture is maintained by the antagonistic pull of the posterior cervical muscles against the force of gravity and the anterior neck muscles.[6]

An important group of muscles in the determination of head position are the suboccipital muscles, which have their origin as well as their insertion between occiput and atlas, occiput and axis, or between atlas and axis. These are short, deep muscles that run in oblique directions and have a high innervation ratio (three to five fibers per neuron), signifying that the number of muscle fibers per motor neuron is small.[7] Consequently, the potential rate of contraction of these muscles is similar to that of the extrinsic eye muscles. Therefore, they are well suited to their role of producing rapid movements as well as fine-tuning action capable of elimination of undesirable components of movement derived from the lower vertebral column.[6,7]

By design, the mobility of the cervical spine allows for its component parts to function unimpaired; that is, the discs are allowed to distort and recover, the ligaments have sufficient ability to permit movement, the apophyseal joints are free of bony disturbance and possess adequate capsular elasticity to permit their freedom of motion, and the soft tissues and muscles have adequate length to allow the bony structures free movement. Loss of movement of any part of the cervical spine may result in pain or disability in the upper quarter.

ABNORMAL POSTURE

Relaxed Postural Position

The relaxed postural position typifies a postural deviation reflective of inhibition of muscle activity. In this abnormal postural position, responsibility for the maintenance of upright spinal posturing is transferred from the contractile muscle unit to the noncontractile structural unit. The contractile unit consists of the muscle and muscle tendon, whereas the noncontractile unit consists of bone, ligaments, cartilage, and connective tissue. By their inherent design, the contractile units are well suited to their postural and movement roles. However, the noncontractile units, as a result of increased postural stress, tend to deform over time, which may result in dysfunction such as pain or instability.

An observable structural deviation that occurs with the relaxed postural position is an anterior displacement of the head relative to the thorax when compared with the anatomic points of reference that occur in standard posture.[3] With the head moving forward, the occipital condyles slide anteriorly on the oval-shaped articular facets of the atlas into a position of increased backward bending. Consequently, the occipital bone moves closer to atlas, resulting in the approximation of the posterior arches of atlas and axis. This position may be a factor in the mechanical production of headaches (Rocobado, course notes, Institute of Graduate Health Science, 1981). This postural position produces suboccipital muscle shortening at the atlanto-occipital joint of the rectus posterior minor and the superior oblique muscles and at the atlantoaxial joint of the rectus posterior major and the inferior oblique muscles. The position of increased backward bending of the head on the upper cervical spine will shorten the muscles forming the suboccipital triangle—the rectus posterior major and the superior and inferior obliques. This shortening may cause irritation to, or interfere with the normal physiology of, the structures passing through this triangle, namely, the dorsal root of the first cervical nerve as well as the vertebral artery.[8] The decreased suboccipital mobility has far-reaching conse-

quences because this region plays a significant role in the production of ar-
throkinetic reflexes. Specialized mechanoreceptors are numerous in the
cervical facet joint capsules as well as in the skin overlying these joints, and
contribute to the consciously perceived system subserving postural and kinesthetic sensations. A disturbance in mobility may lead to degenerative
changes, possibly altering these afferent impulses and decreasing their reflex-
ogenic efficiency.[5,7]

Abnormal Mechanics and Dysfunction

According to biomechanical principles, when a force is applied to a curved
structure, the area on the convex side is stretched while that on the concave
side is compressed.[9] With the increased concavity in the suboccipital region
as a result of shortening of the suboccipital muscles, one would anticipate
lengthening on the convex side of this curve. Because tight muscles tend to
inhibit their antagonists,[1] weakness of the anterior vertebral cervical flexors
may be anticipated. The increased suboccipital backward bending, coupled
with the diminished stabilizing role of the anterior prevertebral cervical stabilizers, results in lengthening of the middle and lower portions of the cervical
spine. As a result, the apex of the cervical lordosis moves cephalad, possibly
to the posterior–inferior portion of C1. Consequently, there is a forward displacement in the active segment of the vertebral column, consisting of the
intervertebral disc, the intervertebral foramen, the articular processes, the ligamentum flavum, and the interspinous ligament.[6] The passive segment of the
vertebral column consists of the vertebra itself. The mobility of the active
segment underlies the movement of the vertebral column.[6] Due to loss of middle
and lower cervical lordosis, an increased compression force is applied to the
posterior aspect of the active segment and a tilting or tension force on its
anterior portion, which shortens the interspinous ligament as well as the posterior portion of the apophyseal capsules while lengthening the ligamentum
flavum and the anterior portion of the apophyseal capsule. This may interfere
with the role of the ligamentum flavum in the prevention of impingement of
the apophyseal capsule between its two articular surfaces during movement.
In addition, one would expect an increase in compression on the posterior
surface of the vertebral bodies,[10] which may result in increased tension anteriorly. Posteriorly, this may lead to early degenerative changes,[10] whereas
traction spurs may be seen anteriorly, particularly on the anterior–inferior portion of the superior vertebral segment and on the anterior–superior position of
the inferior segment.

Changes occur in the muscles and soft tissue in response to the forward
head position.[11] Shortening of the suboccipital muscles moves the occiput posteriorly–inferiorly, which results in an upward and backward displacement of
the mandible in the glenoid fossa. As a result, there is shortening of the suprahyoid muscles, which are the digastric, stylohyoid, geniohyoid, and my-
lohyoid muscles, while there is lengthening of the antagonistic infrahyoid mus-

cles, consisting of the sternohyoid, sternothyroid, thyrohyoid, and omohyoid muscles, resulting in elevation of the hyoid bone.[11] These positions would leave the mouth open if not for excessive contraction of the supramandibular muscles—the masseter and temporalis muscles.[11] Therefore, the relaxed postural position appears to disrupt the normal synergism of the mandibular elevators versus the mandibular depressors. As a result of these positional and muscular changes, the patient may adopt mouth breathing instead of the more desirable nasal breathing.[11] The changes are significant when one views these muscles as links in a chain that joins the cranium with the mandible by the temporalis and masseter muscles, the mandible with the hyoid bone by the suprahyoid and infrahyoid muscles, and the hyoid bone with the scapula by the omohyoid muscle[12] (Fig. 4-1).

With the head moving anteriorly, and the posterior aspect of occiput moving posteriorly–inferiorly, there is shortening of the upper trapezius muscle, which attaches to the superior lateral portion of the scapula, as well as of the levator scapula, which attaches to the superior medial portion of the scapula. Therefore, shortening of these muscles results in scapular elevation. Shortening of the levator scapula muscle is considered clinically significant because this muscle originates from the first four cervical transverse processes and, consequently, is capable of movement in the suboccipital region, especially when the shoulder is fixed. In addition, levator scapula dysfunction may refer pain to the superior medial border of the scapula.[13]

In response to the loss of the midcervical lordosis, more weight and tension

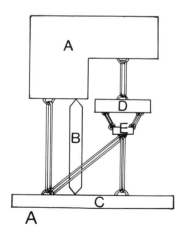
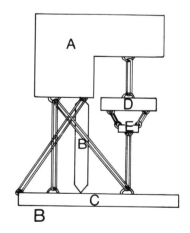

Fig. 4-1. (A) Schematic representation of the interdependent relationship of the upper quarter structures. The elastics show the posterior cervical, supramandibular, suprahyoid, and infrahyoid muscles. The omohyoid muscle is displayed to demonstrate the connection between the hyoid bone and the scapula. (B) Same as in Fig. A, with the addition of the levator scapula muscle and the sternomastoid muscle. The omohyoid muscle has been omitted. A, occiput; B, cervical spine; C, shoulder girdle; D, mandible; E, hyoid bone.

is exerted at the cervical–thoracic junction, resulting from the development of a torque force at the base of the cervical spine, which no longer acts as a weight-bearing column as when the standard posture is assumed.[14] Subsequently, there is a proportionate increase in thoracic kyphosis. The increased thoracic convexity tends to abduct the scapulae and lengthen the rhomboid and lower trapezius muscles, while shortening the serratus anterior, latissimus dorsi, subscapularis, and teres major muscles.

In addition, the increased scapular abduction shortens the pectoralis major and minor muscles, which, by their attachment to the coracoid process of the scapula, tend to pull the scapula over the head of the humerus. In an effort to maintain its resting position in the glenoid, the humerus moves into internal rotation, which shortens the glenohumeral ligament. This may result in contracture of the anterior shoulder capsule, causing diminished shoulder abduction, lateral rotation, and extension. Because a tight muscle inhibits its antagonists,[1] numerous muscle imbalances may result. Weakness of the lower trapezius muscle may result from shortening of the upper trapezius, levator scapula, and serratus anterior muscles, whereas inhibition of the rhomboid muscles may occur in response to the shortening of the teres major muscle. Increased glenohumeral internal rotation will shorten the humeral head medial rotators, resulting in lengthening and inhibition of the lateral rotators. These changes in normal muscle length may result in alteration in the normal scapulohumeral rhythm.

The movement of the scapula into abduction may result in increased acromioclavicular joint compression and may shorten the conoid ligament while lengthening the trapezoid ligament. As a result, the sternoclavicular joint slides posteriorly, shortening the anterior portion of the sternoclavicular capsule. This altered clavicular position may diminish the actual rotation at the clavicular joint and diminish total scapular rotation. The possibility of shoulder impingement is increased by the upper quarter changes seen with the relaxed postural position. The coracoacromial arch is described as an unyielding structure consisting of the coracoid anteriorly, the coracoacromial ligament running from the coracoid to the anterior edge of the acromion, and the acromion itself. Impingement may be caused by the close relationship of the tendon of the long head of the biceps and supraspinatus muscle to the coracoacromial ligament and the anterior portion of the acromion during overhead elevation. Impingement may result in a painful arc syndrome.[15] Because of limited space beneath the coracoacromial arch, rotator cuff impingement may occur if the volume of the structures passing beneath the coracoacromial arch is increased. Owing to the change in length of the rotator cuff muscles and the resulting dyskinesia, abnormal thickening of these tendons may occur, resulting in less space under the coracoacromial arch. The increased glenohumeral internal rotation stretches the rotator cuff and biceps tendon over the humeral head and may be a factor in their diminished blood supply. The vascularity of the rotator cuff is most compromised when the arm is adducted.[15] Degenerative changes of the rotator cuff are frequent because of diminished blood supply at the watershed area, which translates to the distal portion of the supraspinatus tendon, proximal to its insertion into the humeral head.[16] Although the supraspinatus tendon is most involved, the infraspinatus and teres minor tendons are also implicated. Owing to the increased length and subsequent angulation of the tendons over the head of the humerus, ischemia may occur; therefore, small attritional tears have less capacity for repair. This may occur in such a way that, with active contraction of the supraspinatus muscle, the humeral head acts as a compressive force, occluding the vessels coursing longitudinally through the substance of the tendon.[15] The prime movement muscles are largely ineffectual without the help of the rotator cuff muscles to steer the humeral head through the complex motions of roll and glide required to produce the full range of shoulder motion.[17] Repeated microtrauma in this area results in an inflammatory response with edema and increase in volume of the tendinous structures. The inflamed tissues are aggravated by their impingement during abduction. Further impingement occurs if there is a partial tear of the supraspinatus muscle involving its inferior surface, which allows a "buckling" of the tendon as it passes beneath the coracoacromial arch, resulting in a painful catching sensation.[15]

Impingement may also occur because of the formation of osteophytes on the inferior and anterior aspect of the acromion, as a result of traction by the coracoacromial ligament.[18] The shortening of the pectoral muscles pulling the scapula anteriorly, as well as inferiorly, may approximate the acromion and humerus, decreasing the suprahumeral space. Activities such as abduction and shoulder elevation may impinge into this already compromised region and may, over time, lead to the formation of osteophytes, as described by Neer.[18]

The acromioclavicular joint may degenerate in a secondary phenomena because the subacromial bursa extends under the coracoacromial ligament and may be involved as an extension of the inflammatory response.[15] The increased scapular rotation required by a patient with a painful shoulder may result in recurring stress at the acromioclavicular joint, with resultant degeneration.[15,19] Owing to the close proximity of the acromioclavicular joint to the supraspinatus tendon in abduction, degenerative osteophyte lipping of this joint may further mechanically irritate the supraspinatus muscle.[15,18]

The long head of the biceps muscle is subject to impingement because of its close proximity to the coracoacromial ligament during shoulder flexion.[15] Because the biceps tendon undergoes the same motions as the tuberosities, rotator cuff, and subacromial bursa, an alteration in the normal movement patterns of this muscle may result from the relaxed postural position. Because the sheath of the biceps tendon is an extension of the shoulder joint's synovial lining and the synovium is intimately related to the rotator cuff, an inflammatory process involving one of these structures may affect the other. The coracoacromial ligament and the anterior inferior surface of the acromion are known to contribute to the irritation of these tendons.[20,21] Inflammatory processes that constitute the painful arch syndrome can originate anywhere within the arch, including the acromioclavicular joint, the acromion, the rotator cuff, and the biceps tendon.[21]

Entrapment Neuropathies and Abnormal Posture

Nerve entrapment may result from the postural changes that occur with the relaxed postural position.

Suprascapular Nerve

The suprascapular nerve is derived from the upper trunk of the brachial plexus, which is formed from the roots of C5 and C6. Occasionally, the nerve may pass through the body of the scalenus medius muscle and, at the upper border of the scapula, it passes through the suprascapular notch. The notch is roofed over by the transverse scapular ligament, which thus converts it to a foramen. After it passes through the notch, the nerve reaches the posterior aspect of the scapula, in the supraspinous fossa. It supplies the supraspinatus muscle, the glenohumeral and the acromioclavicular joints, and the infraspinatus muscle. The relaxed postural position may cause traction, which in turn induces tension in the brachial plexus where the suprascapular nerve is given off.[22] Fixation of the suprascapular nerve by the foramen can cause tension in the nerve, with abnormal cervical spine–scapula relationships.[22] The relaxed postural position may move the scapula laterally, forward, and medially in relation to the thorax. This protracted position increases the total distance from the origin of the nerve to the suprascapular notch, thus placing stress on the suprascapular nerve.[22] This becomes increasingly important in individuals whose suprascapular notch is less spacious. The relaxed postural position induces shortening of the scalenus medius muscle, which in turn may irritate the suprascapular nerve. The forward head position also increases the distance between the C5-6 cervical segment and this nerve's insertion into the acromioclavicular joint and the infraspinatus muscle. The increased scapular protraction tends to create nerve tension, which may cause pain at the lateral and posterior aspects of the shoulder as well as at the anterior aspect of the acromioclavicular joint.[22]

Dorsal Scapular Nerve

Entrapment of the dorsal scapular nerve can occur because this nerve pierces the scalenus muscle. Conditions such as scalenus anticus syndrome, scalenus medius syndrome, and thoracic outlet syndrome may lead to irritation of this nerve. The relaxed postural position may shorten the scalene muscles, inducing abnormal tension on the dorsal scapular nerve. The scalenus muscles are accessory respiratory muscles. Hypertrophy of these muscles may be seen with abnormal breathing patterns. The relaxed postural position may induce mouth breathing as well as upper respiratory breathing and resultant scalene hypertrophy. Abnormal tension may result as these muscles are stretched with the increased scapular protraction. In addition, hypertrophy of the scalenus medius muscle may result from inadequate stabilization of the spine. This may be caused by ligamentous laxity owing to the increased tension on the anterior cervical spine, as observed in the forward head posture.[22] When the dorsal scapular nerve is hung up at its entrapment point in the scalenus medius muscle, the slack necessary to compensate for head and arm motion is prevented. A tense nerve moving against taut muscles (muscle fibers) can set up the initial mechanical irritation in the nerve that results in a neuropathy.[22] A dorsal scapular nerve neuropathy can cause scapular pain. Irritation to the upper trunk will cause pain along the radial C5-6 axis. In addition, an anomalous cervical rib may induce mechanical irritation to the nerve. According to Kopell,[22] the most frequent cause of upper extremity disability based on a scalene (neurologic type) mechanism is an entrapment neuropathy of the dorsal scapular nerve.

CONCLUSION

Dysfunction of any upper quarter structure may be related to abnormal posture. However, the motor system tends to function as an entity in that a local dysfunction produces a chain of reflexes that may involve the whole motor system and vice versa. Therefore, although upper quarter dysfunctions may be apparent locally, the subsequent solution to pathology may necessitate evaluation of the motor system as a whole.

REFERENCES

1. Janda V: Muscles as a pathogenic factor in back pain. In Buswell J, Smith MD (eds): The Treatment of Patients: Proceedings of the International Federation of Orthopaedic Manipulative Therapists, 4th Conference, Christchurch, New Zealand, 1980
2. Stoddard A: Manual of Osteopathic Technique. 3rd Ed. Hutchinson and Co, London, 1980
3. Kendall HO, Kendall FP, Boynton DA: Posture and Pain. Robert E. Krieger Publishing Co, Huntington, NY, 1977
4. Cyriax J: Textbook of Orthopaedic Medicine. 7th Ed. Vol. 1. Bailliere Tindall, London, 1978
5. Wyke B: Conference on the aging brain. Cervical articular contributions to posture and gait; their relation to senile disequilibrium. Age Ageing 8:255, 2979
6. Kapandji IA: The Physiology of the Joints. Vol. 3. Churchill Livingstone, Edinburgh, 1974
7. Grieve GP: Common Vertebral Joint Problems. Churchill Livingstone, Edinburgh, 1981
8. Warwick R, Williams P (eds): Gray's Anatomy, 35th British Ed. WB Saunders, Philadelphia, 1973
9. Radin E, Simon SR, Rose RM, Paul IL: Practical Biomechanics for the Orthopedic Surgeon. Churchill Livingstone, New York, 1979
10. Cailliet R: Neck and Arm Pain. FA Davis, Philadelphia, 1975

11. Ayub E, Glasheen-Wray M, Kraus S: Head posture: a case study of the effects on the rest position of the mandible. J Orthop Sports Phys Ther 5:179, 1984
12. Brodie AG: Anatomy and physiology of head and neck musculature. Am J Orthop 36:831, 1950
13. Gould JA, Davies GJ: Orthopaedic and Sports Physical Therapy. CV Mosby, St Louis, 1985
14. Saunders HD: Orthopaedic Physical Therapy. Evaluation and Treatment of Musculoskeletal Disorders. Viking Press Inc., Minneapolis, 1982
15. Penny JN, Welsh MB: Shoulder impingement syndromes in athletes and their surgical management. Am J Sports Med 9:11, 1981
16. Rathburn JB, Macnab I: The microvascular pattern of the rotator cuff. J Bone Joint Surg 528:540, 1970
17. Saha AK: Dynamic stability of the glenohumeral joint. Acta Orthop Scand 42:491, 1971
18. Neer CS: Anterior acromioplasty for the chronic impingement syndrome in the shoulder. A preliminary report. J Bone Joint Surg 54:41, 1972
19. Macnab I, Hastings D: Rotator cuff tendinitis. Am Med Assoc J 99:91, 1968
20. Bateman JE: Cuff tears in athletes. Orthop Clin North Am 4:721, 1973
21. Neviaser TJ, Neviaser RJ, Neviaser JS, Neviaser JS: The four-in-one arthroplasty for the painful arc syndrome. p. 107. In Omer GE (guest ed), Urist MR (ed in chief): Clinical Orthopedics and Related Research, No. 163. JB Lippincott, Philadelphia, 1982
22. Kopell HP: Peripheral Entrapment Neuropathies. 2nd Ed. Robert E. Krieger Publishing Co, New York, 1976

5 | Management of Frozen Shoulder

Helen Owens-Burkhart

Patients with a diagnosis of *frozen shoulder* are commonly seen in the physical therapy department. Unfortunately, frozen shoulder is often a "catch-all diagnosis"[1,2] that can imply myriad shoulder problems. In the literature, confusion abounds on the subject of frozen shoulder. First, there is no consensus on the name of this clinical entity. Some of the more common terms that are synonyms for frozen shoulder are adhesive capsulitis, periarthritis, stiff and painful shoulder, periarticular adhesions, Duplay's disease, scapulo-humeral periarthritis, tendinitis of the short rotators, adherent subacromial bursitis,[3] painful stiff shoulder, bicipital tenosynovitis, subdeltoid bursitis, humeroscapular fibrositis, shoulder portion of shoulder-hand syndrome, bursitis calcarea, supraspinatus tendinitis, periarthrosis humeroscapularis, and a host of foreign language terms.[4]

Confusion in terminology probably reflects the confusion in the definition, pathology, etiology, and treatment of this clinical entity that is so evident in the literature. One of the difficulties in reviewing the literature of evaluation and treatment of frozen shoulder, the main thrust of this chapter, was that few studies defined frozen shoulder in the same way. As a result, inconsistencies in patient selection based on their varied definitions made it difficult to assess the value of the treatment being examined. In addition, most studies did not discuss the evaluative procedures used to reach the diagnosis of frozen shoulder. The goals of this chapter are (1) to present a literature review of the pathology, etiology, and clinical features of frozen shoulder; (2) to establish a working definition of frozen shoulder; and (3) to present evaluative and treatment procedures for frozen shoulder. I hope that the reader can readily apply this information to clinical practice, thereby improving patient care.

LITERATURE REVIEW

Frozen shoulder is loosely defined as a painful stiff shoulder.[1] This definition appears to be more of a description of symptoms than a diagnosis. McLaughlin states that frozen shoulder is a popular medical colloquialism and not a diagnosis.[5] In this literature review, a working definition of frozen shoulder will be established.

Pathology and Definition

Historically, Duplay[6] in 1872 was first credited with describing the painful stiff shoulder, referring to the condition as *humeroscapular periarthritis* (periarthritescapulohumerale) secondary to subacromial bursitis. In 1934, Codman[7] coined the term *frozen shoulder,* attributing the painful stiff shoulder to a short rotator tendinitis. Codman devoted only nine pages of his textbook on the shoulder to frozen shoulder, summarizing this condition as difficult to define, explain, and treat. In 1945, Neviaser[3] surgically explored 10 cases of frozen shoulder, finding absence of the glenohumeral synovial fluid and the redundant axillary fold of the capsule, as well as thickening and contraction of the capsule, which had become adherent to the humeral head; thus, he used the term *adhesive capsulitis.* As Neviaser rotated these shoulders, it appeared at first as if the humeral head and capsule were glued together but could be separated with one or two rotational movements, thus freeing joint movement. Microscopic examinations in all 10 cases revealed reparative inflammatory changes in the capsule. Based on this work, Neviaser suggested that *adhesive capsulitis* described the pathology of frozen shoulder.

In 1938, McLaughlin[5] reported that in surgical exploration of a number of frozen shoulders, he found no histologic evidence of inflammation. He too observed a loss of the inferior redundant fold, but the adhesions between the folds were easily separated and separation did not increase shoulder motion. McLaughlin consistently found that the rotator cuff tendon was contracted and shrunken, holding the humeral head tight in the glenoid and allowing little motion at this articulation. Although unsupported by examination, McLaughlin postulated that the tissue changes in the cuff were related to collagen stiffening. This appeared reasonable since McLaughlin observed that prolonged disuse of the extremity preceded a frozen shoulder. He recognized that the reason for shoulder disuse may be in or removed from the shoulder. Although many studies cite disuse of the extremity as a contributing factor,[1,8-11] McLaughlin's study is one of a few that address collagen changes as a result of immobility in the frozen shoulder. Research documents that changes in periarticular connective tissue collagen result from immobilization. The effects of immobilization and its relationship to frozen shoulder will be addressed later.

In 1949, Simmonds,[12] like Codman, proposed that patients with frozen shoulder exhibited inflammation in the rotator cuff, particularly in the supraspinatus tendon. Inflammation of the supraspinatus tendon is secondary to degenerative changes in the tendon caused by impaired blood supply, as the tendon is repeatedly traumatized by rubbing against the acromion process and coracoacromial ligament. Histologic examination of 4 patients with frozen shoulder confirmed the above clinical findings, showing evidence of degeneration of the supraspinatus tendon with hyperemia, a definite inflammatory reaction.

Similarly, in 1973, Macnab[13] illustrated that degenerative changes in the supraspinatus occurred first at the zone of impaired blood supply where the tendon passes over the humeral head. This area is relatively avascular, as the humeral head pressure on the tendon "wrings out" the blood vessels. The lack of circulation in this area could cause degeneration of the supraspinatus tendon. The degeneration process produces a local irritation of the tendon. In response to tissue inflammation, the body produces antibodies affecting the adjacent rotator cuff tendons. This autoimmune reaction produces a diffuse capsulitis, or frozen shoulder.

Lippmann,[14] in 1943, confirmed both Schrager and Pasteur's theory that bicipital tenosynovitis preceded frozen shoulder. In examining 12 surgical cases of frozen shoulder, Lippmann consistently found tenosynovitis of the long head of the biceps tendon. The tendon sheath was typically thickened and edematous, and the tendon was roughened and adherent to the sheath. Lippmann proposed that the progression of the frozen shoulder could be determined by the extent of tendinous adhesion: the more advanced the condition, the more adherent the tendon. He attributed stiffness of the shoulder to the upward spread of the tenosynovitis into the shoulder joint, causing adherence of the intracapsular tendon to the capsule and the articular surface of the humeral head. Ultimately, the intracapsular tendon would disintegrate and gradual improvement of shoulder function would occur.

Turek[15] theorized that continual trauma of the rotator cuff and biceps tendon as they are forced against the acromial arch results in degeneration and edema. The tendons thicken as a result, creating a barrier to humeral head movement under the arch. If trauma persists, healing by granulation tissue results in fibrous adhesions of the biceps tendon, rotator cuff, subacromial bursa, capsule, humeral head, and acromion. The result is loss of motion at the glenohumeral joint.

DePalma[16] stated that the pathologic process of frozen shoulder primarily involves the fibrous capsule. The normally flexible capsule becomes nonelastic and shrunken. The mechanism responsible for these changes is unknown. As the condition progresses, the synovial fluid, fascial covering, rotator cuff, biceps tendon, biceps tendon sheath, and subacromial bursa can all become involved. DePalma observed involvement of these structures in various stages of frozen shoulder.[16] In the early stages, the capsule becomes contracted, with loss of the inferior capsular fold. In the later phases, increased capsular fibrosis occurs. The synovial membrane becomes thickened and hypervascular. These tissues lose their elasticity and easily tear as the humerus is rotated or abducted. The coracohumeral ligament becomes a thick, contracted cord as it spans the tuberosities to the coracoid process. The subscapularis tendon also becomes fibrotic, thereby limiting shoulder external rotation. In addition to the subscapularis, the supraspinatus and infraspinatus are also tight, resulting in restricted glenohumeral motion as the head is held high in the glenoid by these fibrotic tendons, thereby limiting downward humeral excursion. The biceps tendon was found to be adhered to the sheath and the groove. Like Lippmann,[14] DePalma[16] speculated that once the gliding mechanism of the biceps tendon is gone as the tendon becomes anchored to the humerus by adhesions, shoulder function begins to return.

Cyriax,[17] like Neviaser,[3] states that the term *frozen shoulder* is misused and abused. Cyriax says that *frozen* describes a symptom of stiffness. According to Cyriax, frozen shoulder is *arthritis,* which implies that the entire glenohumeral joint capsule is affected, limiting both active and passive movement.

For clarity's sake, I will explain a point of Cyriax's examination of the shoulder, which ultimately will help to clarify the pathology and definition of frozen shoulder. Cyriax[17] has contributed to a very thorough examination process of the shoulder that is used by many physical therapists. His examination includes selective tension testing of the shoulder complex whereby different structures are stressed by active, passive, and resisted motions to determine the site of the lesion. Both contractile elements (muscle, tendon, tendoperiosteal unit, and musculoperiosteal unit) and noncontractile or inert elements (ligaments, synovial membrane, joint capsule, articular surfaces, bursa, dura, fascia, nerve root, and fat pads) are tested.

In the examination, active shoulder motion is initially tested. Although active motion may incriminate both contractile and noncontractile elements, the results, when correlated with passive and resistive testing, frequently can give additional information about the soft tissue lesion. Second, passive shoulder motion is tested to evaluate the inert tissues, since the contractile elements are totally relaxed during passive testing. Last, with resisted shoulder motion, only the contractile elements are evaluated, since the tests are performed isometrically, thus preventing joint movement. Based on this examination procedure, Cyriax observed that patients with "arthritis" causing glenohumeral stiffness have pain and limitation of movement with active and passive testing only. Resisted testing is negative, thereby ruling out any of the contractile structures previously mentioned as the cause of frozen shoulder.

Limitation in both active and passive glenohumeral movement has been observed by others.[8,9,18-20] Cyriax[17] further clarifies that arthritis exhibits limitation of passive motion in characteristic proportions—what he calls the *capsular pattern.* The capsular pattern of frozen shoulder is most limited in external rotation, followed by abduction, then by internal rotation. Both Neviaser[3] and Kozin[18] noted limitations in these same motions. Others observed loss of glenohumeral movement in all directions[12,15,21,22]; in external rotation and abduction only[23]; and in abduction, external rotation, and flexion.[24]

Reeves[25] substantiated the capsular pattern in arthrograms of 17 patients with frozen shoulder. He consistently noted that more contrast dye was deposited posteriorly than in any other areas of the joint capsule and that the joint capacity was grossly reduced and the inferior capsular fold, subscapularis bursa, and biceps sheath were obliterated. Therefore, based on the arthrokinematics of shoulder motion, it follows that if the anterior capsule were more contracted than the posterior capsule, external rotation would be more limited than internal rotation. In addition, abduction would be limited by the loss of the inferior redundant fold and limited external rotation.

Scientific research and clinical observations point to capsular adhesions as the cause of the glenohumeral stiffness in frozen shoulder. Therefore, frozen shoulder will be defined as a shoulder condition in which active and passive motion is painful and restricted at the glenohumeral joint. Passive mobility is limited in a capsular pattern, with external rotation being limited most, followed by abduction, and then internal rotation. This, however, does not rule out that the patient with frozen shoulder may have had a contractile structure initially involved, as pointed out by the investigators previously mentioned. The frozen shoulder may indeed be the end result of such a lesion.[16] According to this working definition, however, a frozen shoulder does not exhibit objective findings of a contractile lesion unless the lesion is concurrent with a noncontractile capsular lesion.

In summary, various pathologies have been outlined as characteristic in frozen shoulder, including both inert and contractile elements of the shoulder. Based primarily on the work of Neviaser[3] and Cyriax,[17] the frozen shoulder will be defined as glenohumeral stiffness resulting from capsular restrictions.

Etiology

Although much has been reported on the pathogenesis of frozen shoulder, its exact cause remains unknown. However, certain factors—pain, disuse, and a periarthritic personality—are considered to contribute to the development of frozen shoulder.

Pain in the shoulder can result from various intrinsic and extrinsic sources.[10,26–28] Whatever the source, pain usually forces the patient to protect the arm from use. Immobilization of a synovial joint has been shown to have detrimental effects on the periarticular connective tissue.[29–36]

Lundberg[37] examined the synovial membrane and fibrous layer of the anterior–inferior capsule of 14 frozen and 13 normal shoulders. He found an increased amount of hexosamine in the frozen shoulder as compared with normal shoulders. This difference was caused by an increase in the total content of glycosaminoglycans (GAG), namely, an increase in heparan sulfate, chondroitin-6 sulfate, and dermatan sulfate, and a decrease in hyaluronic acid in the frozen shoulders. These changes in GAG content reflect a process of fibrosis occurring in the tissue. There was marked fibroblastic proliferation, indicating remodeling of the collagenous portion of the connective tissue. The cause for the increased collagen production is unknown. The end result of increased fibrosis is a "subsequent loss of biologic properties of the connective tissue" in the shoulder joint, namely, "loss of capsular flexibility and toughness."[37]

Therefore, the clinically observed loss of shoulder motion resulting from disuse is definitely the result of underlying capsular connective tissue changes.

The third factor associated with the development of frozen shoulder is that of the periarthritic personality. Some investigators[5,8,9,16] state that psychological factors, especially depression, apathy, and emotional stress, contribute to frozen shoulder. Patients with periarthritic personalities have a low pain threshold[9]; therefore, any shoulder pain will probably lead to early voluntary immobilization of the extremity. These patients take no active role in any treatment, such as exercise for shoulder pain,[9] and are therefore more likely to develop a more severe case of frozen shoulder. Wright and Haq,[38] however, tested 186 patients with frozen shoulder and found no such personality.

Clinical Features

In the literature, a few clinical features appear consistently in patients with frozen shoulder. These common observations include arthrographic and radiographic findings, age of onset, type of onset, and course of the condition.

Arthrographic findings appear to be one of the most prevalent characteristics of frozen shoulder. So that the abnormal arthrogram may be better understood, the normal shoulder arthrogram is discussed first. The joint capsule normally attaches to the humeral head just proximal to the greater tuberosity, then extends medially at the level of the anatomic neck of the humerus and inserts into the bony rim of the glenoid.[39] The redundant fold of the capsule hangs in the axilla (Fig. 5-1). In addition, the shoulder joint can accept 28 to 35 ml of solution, with 16 ml of contrast fluid allowing the best viewing of the normal joint.[39]

In frozen shoulder arthrograms, the contrast dye is injected posteriorly, since the capsule is usually contracted superiorly, anteriorly, and inferiorly.[40] Abnormal findings include retraction of the joint capsule away from the greater tuberosity[38] (Fig. 5-2), a ragged and irregular outline of the capsule,[39] and absence of the axillary redundant fold[41-44] (Fig. 5-2). The joint volume is markedly decreased to less than 10 ml, and pain is usually experienced as the capacity is reached. Frequently, there is no filling of the subscapularis bursa and bicipital sheath.[41,43,45]

Some investigators believe that arthrography is essential in diagnosing frozen shoulder.[44,46,47] Others find it helpful but not essential to rule out other shoulder lesions in addition to confirming frozen shoulder.[39,41] Arthrography, however, gives no clues to what initiates the capsular changes.

Plain film findings in frozen shoulder are usually negative, except that they occasionally show some osteoporosis from disuse.[22,24,39,40,48,49] Seldom is frozen shoulder encountered in a patient less than 40 years of age.[4,11,16,39,40,47,48] Wright and Haq[38] and DePalma[16] speculate that this age coincides with normal degenerative changes of connective tissue, a factor that may precipitate frozen shoulder. Reeves's study[50] confirms that the strength of the anterior–inferior capsule and capsular ligament decreases with age, especially in the fifth decade.

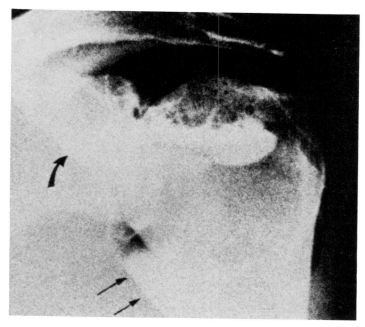

Fig. 5-1. Normal shoulder arthrogram. An external rotation view shows the insertion along the humeral neck, the axillary recess (straight arrows), and the subscapularis bursa (curved arrow). Note that the capsular insertion has a smooth contour. (From Goldman,[39] with permission.)

Some investigators associate frozen shoulder with the postmenopausal stage, when hormonal changes may alter connective tissue also.[7] Most studies of frozen shoulder consider the onset to be insidious.[2,11,15,21] Trauma including minor injuries was only occasionally recalled by some patients.[40]

Although many studies describe frozen shoulder as being self-limiting,[12,19,22,51,52] there are very few documented studies of the natural course of frozen shoulder.[21,51] Reeves[21] studied 41 patients with frozen shoulder for 5 to 10 years (average, 30 months), always to their greatest recovery. He defined frozen shoulder as an "idiopathic condition of the shoulder characterized by the spontaneous onset of pain with restriction of movement in every direction." He noted three consecutive stages of frozen shoulder: pain, stiffness, and recovery. The early painful period lasted from 10 to 36 weeks in Reeves's study. During this stage, arthrographic findings included decreased joint volume and obliteration of the subscapularis bursa and sometimes of the biceps sheath. The painful period gradually subsided, but, at the end of this stage, the shoulder capsule was the tightest and the joint capacity was the smallest. Treatment during this painful period included resting the extremity in a sling and analgesics.

The second phase was the stiff period, lasting between 4 and 12 months,

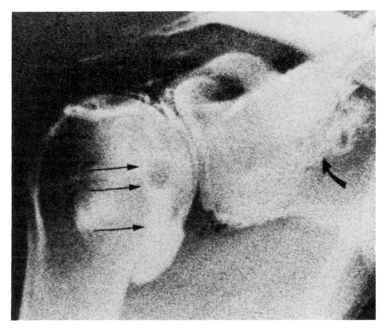

Fig. 5-2. Adhesive capsulitis. The capsule is retracted away from the tuberosities (straight arrows). The axillary recess is small, and extravasation has occurred prior to exercise (curved arrow). (From Goldman,[39] with permission.)

during which there was no improvement in joint mobility. Treatment included encouraging the patient to use the shoulder but to rest the extremity in a sling as discomfort dictated. Pain was generally noted on resumption of activity in this stage.

The last stage noted was spontaneous recovery of motion, lasting from 5 months to 2 years and 2 months. Initially, there was a gradual return of external rotation that coincided with the arthrographic reappearance of the subscapular bursa. Next, there was gradual return of abduction and internal rotation. Treatment during this phase was a home exercise program for external rotation and abduction. This is the same phase that DePalma[16] and Lippmann[14] associated with obliteration of the intracapsular bicipital tendon. The total time for greatest recovery was between 1 and 4 years after the onset of symptoms.

One observation gleaned from this study was that the length of the painful period corresponded to the length of the recovery period. A short painful period was associated with a short recovery period, and a long painful period was associated with a long recovery. More than half of the patients[21] were left with permanent loss of shoulder motion, as compared with the uninvolved "normal" shoulder's range of motion (ROM), but had no limitation in any functional activities. Three patients had functional limitations. Reeves's study[21] contradicts other research indicating full recovery or slight loss of motion in 18 to 24 months from the onset of symptoms.[11,15,19,48,51]

Cyriax also classified frozen shoulder into three stages.[17] The first stage exists when the pain is confined to the deltoid area or at least does not extend distal to the elbow, when the patient can lie on the involved extremity at night, when pain is present only with movement, and when the end-feel is elastic. The second stage is present if only some of the criteria in the first stage are met. The third stage is characterized by severe pain extending from the shoulder to the forearm and wrist, inability to lie on the involved extremity at night, pain at rest and greatest at night, and an abrupt end-feel. Treatment varies according to the stage of the condition and will be addressed later.

In a small series of 21 patients with frozen shoulder, Simmonds[12] observed that after 3 years, only 6 regained normal function, 9 had weakness and pain, and 6 had either weakness or decreased mobility. Gray[51] noted that 24 of 25 patients regained normal glenohumeral motion within 2 years from the onset of symptoms. This success was achieved with treatment of reassurance and occasional simple analgesics and hypnosis.[51] Lipmann and colleagues[48] noted that it is uncommon to outwait the natural course of frozen shoulder without intervention. Simon[22] further emphasized that simply outwaiting the condition does not assure the patient a full painless ROM.

In addition to the previously mentioned clinical features, others are found with less consistency. Opinion varies on their relationship to the incidence of frozen shoulder. These features include sex, side involved, occupation (manual versus sedentary),[19,38] the presence of immunologic factors such as HLA-B27,[46,53,54] serum IgA levels,[55] raised C-reactive protein and immune complex levels,[54] and association with other diseases (hemiparesis,[23,38] ischemic heart disease, thyroid disease,[56,57] pulmonary tuberculosis, chronic bronchitis,[38] and diabetes[49,58–60]).

Diabetes and the incidence of frozen shoulder have been under closer scrutiny, with some interesting results. Lequesne and coworkers[49] tested 60 consecutive patients with frozen shoulder and found that 17 of these had diabetes. In a larger sample, Bridgman[58] found that more than 10 percent of 800 diabetics had frozen shoulder compared with 2 percent of 600 nondiabetic control subjects. These authors contend that the prevalence of diabetes in frozen shoulder is significant.

In summary, the onset of frozen shoulder is usually insidious and occurs in patients more than 40 years of age. The course of the condition has been documented to be as long as 10 years. During this time, the level of pain and restriction can vary greatly. Other typical features of frozen shoulder include abnormal arthrograms with marked capsular changes and normal radiographs.

EXAMINATION

A complete description of the examination of the frozen shoulder is beyond the scope of this chapter. Emphasis will be placed on the physical therapist's objective assessment and the way in which findings relate to treatment of frozen shoulder.

Subjective Findings

In my clinical experience, most patients with frozen shoulder have had the condition for several weeks to several months before seeking treatment. When referred to physical therapy, the patient probably has taken or is currently taking a course of anti-inflammatory medication and has used self-treatment with a heating pad, warm showers, aspirin, and rest of the extremity. Pain motivates the patient to seek medical attention,[9,16] as does decreased function of the extremity.[61] Subjectively, the patient complains of a vague, dull pain over the deltoid that increases with motion[2,40,48] and disturbs sleep.[21,23,24,40,48,62] Functionally, the patient will be unable to sleep on the affected side,[2,6,17] hook a brassiere in the back, comb the hair, or reach for a wallet in a back pocket. The patient usually cannot recall an injury and frequently is unable to determine when the pain and/or loss of function began. If the condition is more advanced, the patient may complain of pain spreading from the shoulder down the forearm,[12,17] up to the cervical spine, and into the ipsilateral scapula, and pain at rest.[17]

These complaints correspond well to Cyriax's stages of capsular lesions.[17] Although Reeves's[21] study documents arthrographic changes in the first and last stages of frozen shoulder, from a practical standpoint Cyriax's division is more clinically applicable. In the patient population that I saw, very few patients were examined arthrographically. It appears that arthrography was reserved for those patients who did not respond to a long-term conservative program of physical therapy and medication. Even if arthrography is performed, Cyriax's stages can also be clinically helpful in treatment planning.

During the interview, it is also important to ask questions concerning the patient's general health to assess any other disease process that may be referring pain to the shoulder. The same applies to pertinent questioning concerning the shoulder complex, cervical spine, and brachial plexus structures, although these areas will be examined.

Objective Findings

Initial observation of the patient frequently reveals a stooped posture with rounded shoulders; the involved extremity is adducted and internally rotated, resting in the patient's lap.[63]

In gait, the arm swing is usually limited or absent on the affected side. A therapist observing the patient disrobe will notice that the patient's shirt is usually removed as though the arm were is a cast. The uninvolved extremity is removed first, with very little movement of the opposite side. The reverse occurs when the patient dresses. The patient usually wears shirts that button down the front and require no overhead action to remove.

The levels of the shoulders are frequently uneven, with the involved side usually elevated in a protective manner. As a result of maintaining this posture, there may be tenderness and trigger points along the ipsilateral upper trapezius, with perceived pain along its course to the suboccipital area. The scapula on the involved side is usually elevated, laterally rotated, and abducted as a result of excessive scapular motion to compensate for the impaired glenohumeral motion. The abnormal scapula position can cause stretch weakness of the rhomboids[63] and levator scapulae tightness, giving rise to local pain. If the condition is longstanding and there has been a long period of disuse, muscle atrophy around the involved shoulder and scapula may be evident.

Because cervical spine dysfunction can refer pain to the shoulder, this area must be assessed.[10,26,27] It is not the objective of this chapter to outline a complete cervical examination, but a few important tests are mentioned. If active cervical ROM is normal, overpressure should be applied at the end of each range.[64] This involves a gentle passive movement at the end of the available range. There should be a slight pain-free increase in the ROM. If active ROM and active ROM with overpressure are negative for provocation of symptoms, the cervical quadrant test can be performed. This involves guiding the head into extension toward one side and then adding cervical rotation to the same side.[64] Gross passive ROM can be performed to rule out any muscular influence in cervical mobility.

Individual cervical segmental mobility should then be tested to ascertain any joint dysfunction. Physical therapists trained in these methods have a variety of testing techniques that can be performed to check segmental mobility in all directions of motion. Cervical compression and traction tests complete the passive cervical spine examination. Additional information concerning the cervical influence on the shoulder pain may be obtained by having the patient elevate the involved shoulder while traction is being applied to the cervical spine and noting if there is any improvement in shoulder pain or ROM.[26] Finally, resistive testing of cervical ROM will provide information concerning the contractile structures of the neck.

The integrity of the brachial plexus must be evaluated in cases of shoulder pain.[26] The standard Addson, hyperabduction, and costoclavicular tests may not be valid with limited shoulder motion. Elvey[26] developed a brachial plexus tension test that can be performed adequately despite restricted shoulder motion. The reader is encouraged to refer to this text for the details.

Acromioclavicular, sternoclavicular, and scapulothoracic dysfunction and first rib syndrome can also give rise to shoulder pain.[26,65] Acromioclavicular joint pain is usually very localized and can easily be pinpointed by the patient.[17] This local pain differs from the diffuse dull pain common with frozen shoulder. Scapulothoracic dysfunction usually results from excessive scapular compensatory motion, and sternoclavicular dysfunction usually results from abnormal shoulder mechanics. First rib dysfunction can result from a variety of problems. The mobility of the sternoclavicular, scapulothoracic,[26,65] acromioclavicular, and first rib[26] should be tested to rule out their involvement in shoulder pain. In summary, careful examination of the cervical spine, brachial plexus, acromioclavicular, sternoclavicular, scapulothoracic joints, and first rib is essential in a complete assessment of shoulder pain.

Much of the remaining objective assessment of the shoulder is based on

Cyriax's[17] examination principles. The entire examination is presented because the negative findings are as important as the positive findings in assessing frozen shoulder. All examination procedures mentioned should be performed bilaterally, using the uninvolved extremity as "normal" for the individual who is being assessed.

Twelve movements are included in the examination, and the order of their performance is important. Active motion assesses both contractile and noncontractile elements, passive motion assesses inert structures, and resisted motion assesses contractile structures.

1. *Active elevation.* Elevation is movement away from the side in the coronal plane, with 180° possible. During active elevation, the patient's willingness to move, the muscular power, and the ROM can be assessed.

2. *Passive elevation.* The ROM, the location in the range in which pain is produced, and the end-feel should be noted. End-feel is the sensation detected by the examiner at the extreme of the passive ROM.[17,66] The normal end-feel of the shoulder is capsular, which is similar to the sensation encountered when two pieces of tough rubber are squeezed together. There is a firm arrest to movement, but some "give" is noted.[17] Both the end-feel and the point in the range where pain is provoked are important in deciding treatment. This will be further discussed in the section on stretching as treatment.

3. *Painful arc.* This can only be tested when 90° of abduction is present actively or passively. Abduction is defined as the amount of movement between the scapula and humerus, with 90° being normal. The patient actively elevates the extremity and notes if there is a painful point in the range bordered on either side by nonpainful motion. The same arc of pain can be felt as the arm is brought down from the elevated position or if elevation is performed passively. A positive finding indicates that a structure is being pinched during the movement.

4. *Passive scapulohumeral abduction.* The scapula is stabilized at its inferior angle as the therapist passively elevates the extremity, noting when the inferior angle begins to move; 90° is the normal range before the scapula moves.

5. *Passive lateral rotation.*
6. *Passive medial rotation.*

As with passive elevation, ROM, the point in the range at which pain is provoked, and the end-feel should be noted.

7. *Resisted adduction.*
8. *Resisted abduction.*
9. *Resisted lateral rotation.*
10. *Resisted medial rotation.*
11. *Resisted elbow extension.*
12. *Resisted elbow flexion.*

All resisted tests are performed isometrically. Both pain and muscle weakness are noted.

As previously mentioned, confusion occurs when more than one lesion exists. With this concise examination, both contractile and inert structures can be assessed.

In summary, because frozen shoulder is a capsular lesion, active elevation and all passive testing is limited and painful. In addition, limitation of passive movement is in a capsular proportion, with most limitation in external rotation, followed by abduction, then internal rotation.

Further information in determining which areas of the capsule are involved in frozen shoulder can be obtained by assessing motions of glenohumeral joint play. Mennel[65] coined the term *joint play* and defines it as small, involuntary movement essential for normal joint motion. He based this definition on joint mechanics, in which rotations, glides, and long axis extension (traction) are normal joint plane motions. Joint play motion is often not more than $\frac{1}{8}$-in movement in any plane. When joint play is lost, joint dysfunction exists. Mennel proposes that manipulation is the preferred treatment to restore joint play.

According to Mennel, there are seven joint play motions at the glenohumeral joint. He recognizes that normal glenohumeral movement depends on normal acromioclavicular, sternoclavicular, and scapulothoracic joint movement. The reader is referred to Chapter 1 on mechanics of the shoulder joint for review of this necessary harmony. All of the joint play motions are actually rolls and glides of the humeral head within the glenoid. In the shoulder, where the convex humeral head is moving on the stationary glenoid, roll and glide occur in opposite directions.[66] Any discrepancies in joint play assessment will direct the therapist with a knowledge of normal joint mechanics to the involved area of the capsule. Furthermore, treatment can be directed to these specific areas.

The normal joint play motions of the glenohumeral joint are anterior glide, posterior glide, lateral glide, inferior and posterior glide, lateral and posterior glide, external rotation of the humeral head within the glenoid fossa, and posterior glide of the humeral head within the glenoid fossa with the shoulder flexed to 90°.[65] Although the joint play motions mentioned above are assessment techniques, they are also treatment techniques that can be used to restore normal shoulder mechanics by stretching the involved portions of the capsule. This will be discussed in the treatment section.

All joint play motions can be quantified using a scale from 0 to 6.[67] Although the assessment of joint play is subjective, grading the movement allows easy documentation of the motion. Again, the uninvolved extremity should be tested to assess "normal" for the patient. Grade 0 indicates no joint movement as in an ankylosed joint; grade 1 indicates marked loss of motion; grade 2, a slight limitation in motion; grade 3, normal mobility; grade 4, a slight increase in mobility; grade 5, a marked increase in motion; and grade 6, joint instability. In frozen shoulder with capsular restrictions, grades 1 and 2 will be encountered most frequently.

A final examination tool is palpation. Cyriax[17] cautions that palpation gives very little information and is often irritating to the involved structures. For these reasons, palpation is reserved until the very end of the examination. In frozen shoulder, palpatory findings are generally negative. There may be tenderness over the acromioclavicular joint as a result of improper shoulder mechanics. In addition, any secondary muscular involvement resulting from posture or abnormal scapular motion may exhibit painful trigger points. In a contractile lesion coexisting with frozen shoulder, there will probably be tenderness over the lesioned structure.

Although this evaluation is lengthy, it is imperative that an accurate assessment of the shoulder lesion be made. Proper treatment is based on an accurate assessment.[25,65,68]

TREATMENT

Prevention is the best treatment of frozen shoulder.[19,40] Although there is little agreement on its treatment when it occurs, there is agreement on the treatment goals: pain relief and restoration of normal shoulder movement.[52,69] Unfortunately, few controlled studies in the literature examine treatment of frozen shoulder. One of the problems in studies of frozen shoulder is the variable patient selection due to the variable definitions of what constitutes frozen shoulder. Another problem, so frequently encountered in any human subject study, is the ethics of the necessity of an untreated control group.

Hazleman[52] studied 130 cases of frozen shoulder retrospectively and found no difference in treatment of local corticosteroid injections, physical therapy consisting of pendulum and pulley exercises with shortwave diathermy, or manipulation under anesthesia. Binder and colleagues[70] followed 42 patients with frozen shoulder for 8 months and found no long-term difference in treatment by intra-articular steroids, Maitland-type passive mobilization, ice, or no treatment. Hamer and Kirk[71] documented no significant advantage in ice or ultrasound treatments, but both were beneficial in decreasing the painful stage and hastening recovery. Lee and coworkers[72] found no difference in patients who received local hydrocortisone and exercises or infrared irradiation and exercises. However, both groups receiving exercises did significantly better than patients receiving analgesics alone. Dacre et al., following 66 cases for 6 months, concluded that local steroid injection, physical therapy with mobilization, or a combination of both were all effective in decreasing pain and increasing shoulder function. They also concluded that the steroid injection was cost-effective.[73]

Biswas and colleagues[61] found that patients receiving intra-articular hydrocortisone, shortwave diathermy, and aspirin as well as active and passive mobilization exercises all benefited. Furthermore, these investigators concluded that exercise is the most important treatment in frozen shoulder. Liang and Lien[74] found no difference in active exercises when combined with intra-articular injection and heat (shortwave diathermy, ultrasound, or moist heat), with heat alone, or with injection alone. Similarly, they concluded that exercises were probably the only useful treatment for frozen shoulder. Rizk and colleagues[75] found that transcutaneous electrical nerve stimulation (TENS) with prolonged pulley traction was superior to a variety of heat modalities and exercises. Pothmann et al.[76] found that one acupuncture treatment of point ST 38 cured acute frozen shoulder.

Transcutaneous Electrical Nerve Stimulation

Various treatments can be used to achieve the goals of pain relief and restoration of mobility, but documentation of their effectiveness in frozen shoulder is lacking. TENS can be used to decrease the symptoms of pain in both the early and later stages of frozen shoulder. Figure 5-3 illustrates an effective TENS application for frozen shoulder.[77] The analgesia provided by TENS allows other therapeutic procedures, such as exercises, to be performed more comfortably. For maximal effectiveness, TENS should be applied before and/or during the exercises.[77] Decreasing the pain during stretching of the frozen shoulder will gain the confidence of the patient as well as facilitate joint relaxation, which is essential for passive joint manipulation.

TENS is significantly more effective in reducing the acute pain.[77] Therefore, TENS is an excellent treatment choice when the patient is in too acute a stage for active treatment. Such is the case in stage 3 of frozen shoulder as defined by Cyriax.[17] If TENS can reduce the discomfort, the patient will use the extremity more and probably avoid the stiffening results of disuse.

Other useful acupuncture points that can be used as electrode sites for

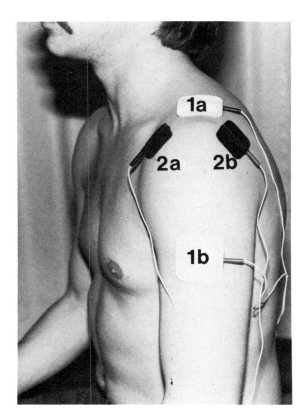

Fig. 5-3. TENS electrode placement for frozen shoulder. (1a) In depression bordered by the acromion laterally, spine of scapula posteriorly, and clavicle anteriorly; acupuncture point LI 16. (1b) Insertion of deltoid at lateral aspect of arm; acupuncture point LI 14 (channel 1). (2a) In depression below acromion anteriorly; acupuncture point LI 15. (2b) In depression below acromion posteriorly; acupuncture point TW 14 (channel 2). (Modified from Mannheimer and Lampe,[77] with permission.)

TENS include a combination of ST 38 and UB 57 or a combination of LI 15, SI 10, GB 34, and LI 11.[78] (See ref. 78 for exact point location.)

Heat

Heat application is a very common treatment used to decrease pain and increase soft tissue extensibility. A variety of modalities, including shortwave and microwave diathermy, ultrasound, moist packs, paraffin baths, whirlpools, and infrared irradiation, create hyperthermia in the tissue.[77] The result of hyperthermia is increased circulation and vasodilation to the tissues.[77] Other investigators recommend heating the joint capsule prior to stretching, since the increased circulation acts as an analgesic.[17] The analgesic effect, however, tends to be temporary.[77]

Ultrasound

Ultrasound research in frozen shoulder began in the 1950s when ultrasound was a new form of therapy. Mueller and colleagues[79] found that ultrasound at 2 W/cm^2 was of no value in treating subacute frozen shoulder. Quin[80] found no difference in groups receiving ultrasound at 0.5 W/cm^2 and exercises and those receiving diathermy and exercises.

Clinically, ultrasound is used for its thermal and mechanical effects on tissue.[80] In frozen shoulder, it is often used prior to stretching of the capsule. Because the sound waves are so focal, the therapist must be very specific as to the target tissue.[81] With the inferior capsule so frequently involved in frozen shoulder, the extremity may need to be positioned in abduction and external rotation to reach the inferior portion effectively. Similarly, any portion of the capsule can be treated specifically with proper positioning of the joint. The therapist may also put the target capsule on stretch as ultrasound is applied.

A home program of heat before exercises can be helpful, especially when the patients can exercise with less discomfort. Warm showers and warm moist compresses are easily applied. Heating pads, especially those with a moist heat feature, are useful as long as the patient does not apply a pad for long periods.[68] Patients frequently abuse heating pads by falling asleep with them. Even with the pad on the lowest setting, the patient should be strictly instructed to apply it only for short intervals. Most of us have seen the mottled skin of a patient who has abused the heating pad.

Cryotherapy

Cryotherapy, like heat application, produces increased circulation and vasodilation to the area. There is, however, an initial vasoconstriction with cold application.[77] Ice packs, ice massage, ice whirlpools, and vapocoolant sprays are all effective cold treatments.

Ice packs can be easily constructed at home with a plastic bag. A proportional amount of rubbing alcohol added to ice keeps it from refreezing solidly. Convincing a patient to use ice at home—especially one who thrives on warm showers and a heating pad—is often difficult. Ice, like heat, before exercises will help the patient perform with less pain. Pain after exercises for more than 1 to 2 hours[17] is abnormal. Ice can prove beneficial in reducing any postexercise soreness.

In the acute phase, when the extremity is generally rested, ice for its analgesic effect is very useful. In addition, if there is a concurrent lesion, such as a rotator cuff tendinitis or bicipital tenosynovitis, ice can combat the inflammation and edema, thereby decreasing pain. With lessened pain, the patient will be more willing to use the extremity and prevent subsequent stiffness.

Exercise

Exercise is the most useful treatment in frozen shoulder.[44,61,74] In the acute stage or stage 3 as defined by Cyriax,[17] all active treatment is contraindicated. Treatment in this stage should be directed at pain relief. As mentioned, rest, ice, and TENS are helpful at this time. In the subacute stage or stage 2, exercises both active and passive may be cautiously initiated, but the patient's reaction must be constantly monitored. Increased pain or pain lasting more than 2 hours after exercise is abnormal.[17] In stage 1, active and passive exercises can be performed, usually safely and vigorously. A good physical therapist must be able to judge when to initiate exercise, the amount and vigor of exercises, and when the patient is aggravated by exercise. Experience helps in this decision making, but each patient is different and must be individually evaluated.

Other guidelines to determine when and to what degree exercise should be used can be based on the end-feel and the pain and resistance sequence.[17] An end-feel other than the capsular resistance is abnormal at the shoulder. With the limited range of frozen shoulder, the end-feel is still capsular only in that it will occur at the end of the reduced ROM.

During passive motion testing, both the location of pain in the range and the end-feel are noted.[17] Combining these two factors will indicate the severity of the condition, thereby guiding treatment. If during passive movement the patient perceives pain before the therapist reaches the end of range, the joint is probably acute and active exercises are contraindicated. During this situation, the therapist will obviously not have a chance to evaluate the end-feel, but this can be done in subsequent visits as the pain subsides. If pain is experienced as the end of range is reached, the patient is less acute and exercises may be cautiously attempted. If exercises exacerbate the pain, they should be delayed. Last, if the end of the limited range is reached and no pain is provoked, exercises will probably be tolerated without problems.[17]

In summary, certain factors can help the therapist determine when and what exercises are indicated for the patient with frozen shoulder. The three stages as outlined by Cyriax, the end-feel, and the pain/resistance sequence are three such guides.[17] A good therapist paces the patient through a graded active and passive exercise program and constantly reassesses the effect of the program on pain and stiffness.

Manipulation

Manipulation, or mobilization as it is frequently called, is a form of passive exercise designed to restore joint play motions of roll, glide, and joint separation.[65] Very few controlled studies involve joint manipulation in the treatment of frozen shoulder. Bulgen and coworkers[82] found no superiority of Maitland-type manipulative techniques in patients with frozen shoulder for more than 1 month over treatment with ice, intra-articular steroid injections, or no treatment. In fact, after 6 weeks of treatment, the group receiving manipulation had greater loss of motion than did the other groups. Bulgen and coworkers explain that the detrimental effect of physical therapy occurred when manipulation was performed during the active stage, an error that must be avoided.[82]

For normal shoulder function, all areas of the capsule must be extensible to allow joint play motion. Capsular extensibility depends on friction-free sliding of the collagen fibers within the capsule.[29] Hyaluronic acid with water is the lubricant between the collagen fibers[29,83,84] that allows this free gliding to occur.

Lundberg's study of the capsular changes in frozen shoulder revealed a marked increase in fibroblastic formation of collagen, a loss of hyaluronic acid, and an increase in sulfated GAGs.[37] The newly formed collagen in the capsule depends on motion for proper alignment and deposition. Without movement, the new collagen is laid down in a haphazard manner. Abnormal collagen deposition occurs between the newly synthesized fibril and pre-existing collagen fibers,[29] resulting in a mechanical block to collagen movement. Multiple adhesions between collagen fibrils and fibers is manifested as joint stiffness. In addition, with the decrease in hyaluronic acid, the lubricant between the fibers is lost, contributing to further impairment of free collagen movement.

Based on these considerations, it seems reasonable to assume that movement of the joint will prevent or limit adhesive formation. Although this is not documented, movement to prevent adhesions is a clinical goal of exercise. In the event that capsular adhesions have formed, manipulation can be used to break the adhesions and restore joint play. Further research is obviously needed in this area.

It is beyond the scope of this chapter to outline every manipulative technique for frozen shoulder. Demonstrations can be found in the texts of Maitland,[64] Mennel,[65] and Kaltenborn.[67] Techniques for each area of the shoulder capsule, acromioclavicular, sternoclavicular, and scapulothoracic joints are illustrated here. Physical therapists benefit by becoming as familiar as possible with as many techniques as possible to afford better treatment to their patients. Any of the techniques illustrated can be adapted as oscillatory or static stretching techniques and can be performed in any part of the range. The goal of

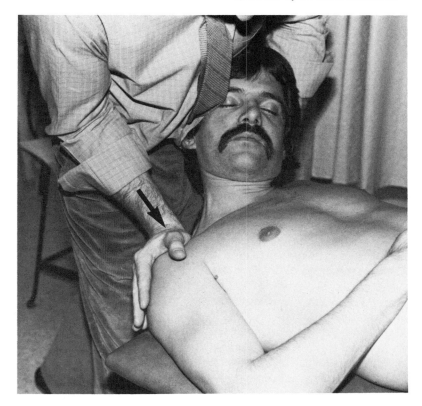

Fig. 5-4. Upper trapezius stretch.

treatment, whether for pain relief or increasing ROM, will influence the choice of treatment technique. The mobilization techniques are illustrated in Chapter 11.

Cervical as well as shoulder pain may be present. This may result from overuse of the upper trapezius and levator scapula with excessive scapular elevation to compensate for the loss of glenohumeral motion.[63] The upper trapezius and levator scapula are usually shortened and will need treatment to decrease pain and restore normal physiologic length. Any of the physical modalities are useful to decrease pain. Massage is relaxing as well as beneficial in moving any excessive fluid accumulation. It also can assist in mobilizing the soft tissue. Stretching of the upper trapezius can be done in a number of ways. Figure 5-4 illustrates a passive upper trapezius stretch.

Patient position: Supine with the head off the edge of the table.

Therapist position: Left hand under the occiput with the head on the forearm stabilizing the head and neck in the desired amount of flexion and sidebending left and rotation right. Right palm over the clavicle and scapula medial to the acromioclavicular joint.

Technique: Left hand maintains head and neck position. Right hand pushes the clavicle and scapula inferiorly.

In a good home exercise for stretching the upper trapezius, the patient simply reaches behind the back and grasps the involved distal humerus. The patient should side-bend away from and rotate toward the involved side and flex the neck to a comfortable position. Once positioned, the stretch is imparted by pulling downward on the involved humerus.

Frequently, pain may be provoked while the shoulder is being manipulated. Although such pain is not desirable, it is often difficult to manipulate a frozen shoulder without some discomfort to the patient. "Shaking" the extremity and momentary pauses will help decrease pain and maintain patient relaxation.[67] Simple gentle shaking of the extremity while in any position will stimulate the joint mechanoreceptors and decrease nociceptive input.[85]

Both Maitland[64] and Kaltenborn[67] offer guidelines to the amount of manipulation to perform in one session. Reassessment is important before and during each treatment session. Treatment can continue as long as pain is decreased and motion is improved.[67] Overtreating can cause increased pain and inflammatory reactions,[63] and may push the patient into an acute stage. The therapist should progress slowly until familiar with the patient's response to treatment. It is well documented that the course of frozen shoulder is slow[21,51]; therefore, the therapist should not expect too much improvement too quickly. A patient who is informed that improvement will be slow will be less frustrated.

Liebolt[86] has recommended four passive stretches that, performed over a period of time, will increase shoulder ROM in frozen shoulder. The four exercises are glenohumeral abduction, external rotation, flexion with external rotation, and flexion performed at the end of the available ROM. These exercises, however, do not deal with the loss of joint play. I have found that these exercises in the cardinal planes often provoke pain and do little to increase ROM.

Mechanical exercises with shoulder wheels, pulleys, and wands are often standard exercises in treating frozen shoulder. Unfortunately, like the stretching in the cardinal plane, these do not address the loss of joint play. Murray[63] outlines three disadvantages of the overhead pulley system: (1) there is no stabilization of the scapula to avoid excessive abduction and upward rotation; (2) there is no force to depress the humeral head; and (3) there is a tendency for the patient to extend the spine to decrease glenohumeral motion. These same three points are applicable to the shoulder wheel, finger ladder, and wand exercises. To improve the use of these apparatuses, stabilization of the scapula can be improved by placing a strap around the scapula and the chair. The therapist or a reliable family member who has been taught the exercises can depress the humeral head while using the apparatus. Last, the patient can be instructed to keep the spine flat against the chair while performing these exercises. Despite these efforts to improve the exercises, Murray[63] contends that these apparatuses should be used only when normal gliding is present.

Active exercises allow more patient control than do mechanical exercises.

Active exercises are essential in maintaining the capsular extensibility obtained through manipulation. They are best performed in a pain-free range to prevent any inflammatory reaction by forcing joint movement. The same principles of mechanical exercises apply to forced active exercises; that is, the active range will not be available if normal joint play is lacking.

Codman or pendulum[7] exercises performed with gravity are usually pain-free. With the patient bent at the waist and the extremity dangling, the weight of the extremity produces joint separation and eliminates a fulcrum at the glenoid or acromion with movement.[7] With traction at the joint, the patient will usually find the exercises more comfortable. For additional traction, the patient can grasp a light weight, such as an iron. The exercises include forward and backward, medial to lateral, and circular motions made with the entire extremity. The object is to have the patient increase the arc of movement within a painful ROM.

Cardinal plane or diagonal active motion can be performed as a home program if the necessary joint play movements are available. Home exercise programs should be kept simple and to a minimum, requiring no special equipment, so the patient will comply with the program, which in frozen shoulder is usually a long course. The number of repetitions as well as the vigor will have to be determined for each patient. As mentioned, for their analgesic effects, preparatory heat or ice may be used prior to performance of exercises.

Last, muscle reeducation and strengthening may be needed to restore normal physiologic balance to the entire shoulder complex and cervical spine. "Muscles cannot be restored to normal if the joints which they move are not free to move."[65] Because there is often excessive scapular motion, stabilization exercises to the scapular area can be performed before full glenohumeral motion is restored. Otherwise, I do not advise strengthening exercises until near normal ROM is achieved. This will avoid strengthening a muscle in a shortened range that may impede the restoration of motion.

Isometric, isotonic (both concentric and eccentric), and isokinetic exercises, free-weights, and proprioceptive neuromuscular facilitation are all useful in restoring muscle strength. Various exercise equipment such as Cybex, Universal, and Nautilus are commonplace in many health clubs, and individual programs should be developed for the patients. After pain abates and ROM is restored, most patients will not continue physical therapy for a strengthening program. Therefore, intermittent follow-up visits should be made to review and alter the exercise program as needed and to assess the patient's progress.

CONCLUSION

In summary, a physical therapy treatment course for frozen shoulder may include preparatory modalities to decrease pain, passive manipulation, muscle reeducation and strengthening, and a home exercise program. The course is long and often tedious to both the patient and therapist since progress is very slow. The goal of treatment is the restoration of normal pain-free shoulder function.

Cortisone injections and manipulation under anesthesia are two other common treatments for frozen shoulder. The literature is filled with arguments for and against manipulations under anesthesia.[87–93] The same varied opinions are documented for treatment by cortisone injection.[69,94–98]

Various manipulative procedures are described in the literature. A common caution, however, is to use short level arms with very gentle force to avoid injury, such as a fractured humerus. Arthrographic studies following manipulation under anesthesia show that the adherent inferior fold of the capsule is torn, allowing the dye to escape into the axillary space and along the medial humerus.[41,42] Some investigators reported rotator cuff tears following manipulation under anesthesia,[43] whereas others did not find any tears of the cuff.[42]

Clinically, if a patient has been treated with manipulation, it is helpful to know the ROM obtained and the complications, if any, that were encountered during the procedure. It is very common for a patient to have less motion following manipulation even if therapy is initiated immediately. This may be owing to an acute inflammatory reaction and muscle splinting due to pain. Pain is frequently increased for several days following manipulation. TENS and ice are very helpful at this stage. Exercises are essential following manipulation under anesthesia. The therapist frequently sees the patient four times a day in the hospital, beginning on the day of the procedure. Reassurance and encouragement are needed to motivate the patient to exercise in the presence of pain.

The physical therapist should be aware of the location, number, and frequency of cortisone injections administered to the patient. Because of reports of spontaneous tendon ruptures following multiple injection, care should be exercised with these patients.

Other treatments reported in the literature include a combination of manipulation under anesthesia and cortisone and arthrographic joint distention to rupture capsular adhesions. Knowledge of any procedure performed on the patient enhances treatment decisions.

In summary, this chapter has presented the varied theories on pathogenesis, definition, etiology, clinical features, and treatment of the frozen shoulder. Physical therapy management, including physical modalities and passive and active exercises, have been presented. Further research in all of the above areas is needed to prevent and better treat the common musculoskeletal complaint of frozen shoulder.

ACKNOWLEDGMENT

I wish to thank Rita K. Owens-Skau, B.S., P.T., for assistance in the preparation of the manuscript, and William Boissonnault, M.S., P.T., and Steve Janos, M.S., P.T., for their assistance with the photographs.

REFERENCES

1. Bateman J: The Shoulder and Neck. WB Saunders, Philadelphia, 1978
2. Neviaser JS: Adhesive capsulitis and the stiff and painful shoulder. Orthop Clin North Am 11:327, 1980
3. Neviaser JS: Adhesive capsulitis of the shoulder: study of pathological findings in periarthritis of the shoulder. J Bone Joint Surg 27:211, 1945
4. Meulengracht E, Schwartz M: The course and prognosis of periarthrosis humeroscapularis with special regard to cases with general symptoms. Acta Med Scand 143:350, 1952
5. McLaughlin HL: The "frozen" shoulder." Clin Orthop 20:126, 1961
6. Rizk TE, Pinals RS: Frozen shoulder. Semin Arthritis Rheum 11:440, 1982
7. Codman EA: The Shoulder. Robert E Kreiger Publishing Co, Malabar, FL, 1934
8. Coventry MB: The problem of the painful shoulder. JAMA 151:177, 1953
9. Cailliet R: Shoulder Pain. 2nd Ed. FA Davis, Philadelphia, 1981
10. Neviaser RJ: Painful conditions affecting the shoulder. Clin Orthop 173:63, 1983
11. Thompson M: The frozen shoulder and shoulder-hand syndromes. Practitioner 189:380, 1962
12. Simmonds FA: Shoulder pain with particular reference to the "frozen" shoulder. J Bone Joint Surg 31B:426, 1949
13. Macnab I: Rotator cuff tendinitis. Ann R Coll Surg Engl 53:271, 1973
14. Lippmann RK: Frozen shoulder; periarthritis; bicipital tenosynovitis. Arch Surg 47:283, 1943
15. Turek S: Orthopaedics. Principles and Their Application. JB Lippincott, Philadelphia, 1977
16. DePalma AF: Surgery of the Shoulder. JB Lippincott, Philadelphia, 1983
17. Cyriax J: Textbook of Orthopaedic Medicine. 7th Ed. Vol. 1. Bailliere Tindall, London, 1978
18. Kozin F: Two unique shoulder disorders. Adhesive capsulitis and reflex sympathetic dystrophy syndrome. Postgrad Med 73:207, 1983
19. Jayson MV: Frozen shoulder: adhesive capsulitis. Br Med J 283:1003, 1981
20. Morgensen E: Painful shoulder. Aetiological and pathogenetic problems. Acta Med Scand 155:195, 1956
21. Reeves B: The natural history of the frozen shoulder syndrome. Scand J Rheumatol 4:193, 1975
22. Simon WH: Soft tissue disorders of the shoulder. Frozen shoulder, calcific tendinitis, and bicipital tendinitis. Orthop Clin North Am 6:521, 1975
23. Bruckner FE, Nye CJS: A prospective study of adhesive capsulitis of the shoulder ('frozen shoulder') in a high risk population. Q J Med 198:191, 1981
24. Flicker PL: The painful shoulder. Prim Care 7:271, 1980
25. Reeves B: Arthrographic changes in frozen shoulder and post-traumatic stiff shoulders. Proc Soc Med 59:827, 1966
26. Elvey RL: The investigation of arm pain. p. 530. In Grieve GP (ed): Modern Manual Therapy of the Vertebral Column. Churchill Livingstone, Edinburgh, 1986
27. Leach RE, Schepsis AA: Shoulder pain. Clin Sports Med 2:123, 1983
28. Neviaser JS: Musculoskeletal disorders of the shoulder region causing cervicobrachial pain. Differential diagnosis and treatment. Surg Clin North Am 43:1703, 1963
29. Akeson WH, Amiel D, LaViolette D: The connective tissue response to immobility: a study of the chondroitin 4- and 6-sulphate and dermatan sulphate changes in

periarticular connective tissue of control and immobilized knees of dogs. Clin Orthop 51:183, 1967

30. Akeson WH, Amiel D, LaViolette D, et al: The connective tissue response to immobility: an accelerated aging response. Exp Gerontol 3:289, 1968

31. Akeson WH, Amiel D, Mechanic GL, et al: Collagen crosslinking alterations in joint contractures: changes in reducible crosslinks in periarticular connective tissue collagen after nine weeks of immobilization. Connect Tissue Res 5:5, 1977

32. Akeson WH, Amiel D, Woo S: Immobility effects of synovial joints: the pathomechanics of joint contracture. Biorheology 17:95, 1980

33. Enneking W, Horowitz M: The intra-articular effects of immobilization on the human knee. J Bone Joint Surg 54A:973, 1972

34. Evans E, Eggers G, Butler J, et al: Immobilization and remobilization of rats' knee joints. J Bone Joint Surg 42A:737, 1960

35. LaVigne A, Watkins R: Preliminary results on immobilization: induced stiffness of monkey knee joints and posterior capsule. In Perspectives in Biomedical Engineering. Proceedings of a symposium of Biological Engineering Society, University of Strathclyde, Glasgow, June 1972. University Park Press, Baltimore, 1973

36. Woo S, Matthews JV, Akeson WH, et al: Connective tissue response to immobility: correlative study of biomechanical and biochemical measurements of normal and immobilized rabbit knees. Arthritis Rheum 18:257, 1975

37. Lundberg BJ: Glycosaminoglycans of the normal and frozen shoulder–joint capsule. Clin Orthop 69:279, 1970

38. Wright V, Haq AMMM: Periarthritis of the shoulder. Aetiological considerations with particular reference to personality factors. Ann Rheum Dis 35:213, 1976

39. Goldman A: Shoulder Arthrography. Technique, Diagnosis, and Clinical Correlation. Little, Brown, Boston, 1982

40. Neviaser JS: Adhesive capsulitis of the shoulder (frozen shoulder). Med Times 90:783, 1962

41. Neviaser JS: Arthrography of the Shoulder. The Diagnosis and Management of the Lesions Visualized. Charles C Thomas, Springfield, IL, 1975

42. Lundberg BJ: Arthrography and manipulation in rigidity of the shoulder joint. Acta Orthop Scand 36:35, 1965

43. Samilson RL, Raphael L, Post L, et al: Arthrography of the shoulder joint. Clin Orthop 20:21, 1961

44. Neviaser RJ: The frozen shoulder diagnosis and management. Clin Orthop 223:59, 1987

45. Neviaser RJ: Arthrography of the shoulder joint. Study of the findings in adhesive capsulitis of the shoulder. J Bone Joint Surg 44A:1321, 1962

46. Rizk TE, Christopher RP, Pinals RS, et al: Arthrographic studies in painful hemiplegic shoulder. Arch Phys Med Rehabil 65:254, 1984

47. Loyd JA, Loyd HM: Adhesive capsulitis of the shoulder: arthrographic diagnosis and treatment. South Med J 76:879, 1983

48. Lipmann K, Bayley I, Young A: The upper limb. The frozen shoulder. Br J Hosp Med 25:334, 1981

49. Lequesne M, Dang N, Bensasson M, et al: Increased association of diabetes mellitus with capsulitis of the shoulder and shoulder-hand syndrome. Scand J Rheumatol 6:53, 1977

50. Reeves B: Experiments on the tensile strength of the anterior capsular structures of the shoulder in man. J Bone Joint Surg 50B:858, 1968

51. Gray RG: The natural history of "idiopathic" frozen shoulder. J Bone Joint Surg 60B:564, 1978

52. Hazleman BL: The painful stiff shoulder. Rheumatol Phys Med 11:413, 1972
53. Bulgen DY, Hazleman BL, Voak D: HLA-B27 and frozen shoulder. Lancet 1:1042, 1976
54. Bulgen DY, Binder A, Hazleman BL, et al: Immuological studies in frozen shoulder. J Rheumatol 9:893, 1982
55. Bulgen DY, Hazleman B, Ward M, et al: Immunological studies in frozen shoulder. Ann Rheum Dis 37:135, 1978
56. Bowman CA, Jeffcoate WJ, Pattrick M, et al: Bilateral adhesive capsulitis, oligoarthritis and proximal myopathy as presentation of hypothyroidism. Br J Rheumatol 27:62, 1988
57. Wohlgethan JR: Frozen shoulder in hyperthyroidism. Arthritis Rheum 30:936, 1987
58. Bridgman JF: Periarthritis of the shoulder and diabetes mellitus. Ann Rheum Dis 31:69, 1972
59. Erhard R: Diabetic capsulitis of the shoulder. p. 101. In Proceedings of the 4th International Federation of Orthopaedic Manipulative Therapists. International Federation of Orthopedic Manipulative Therapists, Christchurch, New Zealand, 1980
60. Fisher L, Kurtz A, Shipley M: Association between cheiroarthropathy and frozen shoulder in patients with insulin-dependent diabetes mellitus. Br J Rheumatol 25:141, 1986
61. Biswas AK, Sur BN, Gupta CR: Treatment of periathritis shoulder. J Indian Med Assoc 72:276, 1979
62. Olsson O: Degenerative changes of the shoulder joint and their connection with shoulder pain. Acta Chir Scand, suppl., 181:104, 1935
63. Murray W: The chronic frozen shoulder. Phys Ther Rev 40:866, 1960
64. Maitland GD: Peripheral Manipulation. 2nd Ed. Butterworths, Boston, 1977
65. Mennel J: Joint Pain. Diagnosis, Treatment Using Manipulative Techniques. Little, Brown, Boston, 1964
66. Warwick R. Williams PL: Gray's Anatomy. 35th British Ed. WB Saunders, Philadelphia, 1973
67. Kaltenborn FM: Mobilization of the Extremity Joints. Examination and Basic Treatment Techniques. Olaf Bokhandel, Oslo, 1980
68. Nelson PA: Physical treatment of the painful arm and shoulder. JAMA 169:814, 1959
69. Valtonen E: Subacromial betamethasone therapy. The effect of subacromial injection of betamethasone in cases of painful shoulder resistant to physical therapy. Ann Chir Gynaecol Fenn 63:suppl. 188, 5, 1974
70. Binder AI, Bulgen DY, Hazleman BL, et al.: Frozen shoulder: a long-term prospective study. Ann Rheum Dis 43:361, 1984
71. Hamer J, Kirk JA: Physiotherapy and the frozen shoulder: a comparative trial of ice and ultrasonic therapy. N Z Med J 83:191, 1976
72. Lee M, Haq AMMM, Wright V, et al: Periarthritis of the shoulder: a controlled trial of physiotherapy. Physiotherapy 59:312, 1972
73. Dacre JE, Beeney N, Scott DL: Injections and physiotherapy for the painful stiff shoulder. Ann Rheum Dis 48:322, 1989
74. Liang H, Lien I: Comparative study in the management of frozen shoulder. J Formosan Med Assoc 72:243, 1973
75. Rizk TE, Christopher RP, Pinals RS, et al: Adhesive capsulitis (frozen shoulder): a new approach to its management. Arch Phys Med Rehabil 64:29, 1983
76. Pothmann R, Weigel A, Stux G: Frozen shoulder: differential acupuncture therapy with point ST-38. Am J Acupuncture 8:65, 1980

77. Mannheimer J, Lampe G: Clinical Transcutaneous Electrical Nerve Stimulation. FA Davis, Philadelphia, 1984
78. The Academy of Traditional Chinese Medicine: An Outline of Chinese Acupuncture. Foreign Languages Press, Peking, 1975
79. Mueller EE, Mead S, Schulz B, et al: A placebo-controlled study of ultrasound treatment for periarthritis. Am J Phys Med 33:31, 1954
80. Quin CE: Humeroscapular periarthritis. Observations on the effects of x-ray therapy and ultrasonic therapy in cases of "frozen shoulder." Ann Phys Med 10:64, 1967
81. Hayes KW: Manual for Physical Agents. 3rd Ed. Northwestern University Press, Chicago, 1984
82. Bulgen DY, Binder AI, Hazleman BL, et al: Frozen shoulder: prospective clinical study with an evaluation of three treatment regimens. Ann Rheum Dis 43:353, 1984
83. Ham A, Cormack D: Histology. 8th Ed. JB Lippincott, Philadelphia, 1979
84. Swann D, Radin E, Nazimiec M: Role of hyaluronic acid in joint lubrication. Ann Rheum Dis 33:318, 1974
85. Wyke BW: Articular neurology—a review. Physiotherapy 58:94, 1972
86. Liebolt FL: Frozen shoulder. Passive exercises for treatment. NY State J Med 70:2085, 1970
87. Haggart GE, Dignam RJ, Sullivan TS: Management of the "frozen" shoulder. JAMA 161:1219, 1956
88. Srivastava KP, Bhan BL, Bhatia IL: Scapulohumeral periarthritis. A clinical study and evaluation of end results of its treatment. J Indian Med Assoc 59:275, 1972
89. Quigley TB: Indications for manipulation and corticosteroids in the treatment of stiff shoulders. Surg Clin North Am 43:1715, 1963
90. Helbig B, Wagner P, Dohler R: Mobilization of frozen shoulder under general anaesthesia. Acta Orthop Belg 49:267, 1983
91. Coombes WN: Frozen shoulder. J R Soc Med 76:711, 1983
92. Quigley TB: Treatment of checkrein shoulder by use of manipulation and cortisone. JAMA 161:850, 1956
93. Weiser HI: Painful primary frozen shoulder mobilization under local anesthesia. Arch Phys Med Rehabil 58:406, 1977
94. Steinbocker O, Argyros TG: Frozen shoulder: treatment by local injections of depot corticosteroids. Arch Phys Med Rehabil 55:209, 1974
95. Murnaghem GF, McIntosh D: Hydrocortisone in painful shoulder. Lancet 1:798, 1955
96. Roy S, Oldham R: Management of painful shoulder. Lancet 1:1322, 1976
97. Cyriax J, Trosier O: Hydrocortisone and soft tissue lesions. Br Med J 2:966, 1953
98. Crisp EJ, Kendall PH: Treatment of periarthritis of the shoulder with hydrocortisone. Br Med J 1:1500, 1955

6 The Shoulder in Hemiplegia

Susan Ryerson
Kathryn Levit

Hemiplegia, a paralysis of one side of the body, occurs with strokes or cerebrovascular accidents involving the cerebral hemisphere or brainstem. Although hemiplegia is the classic and most obvious sign of neurovascular disease of the brain, it can also occur as a result of cerebral tumor or trauma.[1]

One of the most worrisome physical problems for clients with hemiplegia is the shoulder.[2] Shoulder pain, subluxation, loss of muscular activity, and loss of functional use are the most common complaints. These problems can be avoided with proper assessment and treatment and can be ameliorated if they already exist. This chapter reviews biomechanical and motor control impairments and presents a framework for the clinical management of these shoulder problems in hemiplegia.

NORMAL SHOULDER GIRDLE MECHANICS

Before beginning a study of the shoulder girdle in hemiplegia, it is important to review the normal mechanics of the shoulder (see Ch. 1). Three areas of normal shoulder mechanics should be emphasized: (1) the mobility of the scapula on the thorax,[3] (2) scapulohumeral rhythm and the factors influencing both humeral mobility and humeral stability in the glenoid fossa,[4,5] and (3) the muscular attachments of the shoulder–girdle complex.[3,6] Because muscles that move the scapula and humerus have attachments to the cervical, thoracic, and lumbar spine, and rib cage, a loss of motor control and alignment will have multiple effects on the shoulder girdle.

117

ABNORMAL BIOMECHANICS

The loss of motor control of the shoulder in patients with a hemiplegia affects the operation of normal biomechanical principles. In hemiplegia, three factors prevent normal shoulder biomechanical patterns from occurring: loss of muscular control and the develoment of abnormal movement patterns; secondary soft tissue changes that block motion; and glenohumeral joint subluxations. These three factors combine to allow at least three distinct types of shoulder and arm dysfunction.

Loss of Muscular Control and Development of Abnormal Movement

Following the onset of a cerebrovascular accident with hemiplegia, a low tone or flaccid state is present. The length of the lower tone state varies from a short period of hours or days to a period of weeks or months. This state is characterized by a decrease in active postural tone and a loss of motor control in the musculature of the head, neck, trunk, and extremities. Initially, no movement is possible. As motor return occurs, individual muscles gradually become stronger.

In other patients, as motor return occurs, the pattern of control is imbalanced; not all muscles around a joint return at the same strength. Spinal extensor control becomes more evident than spinal flexor control. Early patterns of motor return pull the scapula and arm into abnormal postures. When the scapula and humerus are pulled severely out of alignment, certain muscle groups are positioned in shortened ranges. This results in lengthening or mechanical disadvantage in opposing muscle groups. Because the shortened muscles are available to the patient to use actively, muscle activity in these shortened groups is reinforced cortically with the attempt to move the arm. Muscle firing in these groups may also be reinforced by associated movements.[7] Thus, "functional spasticity" can develop when muscles of the upper extremity are maintained in an almost constant state of excitation.

A third pattern of motor dysfunction in patients is characterized by abnormal coactivation of limb or trunk muscles. These patients get return in both flexor and extensor muscle groups, but have difficulty integrating the firing patterns to produce lateral or rotational movement patterns. These patients also have the ability to recruit distal muscle groups. However, these distal muscle groups are recruited abnormally in what appears to be an attempt to substitute for proximal weakness. As an example, the biceps and wrist flexors may be recruited to help lift the weight of the arm during shoulder flexion while no contraction of the deltoid can be palpated (Fig. 6-1). Over time, a more constant state of excitation develops in the biceps and wrist flexor muscles,

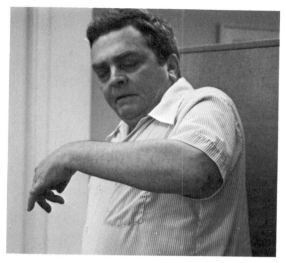

Fig. 6-1.   Left hemiplegia: biceps and wrist flexors recruited to help move shoulder.

leading to muscle shortening. The constant muscle firing in these shortened groups can quickly pull the carpal bones out of alignment, leading to deformities in the forearm, wrist, and hand. The emergence of spasticity will perpetuate abnormal alignment. However, inhibition of spasticity alone will not produce a functional arm. Motor reeducation must be directed toward both the recruitment or strengthening of absent or weak muscle groups and the retraining of available muscles to fire appropriately. Thus, treatment must address the abnormal tonal state, the abnormal movement components, and the abnormal joint alignment to restore normal movement. To restore the normal mechanical relationships of the bones, soft tissue stretching may be necessary.

Soft Tissue Blocks to Motion

Soft tissue blocks to motion can be categorized as loss of scapular mobility, loss of glenohumeral mobility, and loss of the ability to dissociate the scapula and humerus. The loss of scapular stability on the thorax occurs in all but the most minor strokes and is influenced initially by such factors as the pull of the arm into gravity, the development of postural asymmetry, and the influence of patterns of motor return and treatment. As the scapula assumes a position that combines elements of elevation, downward rotation, and abduction, the position of the scapula prevents forward flexion of the arm past 60° to 80°.

Because upward rotation is not available for the scapula, glenohumeral movement greater than 60° is not possible.

Without treatment, the scapula loses its mobility on the thorax and becomes fixed, thus eliminating the scapular component of scapulohumeral rhythm. The loss of this scapular component, consisting of scapular protraction and upward rotation, results in the substitution of scapula elevation. The loss of scapula upward rotation and protraction is important functionally because it is necessary for reach and pain-free elevation of the arm. However, loss of scapular adduction and depression has equal functional importance for resistive tasks such as lifting, pushing, carrying, and upper extremity weight-bearing. The goal in treatment is to restore the normal resting position of the scapula on the thorax and to regain mobility and motor control in all planes of motion.

Changes in scapula position will alter the orientation of the glenoid fossa and affect the resting position of the humerus. In cases of chronic hemiplegia, the humerus is always positioned in some degree of internal rotation, but its position relative to the glenoid fossa will depend on the alignment of the scapula. With a downwardly rotated and depressed scapula, inferior subluxation and internal rotation result (Fig. 6-2). In patients with an elevated, abducted scapula and a hyperextended humerus, the humeral head will be positioned anteriorly in the fossa. In patients with an elevated, abducted scapula and a humerus that postures in abduction and internal rotation, the humeral greater tubercle will impinge under the coracoid process (Fig. 6-3).

Loss of dissociation of the humerus from the scapula is the third block to normal movement. In this case, the scapula has mobility on the thorax and the humerus retains mobility in the glenoid fossa, but any movement of the humerus into flexion or abduction results in simultaneous scapular abduction.

Shoulder Subluxation

Shoulder subluxation occurs in hemiplegia when any of the biomechanical factors contributing to glenohumeral stability are disturbed. The most important factor is the position of the scapula on the thorax. The scapula is normally held on the thorax at an angle 30° from the frontal plane.[3] When the slope of the glenoid fossa becomes less oblique and no longer faces upward, the humerus "slides down" the slope of the fossa and inferior subluxation, the subluxation most frequently mentioned, occurs.[4,6]

Two other forms of subluxation exist in the hemiplegic shoulder: anterior subluxation and superior subluxation. Each of these subluxations have downwardly rotated scapulae, as does the inferior subluxation, but the other scapula and humeral planes of movement vary (Fig. 6-4). These subluxations are discussed in detail in the next section.

Subluxation is not painful as long as the scapula is mobile.[7] However, the

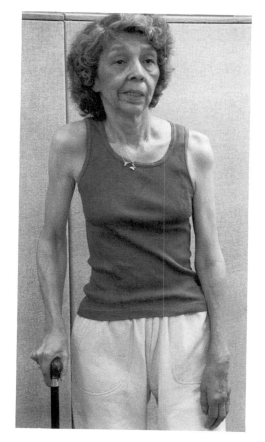

Fig. 6-2. Left hemiplegia: inferior subluxation.

subluxed shoulder should not be allowed to progress into a painful shoulder with loss of passive range of motion (ROM).

Type I Arm

With a severe loss of muscular activity, head and trunk control are virtually absent. This loss of trunk control results in increased lateral trunk flexion on the hemiplegia side.

The scapula in these patients is downwardly rotated for one or more of the following reasons. First, the loss of scapular muscle activity allows the scapula to lose its normal orientation on the thorax and rotate downward (the superolateral angle moves inferiorly). Second, loss of trunk control results in increased lateral trunk flexion. The scapula, moving on this laterally flexed trunk, becomes relatively downwardly rotated, and the glenoid fossa faces

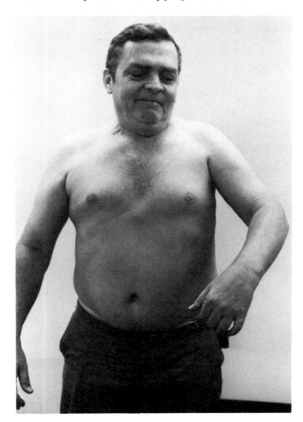

Fig. 6-3. Left hemiplegia: impingement of humeral greater tuberosity beneath acromion.

inferiorly.[3,4] Third, the weight of the arm, if not supported, will pull the weakened scapula downward and place the humerus in relative abduction. With humeral abduction, the shoulder capsule is lax superiorly, and the head of the humerus can slide down the glenoid fossa.[4]

With scapular downward rotation, the glenoid fossa orients downward, and the passive locking mechanism of the shoulder joint, as described by Basmajian, is lost.[6] The loss of this mechanism, the loss of postural tone, and the loss of tension of the shoulder capsule result in an inferior humeral subluxation of the hemiplegic shoulder.

When the body is in an upright position, the weight of the paretic arm and upper trunk will cause the spine to curve with the concavity to the hemiplegic side or to flex forward (Fig. 6-5). This laterally flexed position of the spine places the scapula lower on the thorax, with inferior angle winging. As motor return occurs and the upper trapezius and levator scapular become active, an inferior subluxation may be found with an elevated scapula. In either case, the humerus will hang by the side in internal rotation, the elbow will extend passively, and the forearm will pronate (Fig. 6-6).

With an inferior subluxation, the humeral head is located below the inferior

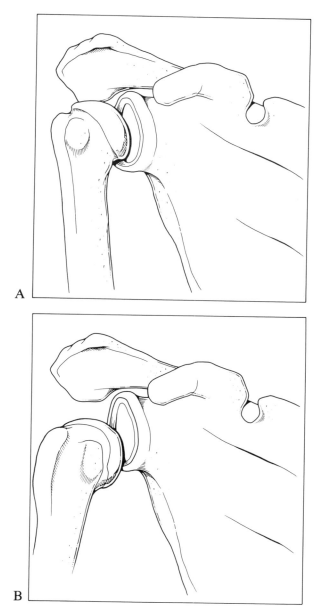

Fig. 6-4. **(A)** Normal glenohumeral alignment. **(B)** Inferior glenohumeral joint subluxation. (*Figure continues.*)

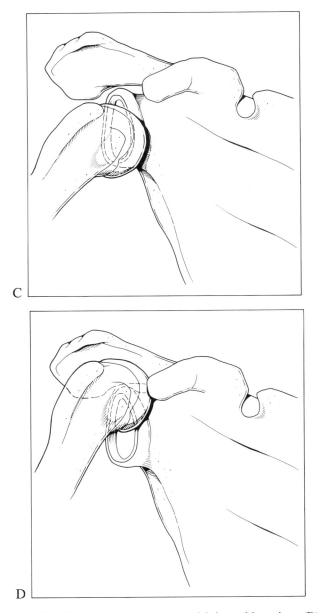

Fig. 6-4. (*Continued*). (**C**) Anterior glenohumeral joint subluxation. (**D**) Superior glenohumeral joint subluxation.

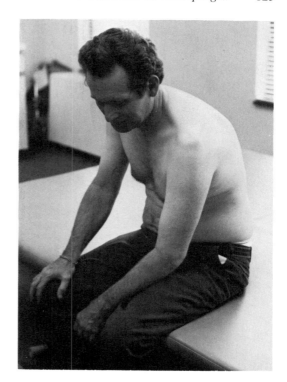

Fig. 6-5. Type I, left hemiplegia: forward flexion of trunk with flaccid arm influencing scapula position.

lip of the glenoid fossa. As subluxation occurs, the shoulder capsule is vulnerable to stretch, especially when the humerus is hanging by the side of the body. In this position, the superior portion of the capsule is taut.[4] The weight of the dependent humerus will place an immediate stretch on the taut capsule. Over time, the superior portion of the capsule will become permanently lax.[8]

When subluxation occurs, the movement possibilities are limited owing to the mechanical position of the humeral head. Any movement that occurs will not follow the rules of scapulohumeral rhythm. With an inferior subluxation of long standing, scapular elevation with humeral internal rotation may be the only movement available.

Soft tissue tightness is found in both sections of the pectoral muscles, and posteriorly in the rotator cuff and the insertion of the latissimus dorsi muscle.

Reduction of Inferior Subluxation. To reduce an inferior subluxation, the scapula must first be upwardly rotated to neutral and moved to its normal position in the frontal plane (elevated if low on the rib cage and depressed if high on the rib cage). The humerus is then moved to neutral from internal rotation and lifted up into the fossa. Care must be given to keep the spine aligned vertically during the subluxation reduction.

Biomechanical shoulder problems resulting from this type of arm include

1. downward rotation of the scapula,

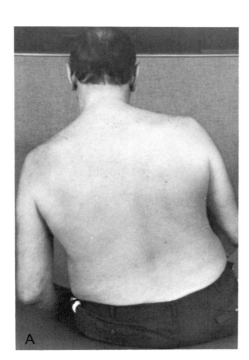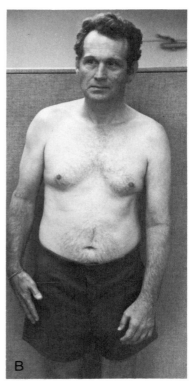

Fig. 6-6. **(A)** Type I, left hemiplegia: left side of body falling laterally into gravity, scapula lower on thorax. **(B)** Type I, left hemiplegia: humerus hangs by the side in internal rotation, elbow extension, and forearm pronation.

    2. vertebral border and/or inferior angle winging of the scapula,
    3. inferior glenohumeral joint subluxation, and
    4. humeral internal rotation.

Type II Arm

    The second pattern develops as the trunk gains more extension control than flexion control. An increase in cervical and lumbar extension is evident. The head and neck assume a position of ipsilateral flexion and contralateral rotation. At the thoracic level, this imbalance results in a unilateral loss of control of the abdominals. Therefore, the rib cage loses its abdominal "anchor" and will flare laterally and/or rotate (Fig. 6-7). The scapula and humerus are strongly influenced mechanically by this rib cage deviation. The downwardly rotated scapula begins to move superiorly on the thorax, and the humerus

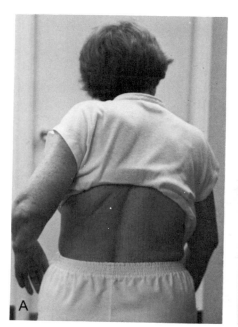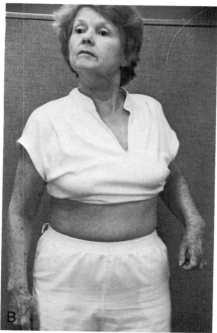

Fig. 6-7. (**A** and **B**) Type II, left hemiplegia: loss of rib cage anchor with rib cage rotated backward and humeral hyperextension with internal rotation.

hyperextends with internal rotation. The glenohumeral joint will sublux anteriorly. With an anterior subluxation, the humerus is internally rotated and positioned inferior to and forward of the glenoid fossa (Fig. 6-4B). The humeral head appears aligned with the acromion in the sagittal plane, resulting in an apparent shortening of the length of the clavicle. As the humeral head moves forward out of the socket, the distal end of the humerus moves into hyperextension. Inferior angle or vertebral border winging of the scapula will occur.

This combination of rib cage rotation and humeral hyperextension allows the elbow to flex and the forearm to pronate (Fig. 6-8). As the scapula continues to elevate on the thorax, and the subluxed, internally rotated humerus moves into stronger hyperextension, the humeral head protrudes forward against the proximal end of the biceps tendon. This forward pressure of the humerus against the already shortened biceps tendon will mechanically move the forearm into a supinated position (Fig. 6-9). The wrist may appear to be less flexed as the carpals move dorsolaterally.

This anterior subluxation will limit movements that require the humerus and hand to be in front of the body. If the patient is asked to lift the arm, shoulder elevation with humeral internal rotation, hyperextension, and elbow flexion will be the movement pattern available.

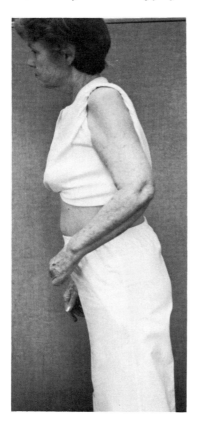

Fig. 6-8. Type II, left hemiplegia: humeral hyperextension with forearm pronation.

Soft tissue tightness will be present in the pectoral muscle groups, rotator cuff, biceps, and forearm and hand.

Reduction of Anterior Subluxation.   To correct this subluxation, the rib cage is derotated and spinal alignment is corrected; the scapula can then be realigned on the rib cage. To realign the scapula on the rib cage, it must be moved down from its elevated position and upwardly rotated to neutral. While stabilizing the scapula in its corrected position, the humerus is moved from internal rotation to neutral. The humeral head can then be moved back as the distal end of the humerus is brought forward out of hyperextension, then lifted up into the fossa.

Biomechanical shoulder problems resulting from this type of arm include

1.   downward rotation and elevation of the scapula,
2.   scapular inferior angle and/or vertebral border winging,
3.   anterior subluxation, and
4.   humeral internal rotation.

In chronic cases of anterior subluxation, elbow flexion becomes more dom-

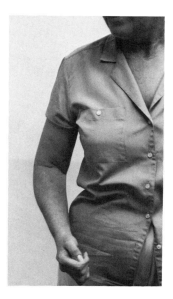

Fig. 6-9. Type II, right hemiplegia: humeral hyperextension with forearm supination.

inant and the forearm adducts across the abdomen. Shortening and spasticity in pectoral and biceps groups may develop, and the scapula loses mobility in the direction of depression and upward rotation.

Type III Arm

The third type of arm pattern is characterized by abnormal coactivation of the limb muscles. This gives an appearance of "mass" flexion in the hemiplegic upper extremity. The neck and trunk control in clients with this upper extremity pattern contain elements of both flexion and extension. The control patterns are not sufficiently integrated to allow selective combinations of movement, and rib cage flairing accompanies active movement of the hemiplegic arm. The scapula is usually elevated and abducted on the thorax. The scapula moves superiorly and tilts anteriorly causing the humerus to lie under the coracoid process in a superior subluxation. The humerus is tightly held in internal rotation and abduction, so that the elbow joint lies directly below the shoulder in the frontal plane but is abducted away from the rib cage.

Passive motion of the glenohumeral joint is severely limited because the humeral head is lodged under the coracoid process. Although the deltoid and biceps attempt to initiate humeral motion, no dissociation occurs between the humerus and scapula. During attempts to move, these patients typically "fire" strongly in this elevation–abduction–internal rotation pattern with elbow and wrist flexion (Fig. 6-10). By increasing humeral internal rotation, patients can "lock" their elbows into elbow extension. When distal movement exists, it is used to reinforce the active shoulder pattern. The wrist assumes a flexed and

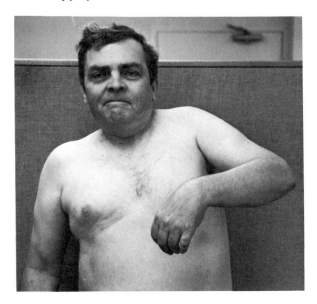

Fig. 6-10. Type III, left hemiplegia: active motion available in shoulder elevation, humeral abduction, internal rotation, and elbow flexion.

radially deviated position. This moves the forearm mechanically from pronation in the direction of supination.

Soft tissue tightness in the deltoids, pectorals, and rotator cuff are frequent secondary complications. Soft tissue tightness in these groups is often mistaken for atrophy from brachial plexus injury.

Reduction of Superior Subluxation. The superior subluxation is the most difficult to reduce. The scapula is returned to a neutral position; it must be lowered, upwardly rotated, and adducted. The humerus is externally rotated to neutral, using slight traction if necessary. External rotation of the humerus is then combined with horizontal adduction of the distal humerus as the humeral head is brought back into the fossa.

Biomechanical shoulder problems resulting from this type of arm include

1. scapula elevation and abduction with vertebral border winging,
2. superior subluxation,
3. humeral internal rotation, and
4. lack of dissociation between scapula and humerus, and between scapula and rib cage.

Relationship of Subluxation to Control

The type of shoulder subluxation and the motor control available affect the hemiplegic patient's ability to move the arm functionally in three ways. First, the loss of antigravity postural tone and the subsequent patterns of motor return will change the relationship of the scapula to the trunk and the relationship of the distal arm to the scapula. This change in position will alter the anatomic relationship of the joints. Second, the changes in bony alignment will change the resting length and direction of pull of the major muscle groups of the shoulder and arm. Biomechanically, this will lead to muscle imbalance and problems of motor control. Third, changes in muscle excitation and recruitment patterns may occur in these muscles, in which resting lengths have been altered. Patterns of spasticity or abnormal coactivation of muscles may result in problems in any or all of these areas and will contribute to the abnormal and inefficient motor patterns associated with hemiplegia. Clinically, it is necessary to analyze the patient's motor patterns to identify the segments of abnormal motion. This will facilitate more effective treatment.

MUSCULOSKELETAL CONSIDERATIONS

Shoulder Pain

Shoulder pain is one of the major problem areas in hemiplegia.[2] Pain occurs in the hemiplegic shoulder as a result of muscle imbalance with loss of joint range, impingement of the shoulder capsule during improper ROM, improper muscle stretching, tendinitis, hypersensitivity, or hyposensitivity; pain also is caused by sympathetic changes.

To plan a treatment program, the nature of the pain, the precise anatomic location of the pain, the duration of the pain, and the body position during the movement that causes the pain must be assessed. Four categories of shoulder pain can be identified: joint pain, muscle pain, pain from altered sensitivity, and shoulder–hand pain syndrome.

Joint Pain

Joint pain in hemiplegia occurs when a joint is placed in a biomechanically compromised position as a result of either shoulder muscle imbalance or improper movement patterns. When the joint is improperly aligned, passive or active motion either with or without weight-bearing will result in joint pain. This pain is sharp and stabbing in nature. It is relieved immediately when joint alignment is corrected. At the shoulder, joint pain occurs when glenohumeral alignment and rhythm is not maintained. The most frequent reasons for poor alignment occuring are (1) lack of appropriate humeral rotation during forward flexion, and (20 improper placement of the humeral head in the glenoid fossa.

Treatment for this type of pain begins with immediate cessation of the movement pattern. Forced motion with pain must *never* be allowed. The movement should STOP; the limb should be lowered and the bones must be correctly realigned before treatment begins again. If soft tissue or joint tightness exists, realignment may not be possible unless soft tissue or joint mobility is improved or increased.

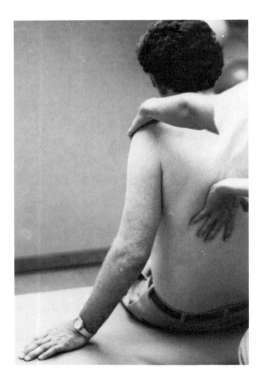

Fig. 6-11. Left hemiplegia: body moving on weight-bearing upper extremity.

Muscle Pain

Muscle pain occurs as a shortened or spastic muscle is lengthened too fast or lengthened beyond the range to which the shortened muscle is "accustomed." Often, this type of pain occurs when the upper extremity is in a weight-bearing position and the patient is asked to move the body on the limb (Fig. 6-11). Muscle pain is perceived as a "pulling" sensation and is localized to the region of the muscle belly that is being stretched. The pain is immediately relieved if the amount of severe stretch is decreased a few degrees. Because lengthening shortened muscles is a goal of treatment, the muscle is not allowed to move back to the shortened range, but is allowed to shorten until the pain is relieved. Treatment can proceed with careful attention given to speed and progression of movement.

The pain that accompanies tendinitis is related to muscle pain, for it is caused by the same mechanims. Overstretching of a limb muscle followed by overaggressive weight-bearing with poor joint alignment results in tendinitis. The pain is described as aching or sharp, remains after the weight-bearing is stopped, and is referred to other locations. In the hemiplegic upper extremity, the two most common types are bicipital groove tendinitis with pain referred down into the muscle belly, and bicipital tendinitis across the elbow with pain referred down the volar aspect of the forearm.

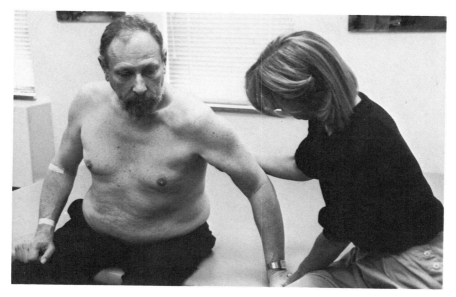

Fig. 6-12. Left hemiplegia: weight-bearing with improper alignment.

The inappropriate weight-bearing pattern that leads to tendinitis in these cases is severe humeral internal rotation with forced elbow extension, along with an inactive trunk and "leaning" on a weak scapula (Fig. 6-12).

The weight-bearing extended arm activity should be stopped until the pain subsides. When weight-bearing treatment is resumed, particular care should be given to proper joint alignment and active trunk scapular pattern (Fig. 6-13).

Altered Sensitivity

The pain that occurs because of altered sensitivity of the central nervous system (CNS) to sensory input is found at the acute stage of recovery following an insult.

This pain occurs in the upper extremity and is described as both diffuse and aching and localized to the shoulder and sharp. It typically occurs during the middle of a treatment session that has included tactile, sensory, kinesthetic, and proprioceptive stimuli. One expalnation for its occurrence is that the levels of "tolerance" of the impaired CNS have been reached. The treatment should stop for that session, and the duration of treatment and the nature of the treatment should be noted. Subsequent treatment should be graded to allow movement to continue but not to exceed the patient's sensory tolerance. If treatment is stopped completely, these patients may proceed to **Shoulder–Hand Syndrome.**

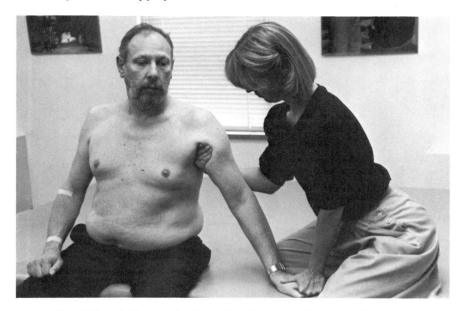

Fig. 6-13.   Left hemiplegia: weight-bearing with proper alignment.

Shoulder–Hand Syndrome

Shoulder–hand syndrome begins with diffuse ''aching pain'' in the shoulder and entire arm. Because this pain interferes with the desire to move the arm, the hand soon becomes swollen and tender. If passive motion is forced on a swollen wrist and hand, the joints will become sharply painful.

The second stage is characterized by decreased ROM of the shoulder girdle, hand, and fingers. Skin changes are also present because of the lack of motion and loss of tactile input.

The syndrome culminates with presence of atrophied bone and severe soft tissue deformity and joint contractures. Shoulder–hand syndrome can be prevented by a program that

1.   grades the motor program in stages with increasing sensitivity to movement,

2.   gradually but consistently uses weight-bearing activities for the entire shoulder girdle and upper extremity,

3.   reeducates open-ended activities (non-weight-bearing) with appropriate scapulohumeral rhythm,

4.   prevents edema, and

5.   teaches patients how to care for their arms.

TREATMENT PLANNING

The treatment of the deficits in motor control in the patient with hemiplegia focuses on the improvement of function and the prevention of further disability from secondary complications. In this section, treatment objectives for the hemiplegic shoulder will be presented in three major categories. The first category of objectives is designed to help the patient relearn basic postural control. The second set of objectives focuses on the neuromuscular deficits of hemiplegia: loss of extremity motor control and function. In the third category, the objectives for the secondary complications of hemiplegia—subluxation, pain, loss of motion, and spasticity—will be discussed.

Reestablishment of Postural Control

The objectives for establishing postural control include

1. the facilitation of righting reactions, equilibrium reactions, and protective reactions, and
2. the provision of normal tactile, proprioceptive, and kinesthetic input.

Before specific retraining of the shoulder in patients with hemiplegia can begin, postural control of the head, neck, and trunk must be present. This postural trunk control provides the body with the ability to shift weight. The ability of the body to shift and bear weight to one side frees the opposite extremity for the functions of reaching, grasping, and releasing. Along with sensory feedback (tactile, proprioceptive, kinesthetic, visual, and vestibular), movement requires a base of stability or base of support, a point of mobility, and a weight shift. Weight shift, either anterior, posterior, lateral, or diagonal, is followed by one or more of the following: righting reactions, equilibrium reactions, protective reactions, or falling. The establishment of head and neck control allows the shoulder girdle to dissociate or move freely from the thorax and the humerus to dissociate from the scapula. To establish good motor control, the body (trunk) must be able to adjust posture automatically so that an upper extremity movement may achieve its purpose.

Neuromuscular Deficits

Objectives for reestablishing motor control and function of the hemiplegic arm include

1. reestablishing normal alignment,
2. establishing normal weight-bearing patterns in the upper extremity,

3. initiating and "holding" proximal non-weight-bearing patterns, and
4. reeducating distal movement for functional skills.

Reestablishing Normal Alignment

It is necessary to reestablish normal alignment before attempting to reeducate motor control. The shoulder girdle must be properly aligned either by lengthening shortened or spastic muscles or by supporting body parts that do not have sufficient muscular activity.

Establishing Weight-Bearing

The ability to accept and bear weight on the affected arm following a stroke is one of the most important goals of a therapeutic program. Active weight-bearing on either a partially flexed or extended upper extremity is used as a means of increasing mobility; increasing postural control of the trunk; improving motor control of the affected arm; introducing and grading tactile, proprioceptive, and kinesthetic stimulation; and preventing edema and pain. Positions that provide weight-bearing for a hemiplegia shoulder and arm include (1) rolling onto the affected side in preparation for getting out of bed (Fig. 6-14A&B), (2) supporting the forearm on a pillow placed in the lap or on a lap board or on a table when sitting (Fig. 6-14C), and (3) extending the weight-bearing arm down onto a countertop while standing (Fig. 6-14D).

An active weight-bearing program for the paretic arm stresses "active" patterns in the trunk and does not allow the patient to lean or "hang" on the ligaments of the affected extremity (Fig. 6-15). This active participation of the trunk is accomplished by placing the upper extremity in an aligned weight-bearing position and asking the trunk or "body" to move on the stable arm in anterior–posterior, lateral, and rotational directions.

In the acute stage of hemiplegia, when very little postural control is present, upper extremity weight-bearing is used to facilitate proximal motor control. When the upper extremities are "fixed" onto the supporting surface through forearm weight-bearing activities, the arm becomes a point of stability for movements of the trunk and pelvis. As the body moves away from the arm, scapular protraction and upward rotation, humeral flexion, and upper trunk flexion are encouraged (Fig. 6-16A). As the body moves toward the arm, scapular adduction and trunk extension are encouraged as the humerus moves into more extension (Fig. 6-16B). When the pelvis and trunk move laterally, the scapulae move in opposite directions, one into more abduction and one into more adduction. The humerus on the side of the lateral weight shift becomes more externally rotated, while the other humerus becomes more internally rotated (Fig. 6-17).

For patients with available but synergistic movement patterns, upper extremity weight-bearing can be used to lengthen or inhibit tight or spastic muscles

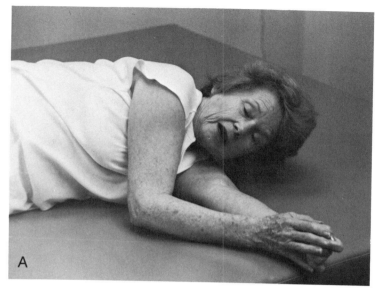

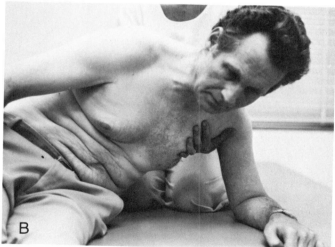

Fig. 6-14. Weight-bearing positions for the upper extremity. **(A)** Left hemiplegia: rolling onto affected side. **(B)** Left hemiplegia: moving onto affected forearm. (*Figure continues.*)

while simultaneously facilitating muscles that are not active. When the person sits with hands down and open, a rotational movement of the body toward the affected upper extremity will lengthen tight shoulder depressors and downward rotators, tight humeral internal rotators, and elbow flexors, while simultaneously activating the opposing groups (Fig. 6-18).

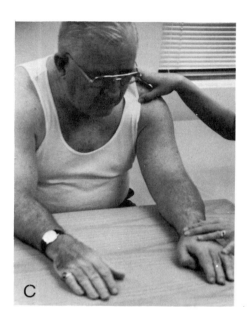
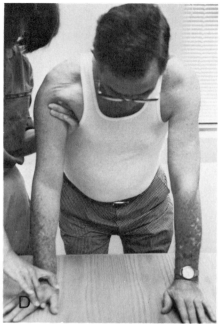

Fig. 6-14. (*Continued*). (**C**) Left hemiplegia: supporting forearm on table. (**D**) Right hemiplegia: extended arm weight-bearing.

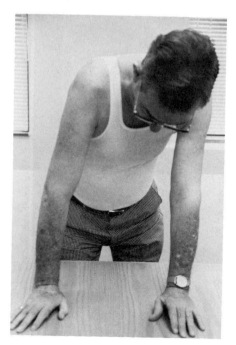

Fig. 6-15. Right hemiplegia: improper weight-bearing on extended arm—"hanging" on shoulder and mechanically locking elbow.

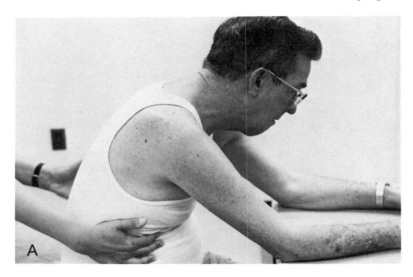

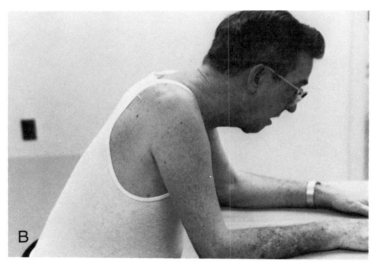

Fig. 6-16.   Right hemiplegia: (**A**) moving body away from weight-bearing arm; (**B**) moving body toward weight-bearing arm.

Initiating and "Holding" Proximal
Non-Weight-Bearing Patterns

When the hand or arm is placed in a position of weight-bearing, the motions of the shoulder girdle occur as a reaction to the body's movement over the fixed extremity. When the arm is taken out of weight-bearing and is asked to move in space, the demands on the shoulder girdle are different from weight-bearing demands. The motor demands on the shoulder for non-weight-bearing

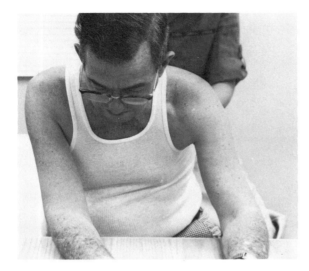

Fig. 6-17. Right hemiplegia: weight shifting to right moves right humerus into more external rotation while left humerus begins to move into the direction of internal rotation.

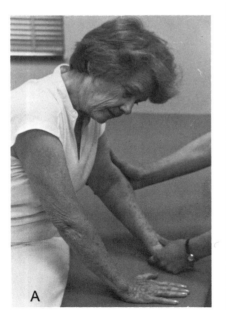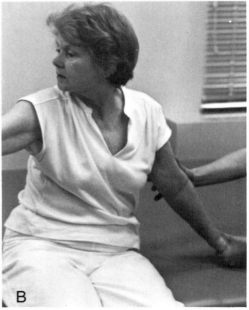

Fig. 6-18. (**A** and **B**) Left hemiplegia: rotational body movements over a weight-bearing upper extremity.

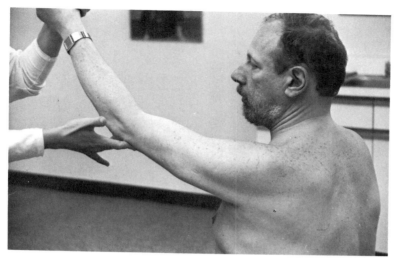

Fig. 6-19.   Left hemiplegia: place and hold position.

(open-ended) activities can be divided into (1) the ability to hold the weight of the limb against gravity; (2) the ability to initiate antigravity movement patterns, including the ability to switch from glenohumeral to scapulohumeral movement as needed; and (3) the ability to reciprocate and coordinate the combinations of mobility and stability needed for reaching, grasping, carrying, and releasing.

Motor reeducation aimed at training the hemiplegic arm to move against gravity will vary according to the patterns of return present and variables such as pain, spasticity, or malalignment. Techniques for managing pain and spasticity are discussed separately (see Treatment of Secondary Complications) and should be used before treatment of motor control proceeds. Orthopaedic changes, particularly those that are longstanding, represent a particular treatment challenge because although orthopaedic malalignment at the shoulder will necessitate compensation or abnormal movement, it is frequently impossible within a treatment session to reposition the scapula or humerus in normal alignment before proceeding with movement reeducation. In these cases, the goal is to gain some increase in mobility in the direction of normal alignment, followed immediately by a movement pattern that uses this new mobility. Over successive treatments, as soft tissue mobility is increased and passive resting positions become closer to normal alignment, the types and combinations of movement can be increased.

When pain, spasticity, and malalignment of the shoulder joints are not problems, treatment can be directed immediately to improving motor control. In the acute stage, in which muscle tone is low and little motion is present, teaching the patient to manage the weight of the arm against gravity is the first stage of motor control to be introduced. This is done by teaching the patient to "hold" the scapula and humerus in an antigravity position (Fig. 6-19).[7,9]

"Place and hold" activities are practiced in supine and, later, in sitting positions until the patient develops control of the arm in various combinations of scapula and humeral patterns.

The patient is then taught to move actively within his or her range of control. When the concept of holding has been achieved, the patient is asked to initiate patterns at the shoulder. This is done by moving the hemiplegic arm in many functional patterns combined with strong sensory stimulation during each treatment session. Muscle groups that are unable to contract after the joint has been realigned need to be stimulated. The techniques of stimulation have been described by Bobath and others. The techniques are the same, although they have been ascribed different names:

joint compression (pressure tapping, joint approximation),
resistance with proper alignment maintained,
quick stretch (inhibitory tapping, "pull-push"),
sweep tapping (brushing, icing), and
repetition.

When the patient has movement available, but efforts to move the arm produce abnormal patterns, treatment is directed toward establishing more normal coordination. This may involve both inhibiting the abnormal way in which muscles are recruited and retraining in the correct pattern of motor recruitment. Problems in motor recruitment can best be addressed by teaching the patient to identify and quiet muscles that are firing inappropriately through techniques of inhibition or biofeedback. The patient is then taught to allow passive motion of the arm without firing muscles inappropriately or allowing muscle tone in the arm to increase. The patient is then encouraged to try to "follow" the movement and finally to perform it actively with less assistance from the therapist. Place and hold exercises are useful in helping the patient use the correct muscles at the shoulder girdle without inappropriately firing distal muscle groups. While new recruitment patterns are being established, the patient is also taught appropriate control of the previously "overused" muscles. Thus, the patient learns to inhibit biceps activity when reaching, but to use the biceps appropriately to bring the hand to the mouth.

Patients who have less spasticity or more complete motor return have fewer problems with abnormal recruitment but more problems with motor control. This category of patients has missing components of motor activity. Compensatory motions resembling an abnormal pattern result. For example, lack of active external rotation of the humerus will lead to a substitution pattern of abduction, internal rotation of the humerus, and scapula elevation (Fig. 6-20). If this motor pattern is being used because the patient cannot actively externally rotate the humerus, the goal of treatment must be to make external rotation available during active shoulder movement and to establish the ability to hold the humerus in external rotation while moving distally. Similarly, other patients may have difficulties with protraction and upward rotation of the scapula. In this case, the therapist must control the motion of the scapula proximally to

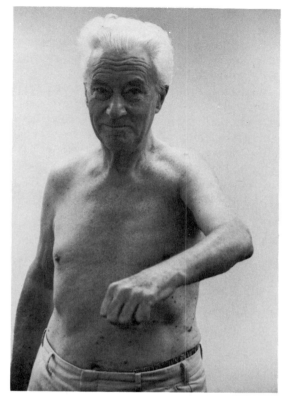

Fig. 6-20. Left hemiplegia: lack of active external rotation results in compensation pattern of humeral abduction and internal rotation.

facilitate the correct motion of the scapula while the patient works on upper extremity placing or movement sequences.

Reeducating Distal Movements

Distal motor control, to be accurate, must be based on normal patterns of mobility and stability in the scapula and glenohumeral joint. Once the patient can initiate normal motion at the glenohumeral and scapulothoracic joints and can maintain the shoulder in positions against gravity, the patient must learn to add combinations of elbow position and forearm rotation to the control established at the shoulder. To use the hand functionally for grasping, carrying, and releasing, the hemiplegic patient must be able to position the hand appropriately for grasp by selecting appropriate forearm and wrist positions, hold the hand in position while the fingers move, and sustain grasp while moving proximally. Problems in any of the above may interfere with adaptive grasp.

As shoulder girdle control builds, the positions and movements of the distal segments must be added in treatment so that various distal positions are available to the patient to use functionally. As new combinations of motor behavior are learned, the patient should be taught a functional task using this pattern to ensure carry-over from exercise into everyday life.

Different grasp patterns require varying wrist and forearm positions. In addition, the transition from grasp to manipulation involves the addition of complex fine motor patterns that are often task-specific. Improving the level of hand function is thus a separate treatment process that requires good motor control of the shoulder, elbow, forearm, and wrist as a precursor of success.

When the hemiplegic patient has biomechanical shoulder girdle problems, accurate positioning of the hand for function is difficult as the patient attempts to hold the shoulder against gravity and initiate appropriate antigravity movement patterns.[10]

Treatment of Secondary Complications

The objectives for each of the secondary complications—subluxation, pain, loss of motion, and spasticity—are discussed separately.

Subluxation

Acutely, if subluxation is not present, treatment follows the objectives listed under Treatment Planning. If subluxation has occurred, treatment must be preceded by careful assessment, reduction of subluxation, and proper support.

Proper assessment of subluxation includes determination of

1. the exact position of the humeral head, scapula, ribcage, and spine;
2. mobility or passive range of motion;
3. tone;
4. amount and location of motor control.

The assessment will reveal the cause of the subluxation (i.e., loss of motor control of scapula and/or humerus, soft tissue tightness, and hypotonus or hypertonus). Appropriate treatment can then begin.

Treatment of subluxation includes the following goals:

1. manual alignment and support of scapula on the thorax and humerus in the glenoid fossa during treatment,
2. increase in motor control in shoulder girdle muscle groups,
3. inhibition of spasticity or stretching of soft tissue tightness,
4. maintenance of pain-free ROM with proper glenohumeral rhythm, and

5. prevention of stretching of shoulder capsule through proper positioning and/or shoulder supports.

Proper positioning can be achieved through the use of lapboards, tables, armrests, or pillows when sitting; self-assisted motion during functional activities; and weight-bearing on the forearm or hand.

Shoulder Subluxation Supports. The shoulder should be supported in the acute stage of hemiplegia to prevent stretch on the capsule or to eliminate pain. In the 1950s and 1960s, orthopaedic slings were given to patients with hemiplegia. These slings held the humerus against the body in internal rotation and kept the elbow in flexion. The arm was immobilized and the patient was unable to see the arm or try to use the arm even for support. In the 1970s and 1980s, alternative slings were produced: the Rolyan hemi arm sling, the shoulder saddle sling, and variations on the axillary support as described by Bobath.[7]

Rolyan hemi arm sling (Rolyan Smith and Nephew, Inc., Menomonee Falls, WI): This sling has a humeral cuff and a figure eight suspension. It will provide moderate support to the humerus and allows the elbow to be extended. The arm is free to be moved and used for support (Fig. 6-21A).

Shoulder saddle sling (Fred Sammons, Inc., Brookfield, IL): This sling has a forearm cuff and a shoulder saddle suspension. It provides maximum support to the entire arm and prevents the arm from "banging" around during functional activities. This sling is excellent for the flaccid limb with pain. It allows moderate humeral and elbow movement (Fig. 6-21B).

Axillary support (All Orthopedic Appliances, Inc., Miami, FL): This support elevates the scapula and provides minimal inferior support for the humerus. It should not be used in patients with elevated scapulae. It has been criticized for placing pressure on the brachial plexus when inappropriately donned (Fig. 6-21C).

Since no device is available that upwardly rotates the scapula, no shoulder support will correct glenohumeral joint subluxation. Shoulder supports will help support and/or maintain position on the rib cage once the correction has been made. Shoulder supports will also prevent the flaccid arm from banging against the body during functional activities, thus decreasing shoulder joint pain. They also help to relieve downward traction on the shoulder capsule caused by the weight of the arm.

Therapy clinics should have different types of shoulder supports available and evaluate which support provides the best protection for each patient.

Pain

The causes of shoulder pain have been described in detail. Treatment of the painful shoulder and arm should include

1. immediate cessation of any movement or activity that causes or increases the pain,

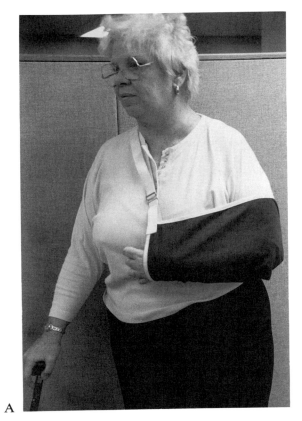

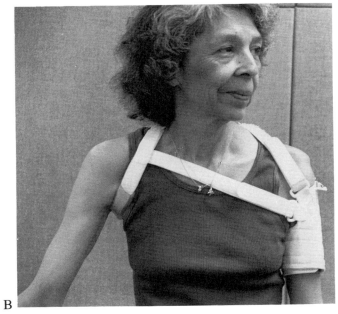

Fig. 6-21. **(A)** orthopaedic sling. **(B)** Rolyan hemi arm sling. (*Figure continues.*)

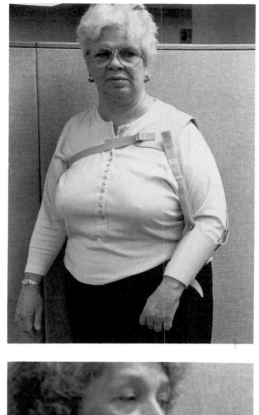

C

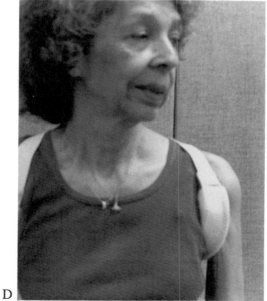

D

Fig. 6-21. (*Continued*). (**C**) Shoulder saddle sling. (**D**) Axillary strap.

2. removal of edema, if present,
3. realignment of the shoulder girdle/trunk complex either by the therapist manually (passively) or by the client actively (this includes lengthening or inhibition of the shortened or spastic muscle groups and realignment of maligned joints),
4. reeducation of the inactive muscle groups, and
5. a graded program of weight-bearing through the shoulder, forearm, and hand

Loss of Range

Loss of ROM at the shoulder can lead to decreased arm function and impaired balance in patients with hemiplegia. Although classic stretching procedures (non-weight-bearing) are often used for loss of shoulder motion in hemiplegia, slow maintained stretching or elongation through weight-bearing (i.e., functional stretching in conjunction with retraining motor control) is more effective.

Spasticity

The importance of spasticity in the treatment of hemiplegia is a controversial subject.[11,12] Spasticity is one of the positive symptoms of hemiplegia, along with clonus and disinhibition of primitive reflexes. Although spasticity must be dealt with during the treatment of the hemiplegic shoulder, the negative symptoms, paresis, loss of force production, delayed initiation of movement, and pathologic cocontraction of muscles, must also be addressed.[13]

While inhibition of spasticity alone will not result in a functional upper extremity, persistent muscle activity or muscle shortening will block normal movements from occurring. It is only when tone is inhibited that a true assessment of the patient's motor abilities can be performed. The presence and distribution of spasticity in the upper extremity is often influenced by the patient's ability to control the trunk and lower extremity in transitional movements and in standing and walking.

Campbell[11] hypothesizes that by preventing the development of abnormal compensatory motor patterns through activation of normal motor control, therapists may decrease or even prevent the development of spasticity. From a movement point of view, existing spasticity in the upper extremity can be inhibited by (1) maintained elongation or lengthening in the pattern of shortened muscle groups, (2) activation of the trunk musculature through upper extremity weight-bearing or (3) reeducation of the pelvis and lower extremity. We believe that in stroke patients who have not developed spasticity, effective treatment can guide motor return and prevent the development of abnormal motor patterns.

CONCLUSION

The importance of identifying the exact location and nature of shoulder girdle dysfunction in hemiplegia has been stressed in this chapter. Because the abnormal motor patterns of hemiplegia can arise from a combination of abnormal alignment, unbalanced motor return, and abnormal patterns of muscle excitation and recruitment, treatment strategies must be based on a thorough understanding of the interrelationships between orthopaedic and neurologic factors. The presence of subluxation and pain are additional problems that must be addressed before neuromuscular reeducation can begin. The positive results of any treatment regimen will ultimately depend on the clinician's systematic evaluation and skill in implementing appropriate treatment of the shoulder girdle complex.

REFERENCES

1. Adams RD, Victor M: Principles of Neurology. McGraw-Hill, New York, 1981
2. Davis PM: Steps to Follow. Springer-Verlag, Berlin, 1985
3. Kapandji IA: The Physiology of the Joints: Upper Limb. Churchill Livingstone, Edinburgh, 1970
4. Cailliet R: The Shoulder in Hemiplegia. FA Davis, Philadelphia, 1980
5. Codman EA: The Shoulder. Thomas Todd, Boston, 1934
6. Basmajian JV: Muscles Alive. Williams & Wilkins, Baltimore, 1979
7. Bobath B: Adult Hemiplegia: Evaluation and Treatment. 2nd Ed. William Heinneman Medical Books, London, 1979
8. Jensen M: The hemiplegic shoulder. Scand J Rehabil Med (Suppl) 7:113, 1980
9. Carr JH, Shepherd R: A Motor Relearning Programme for Stroke. Aspen Systems, London, 1983
10. Rubiana R: Examination of the Hand and Upper Limb. WB Saunders, Philadelphia, 1984
11. Campbell S: Pediatric Neurologic Physical Therapy. Churchill Livingstone, New York, 1984
12. Sahrmann S, Norton BJ: The relationship of voluntary movement to spasticity in the upper motor neuron syndrome. Ann Neurol 2:460, 1977
13. Lance JW: The control of muscle tone, reflexes and movement: Robert Wartenberg lecture. Neurology 30:1303, 1980

7 | Evaluation and Management of Thoracic Outlet Syndrome

Julianne Wright Howell

Thoracic outlet syndrome represents a multitude of syndromes involving the upper quarter and hand that are believed to be caused by proximal compression of the subclavian artery, vein, and/or brachial plexus.[1-5] Most investigators agree that at least one of these structures must be compressed at some point between the superior opening of the thorax and the axilla to qualify as thoracic outlet syndrome.

This chapter focuses on this diagnosis; however, I have elected not to perpetuate the use of the term *thoracic outlet syndrome,* because "thoracic outlet" is anatomically incorrect when used to describe the superior opening of the thoracic cavity. According to the classic anatomists, the superior opening of the thorax is the thoracic inlet, and it is simply an anatomic misnomer to refer to the superior opening as the outlet.[6,7] Therefore, for the sake of anatomic correctness, the area bordered anteriorly by the clavicle and first thoracic rib and posteriorly by the first thoracic vertebra is the inlet, not the outlet, of the thorax. I recognize that most of the literature refers to this area as the outlet; however, the reader should take note of the change in nomenclature from thoracic outlet syndrome to thoracic inlet syndrome (TIS) in this chapter.

The amount of literature on TIS available to the clinician is overwhelming and relates primarily to etiology, differential diagnosis, and the surgical management of the TIS patient. Because of the vast number of reports on TIS, the reader may be totally unaware that many investigators question the frequency of its occurrence, and that some even doubt the existence of the syndrome![8-10] Those who doubt the existence of TIS cite as evidence (1) the lack of "proof positive," since there is no single diagnostic test or battery of tests; (2) the failure of surgical intervention to relieve the patient's symptoms consistently, as well as the high percentage of patients whose symptoms consistently reoccur postsurgically; and (3) 50 to 90 percent of these patients respond to physical therapy without surgical removal of a muscle and/or rib.

In addition to the above factors, the risk of surgical complications, such as brachial plexus palsy, pneumothorax, and recurrence of symptoms, has convinced many practitioners to take a more conservative approach in their management of these patients.[5]

As a result of this change in philosophy, physical therapy is often the first line of treatment prescribed for these patients. Unfortunately, for the physical therapist who desires more information on this topic, documentation of physical therapy evaluation, treatment, and results of therapeutic intervention is scarce and, at best, sorely lacking in scientific organization.

Therefore, it is the purpose of this chapter to provide the reader with background information relative to special testing for TIS, a review of the existing literature on physical therapy management of TIS, and suggestions that I have found helpful in the evaluation and treatment of these patients. I hope that this chapter will provide food for thought and persuade readers that only by careful documentation of their clinical findings and results of treatment will the understanding of this syndrome improve.

CLINICAL PRESENTATION

Characteristically, individuals who develop TIS are usually women (outnumbering men three to one) and middle-aged. The onset of symptoms is generally insidious, but has been reported by some investigators to follow trauma involving the shoulder girdle.[11-13] Patient complaints include inability to raise or maintain the arm in a static posture for short periods of time without the onset of their symptoms. Typical examples of activities which evoke symptoms include styling hair, driving, needlework, lifting, overhead use of the arm, carrying a briefcase, and typing. The patient's symptoms may include pain involving the neck, upper extremity, and hand; the feeling that the upper extremity is heavy, tired, and swollen; and that the skin is blotchy, discolored, and a different temperature.

The symptoms of TIS are assumed to be of neurovascular origin, involving compression of the subclavian artery, vein, and brachial plexus. Generally, these structures are compressed in combination, but cases of single structure compression have been reported.[14,15] Symptoms related to compression of the brachial plexus have been documented in 90 percent of all TIS cases.[13,16,17] Those symptoms, as reported in frequency of occurrence, include pain, paresthesia, and paresis of the neck, upper extremity, and hand. Roos, in a ret-

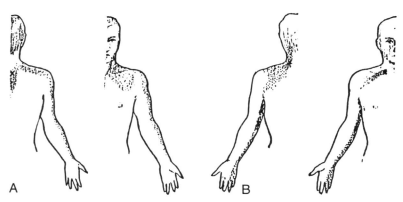

Fig. 7.1.   Thoracic inlet syndrome symptom patterns for (**A**) upper plexus involvement and (**B**) lower plexus involvement.

rospective analysis of 3,630 TIS patients, identified two distinct neurologic symptom patterns in these patients.[16] One pattern involves the upper roots of the plexus (C5–C7), and the other involves the lower roots of the plexus (C8 and T1). Some patients within the sample were found to have atypical symptoms that involved both upper and lower plexus compression[16] (Fig. 7-1).

Symptoms of vascular origin occur in 5 to 10 percent of all cases and are rarely the only complaint.[18] The most widely reported complaints that suggest vascular involvement include edema, heaviness or weakness of the upper extremity, and the triad of cyanosis, blanching, and erythema mimicking Raynaud's phenomenon.[4,19]

ETIOLOGY

The list of probable etiologies for compression of these neurovascular structures is endless (Table 7-1). Those causes most commonly implicated and surgically removed include an anomalous cervical rib,[20] the first thoracic rib,[21]

Table 7-1. Suggested Etiologies of Neurovascular Compression Against First Thoracic Rib

Primary TIS		Secondary TIS
Soft Tissue	Bony	
Anterior scalene		
Middle scalene		
Pectoralis minor		Trauma
Subclavius		Occupational stresses
Costocoracoid fascia	Cervical rib	Shoulder girdle descent
Fibromuscular bands	Clavicle malunion	Overweight conditions
Pancoast's tumor	Transverse processes	Pendulous breasts

Primary TIS has an anatomic basis and secondary TIS is situational.

the scalene anticus,[22] and anomalous fibromuscular bands.[23] I have found the classification scheme of primary and secondary TIS useful to simplify this confusing list of etiologic mechanisms.[24] According to Jaeger et al., the primary form of TIS is caused by compression from a bony or soft tissue abnormality. These structures may include, but are not limited to, a cervical rib, a malunion of the clavicle, anomalous fibromuscular bands of the scalene muscles, or a Pancoast's tumor of the apex of the lung. Secondary TIS, on the other hand, occurs in the absence of any anatomic variation, and is the direct result of trauma to the upper extremity or cervical spine. As a result of this trauma, cervicothoracic posture is altered and, in turn, produces intermittent compression of the plexus and subclavian vessels.[24] Although this classification scheme has helped me to simplify the list of etiologies, I have not found that patients with either form of TIS have any different clinical presentation or that this scheme has much predictive value in selecting the most successful management plan for these patients.

SPECIAL TESTS FOR THORACIC INLET SYNDROME

The difficulty in making the diagnosis of TIS is well documented.[5,8] Subsequently, a barrage of tests is used to localize the cause of the patient's symptoms. Among the most familiar are the provocative maneuver tests, which include the scalene anticus, costoclavicular, hyperabduction, and 3-minute elevated arm exercise tests. Although there are many other tests and methods of testing, this chapter will be limited to reviewing the related literature and testing methods performed by the physical therapist.

Provocative Maneuver Tests

The scalene anticus or Adson's test is used to evaluate the muscle's role in the compression of the subclavian artery as it passes between the anterior and middle scalene muscles enroute to the axilla.[22] To compress the artery, the anterior scalene must be stretched from its origins on the anterior tubercles of the transverse processes of C4, C5, C6, and C7 to its insertion on the scalene tubercle of the first thoracic rib. To stretch the anterior scalene, Adson stipulated that the patient must hyperextend and rotate the head toward the affected side and take a deep breath. Meanwhile, the examiner must monitor the radial pulse of the affected upper extremity as it is held in a relaxed position at the patient's side (Fig. 7-2). By definition, a positive test for the anterior scalene is indicated by an obliteration or a decrease in the pulse rate.[22]

The space between the first rib and the clavicle has also been implicated in the compression of these neurovascular structures. Falconer and Weddell[21] described the costoclavicular or exaggerated military position. This test is designed to narrow the space between the first rib and the clavicle, to compress the subclavian vessels and/or the brachial plexus. To perform the test, the

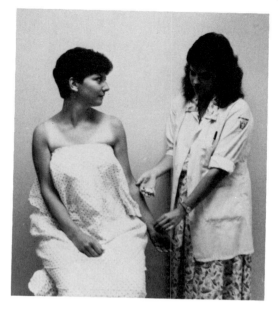

Fig. 7-2.   Left scalene anticus test.

subject is seated with arms held comfortably at the sides. To approximate the anterior surface of the rib to the posterior surface of the clavicle, the subject retracts and depresses the shoulder girdle. Simultaneously, the examiner monitors for a change in the radial pulse. By definition, a positive costoclavicular test is indicated by obliteration or decrease in pulse rate and/or the onset of symptoms[21] (Fig. 7-3).

The hyperabduction maneuver as described by Wright[25] involves passive circumduction of the affected upper extremity overhead while the examiner monitors the radial pulse. It is important that the examiner monitor the pulse while the arm is slowly moved into the overhead position to localize the point in the arc of motion where the pulse changes (Fig. 7-4). Hypothetically, there are two potential sites for compression of the neurovascular bundle during this maneuver. The first site is between 0° and 90° of shoulder abduction when the subclavian vessels and the plexus are stretched around the coracoid process. The other site of compression is at the costoclavicular space as it narrows, with shoulder abduction beyond 90°. The hyperabduction test, by definition, is positive if the pulse rate changes and/or symptoms are elicited.[25]

The 3-minute elevated arm exercise test has gained in popularity since it was described by Roos.[16] This test is performed with the patient sitting, arms abducted 90° from the thorax and the elbow flexed 90° with the shoulders braced slightly. The patient is then asked to open and close his or her fingers slowly and steadily for a full 3 minutes (Fig. 7-5). The examiner watches for dropping of the elevated arms and decreased rate of fisting or the onset of the patient's

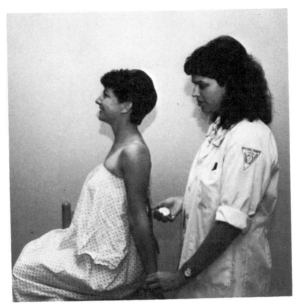

Fig. 7-3. Costoclavicular provocative maneuver.

symptoms. According to Roos, a person can normally perform this test without symptoms other than mild fatigue; however, TIS patients will complain of their usual symptoms. Furthermore, Roos states that this test will evaluate involvement of all three of the neurovascular structures since the test position places the structures in the position for greatest compression. A positive elevated arm exercise test is indicated by the patient's inability to complete the full 3 minutes and the onset of the patient's symptoms.[3]

The four provocative maneuvers discussed above are the most commonly used tests for obliteration of the pulse and reproduction of symptoms when TIS is suspected. However, the reader should realize that there are vascular testing instruments such as the photoplethysmograph (PPG) and the Doppler ultrasound (Doppler) that are often used to monitor blood flow in place of examiner palpation of the radial pulse during the provocative maneuver. I believe that monitoring vascular flow with instrumentation rather than palpation offers several advantages that are worth consideration:

1. Both instruments are noninvasive monitors; therefore, the patient is not at risk, as would be the case with an arteriogram or venogram.
2. Instruments may offer better sensitivity to detect subtle changes in blood flow.
3. A change in the volume of blood flow can be quantitated with instruments, whereas only a change in pulse quality can be detected by palpation.
4. If the examiner is unsure which subclavian vessel is involved, the Doppler can be used to differentiate venous from arterial flow.

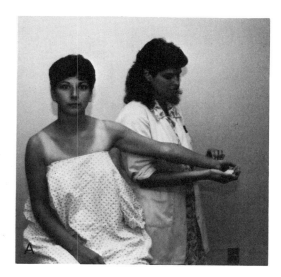

Fig. 7-4. Hyperabduction maneuver at (A) midway position and (B) on completion.

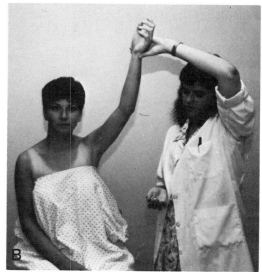

5. A permanent record of the pulse tracing can be produced by both instruments and can then be used as an objective finding in the patient's medical record.

6. For patients whose symptoms are produced by overhead or repetitive motion, the PPG monitor can be attached to the patient while performing the symptom-provoking tasks.

7. The Doppler probe flow detector can be placed externally over the vessel along its entire course through the neck and upper extremity to localize the site of compression.

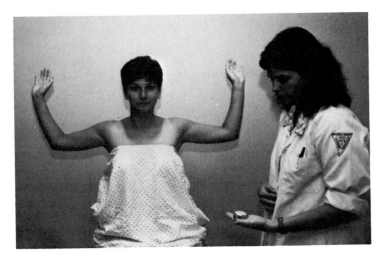

Fig. 7-5. Three-minute elevated arm exercise test.

A few physical therapists are fortunate enough to be trained in vascular testing; for those who are not, there may be a vascular testing center located in the therapist's facility or community with which the therapist can consult. If the therapist is treating several such patients, chances are that many of them will have undergone vascular testing; therefore, the therapist may want to be able to interpret or compare the results of these tests with clinical findings. Similarly, the TIS literature is filled with references to the PPG and Doppler as mechanisms with which to diagnose and evaluate the effectiveness of treatment. To critique these results, the therapist needs some basic background knowledge.

If, at this point, the reader understands that provocative maneuver tests are used for exactly what their name implies—to provoke a change in blood flow and/or to evoke symptoms in a patient suspected of TIS—all is well and good! However, I caution the reader not to assume, without the benefit of additional information, that a positive response to any of these special tests implies that a patient has TIS. Interesting documentation shows that these special maneuvers produce changes in blood flow and evoke symptoms not only in TIS patients, but also in a large percentage of normal asymptomatic individuals. Geroudis and Barnes[19] studied the prevalence of vascular compression during provocative maneuver testing in 130 asymptomatic normal individuals. The PPG was used to monitor digital blood flow during these maneuvers, and the response was categorized by these investigators based on the change in the amplitude of the digital pulse. A response was classified as normal if less than 76 percent reduction in pulse amplitude was noted, and as abnormal if more than 75 percent of the pulse amplitude was reduced or if there was complete absence of the digital pulse. Based on this classification scheme, abnormal responses were noted in 60 percent of the subjects for at least one of the provocative maneuvers; 55 percent of these were abnormal bilaterally. In addition, abnormal flow patterns were recorded in 27 percent of the subjects for two of the three maneuvers. Specific results for each individual test revealed that Adson's test reduced the pulse amplitude in more than half of the sample, and the hyperabduction test occluded the blood flow in 10 percent of the sample.[19] This prevalence of false-positive results for provocative maneuver testing of 160 normal individuals was also reported by Pisko-Dubienski and Hollingsworth.[18] These investigators used a Doppler to document alterations in blood flow and the onset of symptoms during performance of the costo-clavicular and hyperabduction tests, Adson's maneuver, and a position of 90° of shoulder abduction.[19]

Occlusion of the subclavian artery with hyperabduction of the arm over-head was shown to be a frequent phenomenon, occurring in varying degree in a sample of 150 normal subjects.[25] Wright found that for positions from neutral to directly overhead, the radial pulse obliterated bilaterally 80 percent of the time in 125 of these normal subjects. These results were obtained provided the head was held in midline or the cervical spine was flexed; however, if the head was rotated or hyperextended to stretch the anterior scalene, the frequency of obliteration was increased. Furthermore, when the provoking position was held for at least an additional 2 minutes, neurologic symptoms were elicited.[25]

Because the validity of these maneuvers is questionable, it behooves the reader to use these tests with this in mind. After provocative maneuver testing of more than 160 asymptomatic undergraduate physical therapy students, I found that it is not unusual to tally approximately 50 percent of the students as responding positively to at least one of the provocative maneuvers! The test that has consistently produced the most false-positive results in these students is the hyperabduction maneuver, followed closely by Adson's test.

The previous information illustrates the frequency of false-positives re-sponses for the provocative maneuvers in a population of normal subjects. At this point, the reader should ask, "What does a positive response to a pro-vocative maneuver in TIS patients signify?" If both symptomatic and asymp-tomatic individuals test positively to these maneuvers, what is the validity of these tests? Taking this question one step further, is there predictive value to these provocative maneuvers? Can a relationship be established between the results of these provocative maneuver tests in TIS patients before and after surgical removal of the offending structure or physical therapy? Do the pre-viously positive tests then become negative? Can a relationship be established between a TIS patient's clinical status and his provocative maneuver tests before and after surgical or physical therapy? The reports by several investi-gators who have documented preoperative and postoperative information for both the patient's clinical status and response to provocative maneuver findings may help to answer these questions. Of 29 TIS patients, Sanders et al.[26] found that all were symptomatic but that only 13 had abnormal preoperative PPG tracings. Following surgery, eight of these 13 patients were reexamined and half of these, despite the fact that they reported relief of symptoms, continued to demonstrate abnormal PPG tracings.[26] In another report, a high percentage of 47 preoperative TIS patients had changes in blood flow as shown by Doppler monitoring for the costoclavicular, hyperabduction, Adson's maneuver, and 90° of shoulder abduction. Postoperatively, none of the patients had residual symptoms despite the fact that five patients still demonstrated minor flow disturbances.[18] Although the results from both of these studies might lead one to conclude that there is no relationship between clinical status and provocative maneuver testing, perhaps the following should be taken into consideration. In these reports, all patients had relief of their symptoms postsurgically. Ninety percent of all TIS patients have neurologic complaints and only 10 percent are known to have vascular symptoms. Because both Sanders and colleagues[26] and Pisko-Dubienski and Hollingsworth[18] noted that the patients' symptoms were relieved, perhaps (1) their complaint was primarily neurologic and was adequately relieved with surgery, since neither group noted the onset of symptoms with postsurgical maneuver testing; and (2) the positive vascular response may have occurred because a large number of individuals normally respond with false-positive results to these tests.

On the other hand, 45 TIS patients were studied with Doppler by Stanton and coworkers, who found that 44 of these patients had positive provocative maneuver responses before surgery.[27] After surgical intervention, only two of the patients' tests remained abnormal, although eight patients still complained of residual and recurrent symptoms.[27] Based on the available information, I believe that there is not enough evidence to come to a conclusion concerning the relationship between a TIS patient's clinical status and his response to provocative maneuver testing.

Motor Nerve Conduction Velocity Studies

Most TIS patients present with neurologic complaints as opposed to the few with strictly vascular symptoms. Many of the symptoms of TIS are also associated with other compression neuropathies of the upper extremity; therefore, motor nerve conduction velocities (MNCVs) are often used to localize the site of compression.[11] The conduction velocity of the ulnar nerve (UNVC) is reported most frequently by investigators who use this test extensively with the TIS patient. This is in keeping with the neurologic symptom pattern outlined by Roos[16] for compression of the lower roots of the brachial plexus. Although many researchers obtain MNCVs in these patients, the information from the test result is often used in very different ways. For instance, Urschel and Razzuk[17] use the velocity of conduction as criteria of whether to operate. This decision was based on a comparison of the clinical status of 79 patients with the patients' preoperative and postoperative UNCVs. Urschel and Razzuk found that the patients who had total relief following surgery also had a presurgical UNCV of less than 60 m/sec as compared with those patients who continued to complain of residual or no change in their symptoms who had an initial UNCV of greater than 60 m/sec. Although a normal UNCV from Erb's point is considered by Urschel and Razzuk to be 70 m/sec, patients with an

Table 7-2. Comparison of Normal Ulnar Nerve Conduction Velocities for Erb's Segment and Measurement Technique

Reference	Measurement Technique	Velocity
London[28]	Calipers	58.9 ± 4.2
Cherington[52]	?[a]	59.0
Daube[53]	?[a]	60.0 ± 5.4
Jebsen[29]	Calipers	61.3 ± 5.4
London[28]	Steel tape	70.2 ± 5.02
McGough et al.[13]	?[a]	70.0
Urschel and Razzuk[17]	?[a]	70.0
Caldwell et al.[12]	Steel tape	72.0

[a] Unknown.
Velocity measured in meters per second.

initial UNCV of more than 60 m/sec are now referred to physical therapy instead of to surgery. On the other hand, the results of MNCV studies are used by others as just one of the many pieces of the diagnostic puzzle. Caldwell and coworkers[12] suggest that to allow MNCV results to dictate the course of management for these patients is a mistake. They recommend that additional evidence be obtained (such as positive electromyographic studies, documentation of sensory loss, and positive provocative maneuvers) before the course of management is decided.

One possible source that may create this apparent disagreement concerning the exact usefulness of conduction velocity studies with TIS is the variability in normal UNCV for Erb's point. Urschel and Razzuk consider 70 m/sec a normal value for this segment. Table 7-2 shows that there is no universal agreement as to what normal value is. The range of UNCV for Erb's point varies from 58.9 m/sec[28] to 72.2 m/sec.[12]

Numerous explanations have been given for the variation in this conduction value. These include (1) different tools such as steel tape are used rather than calipers to measure the distance between the point of supramaximal stimulation and the area under investigation,[28] (2) failure to maintain the ambient temperature constant can produce a difference of 2.4 m/sec for each degree centigrade,[29] and (3) each individual's own MNCVs are known to vary on a day-to-day basis.[30] Because of these inconsistencies, many use standard MNCVs as a guide and establish the normal value for the segment under study for their particular center. London[28] suggested that the subject's contralateral MNCV could be used as the "control" for normal to compare velocities on an individual basis.

Obviously, the diagnosis of TIS is not made any easier by the use of electrophysiologic studies. Jaeger et al.[24] have pointed out that some of the seemingly contradictory results of UNCV may be explained by the fact that Erb's point is the most proximal point of the lower trunk being stimulated. These investigators suggest that the portion of the lower trunk not currently studied is the point where the nerve crosses over the first rib. To assess the entire length of the lower trunk thoroughly, they described the technique of C8 root stimulation. These authors also addressed the importance of reproducing the patient's chief complaint with this technique. Instead of placing the patient in the standard position with the affected upper extremity slightly abducted from the body, various positions are used to provoke the patient's symptoms.

Most of these patients have sensory symptoms (i.e., pain and paresthesia), not motor dysfunction. Evoked somatosensory potential testing has recently been used by several groups for evaluation of the sensory fibers.[31] It is still too early to determine whether evoked somatosensory testing is worthwhile, since data are still being collected. Although not every therapist has such so-phisticated equipment, sensory and sympathetic testing is readily available and is worth including in the evaluation of the TIS patient. I have found that while most of these patients show very little motor involvement, abnormalities appear on sensory and sympathetic tests.

Summary of Special Tests

This section has only scratched the surface of tests available to the physical therapist in the evaluation of TIS; I hope, however, that I have made it very clear why there is no universally agreed-on diagnostic protocol for this syn-drome. A fundamental evaluation scheme for the physical therapist that may be of assistance in establishing which of these tests are useful is presented later in this chapter.

To summarize the discussion regarding the special tests, first, provocative maneuvers are commonly used to diagnose TIS. However, when using them, the therapist must remember that specific positions were originally described for each maneuver. Any modification may change the test's intended purpose. Second, Adson's, Wright's, and the hyperabduction tests were all designed to evaluate the effect of position change of the upper extremity on the blood flow to the limb; however, only 5 to 10 percent of all TIS cases have vascular involvement. Third, although many TIS patients respond positively to the ma-neuvers, many asymptomatic normal persons also respond positively. There-fore, a positive test does not necessarily indicate TIS; other factors should be taken into consideration. Fourth, the relationship between the patient's clinical status and the response to provocative maneuver testing is still uncertain. Last, methods such as Doppler ultrasound and photoplethysmography are often used in place of palpation during provocative maneuver testing with some advan-tages. However, there is no evidence to support the use of instrumentation over palpation.

Because 90 percent of all TIS patients have neurologic complaints, many authorities believe that the site of compression can be better localized with nerve conduction studies. The information obtained from MNCVs was used in various ways by different researchers. Urschel and Razzuk[17] establish the diagnosis and select the course of treatment based on conduction velocity. Others use the information as a mechanism of differential diagnosis.[2,5,12,32]

In addition, what is considered a normal conduction velocity for the segment from Erb's point distally is widely variable, and multiple factors have been cited for the discrepancy. As in provocative maneuver testing, no relationship has been confirmed between the patient's clinical status and the conduction velocity of the nerve.

CONSERVATIVE MANAGEMENT OF THORACIC INLET SYNDROME

Historic Perspective: The Role of the Physical Therapist

In the literature, and perhaps in personal experience, the physical therapist will encounter varied opinions regarding the role of physical therapy in the treatment of TIS. The therapist's role as described in one well-known protocol has been to instruct the patient in a standardized set of exercises. The exercises were carried out for a 2- or 3-week period, unless the patient's symptoms worsened.[2,32] All patients were instructed by the therapist in shoulder girdle elevation and stabilization exercises, flexibility exercises for the chest and cervical musculature, and controlled breathing routines. If no symptomatic relief was obtained by the end of the trial exercise period, an additional 1 to 3 weeks of cervical traction was ordered to rule out cervical disc or nerve root involvement.[2,32]

The therapist may also encounter those who believe that specific structures are responsible for the patient's symptoms, and that surgery—not therapy—is preferred as the ultimate treatment. According to Roos,[3] the results of formal physical therapy in the management of TIS are often disappointing except for patients with mild to moderate symptoms. Roos believes that those who experience severe neurologic symptoms have anomalous fibromuscular bands or irregularities of the anterior scalene that irritate the plexus. He also believes that for these patients to feel better, those structures must be surgically removed. In Roos's experience, exercise, transcutaneous electrical nerve stimulation, and biofeedback only aggravate the symptoms to make the patient worse. Physical therapy involvement in the treatment of this physician's patients is limited to the use of heat and massage to reduce the severity of the symptoms for patients awaiting surgery, and for postural exercises in those patients with mild to moderate symptoms.[3,16,33]

Until recently, the role of the physical therapist has been either one of instituting a prescribed exercise protocol or of providing comfort for the patient awaiting surgery. However, over the last decade, many physicians have elected to postpone surgical intervention in favor of a more exhaustive trial of conservative management.[5,13] McGough et al.[13] extended medical management for as long as 2 years before surgical intervention. As a result, 90 percent of their 1,200 patients were successfully relieved without surgery. In addition, these investigators also reported a higher success rate for those patients who ultimately required surgery.

The rise in popularity to exhaust conservative treatment before surgical intervention affords the physical therapist the opportunity to redefine the role of physical therapy in the management of the TIS patient. The door is open for the therapist to use specialized upper quarter musculoskeletal evaluation skills to localize the patient's problem. The therapist can then consult with the physician on these findings and together they can develop treatment tailored to the patient's needs instead of using treatment dictated by standard protocol. Perhaps in time, the results of treatment tailored to a patient's requirements will be reflected in a consistently high percentage of successful outcomes rather than the 50 to 90 percent success now anticipated from physical therapy management.

Philosophy of Physical Therapy Management

Unlike the surgical literature, which is flooded with possible etiologies for this syndrome, those who conservatively manage TIS patients contend that faulty posture of the cervicothoracic spine and shoulder girdle provokes the patient's symptoms. According to many researchers, this altered posture places the brachial plexus and subclavian vessels in a position that makes them more vulnerable to being stretched, compressed, and rubbed by surrounding structures.[34–40] Although it is unknown whether faulty posture is the cause or the effect, the observation has been made that the symptoms of TIS correspond to a loss of muscular support and/or increased muscular tautness in the cervicothoracic and shoulder girdle region.[1,13,34–40]

Those who suggest that postural deviations contribute to the symptoms of TIS question whether a bony structure, such as a cervical or thoracic rib, should be held totally at fault for the symptoms, especially considering the fact that most individuals have first thoracic ribs and are asymptomatic, while others have bony abnormalities and never manifest any of the symptoms of TIS. For example, cervical ribs occur in approximately 0.5 percent of the population; of those, only 5 to 10 percent ever become symptomatic.[22] Admittedly, when a cervical rib is identified in a symptomatic person, it has become common practice to implicate the rib as the cause and to excise it. However, several investigators have reported that postural correction has relieved the symptoms of some of these patients even though they have cervical ribs. Peet et al. included both patients with positive and patients with negative cervical radiographs in their treatment regime directed at postural correction. After an intensive program of strengthening and flexibility exercises, these researchers concluded that all of the patients, regardless of x-ray findings, had the same 70 percent chance of achieving relief from their symptoms.[1] Similarly, Haggart reported successful treatment results for a single case study involving a patient with a cervical rib who had followed a program of strengthening for the muscles of the shoulder girdle.[37]

Perhaps, for some patients, it is imperative that a muscle be excised and/or the first thoracic rib removed before they experience symptomatic relief. However, some patients have undergone surgery, and have had recurrence of their symptoms within a short time. Sanders et al. reported recurrence of symptoms in 17 percent of the 239 scalenectomy patients and in 16 percent of the 214 patients who had excision of the first rib.[26] Recurrence of the patient's symptoms following removal of anatomic structures seems puzzling unless something other than the structure created the original symptoms.

The best argument in favor of the hypothesis of faulty posture is the fact that treatment programs for correction of upper quarter posture have successfully relieved the symptoms in 50 to 90 percent of all TIS patients. Therefore, the remainder of this chapter addresses physical therapy evaluation and treatment of the TIS patient.

PHYSICAL THERAPY EVALUATION OF THE THORACIC INLET SYNDROME PATIENT

According to Roos, "thoracic outlet syndrome is a clinical diagnosis that depends on a careful history and physical examination."[16]

Patient History

Generally, the patient with TIS may initially have what appears to be an overwhelming problem. However, if time is set aside at first presentation for a well-organized interview, the acquired information will be an invaluable guide for structuring the treatment plan. The interview will not reveal whether the patient has TIS, but the list of probable diagnoses will be narrowed and the physical examination will be expedited. The first rule of thumb when working with these patients is to not underestimate the importance of the patient interview!

Any interview format for questioning patients with upper quarter dysfunction may be used; however, it is best to choose one with which you are comfortable. I have found that a few key questions are useful when working with TIS patients. The interviewer should not be overly concerned if patients cannot recall an incident or accident that may be responsible for their current condition. Insidious onset of the symptoms of TIS is well documented. I have also found that some persons have conditions generally not considered trauma per se, such as a recent gain in weight and pregnancy. After careful questioning, the weight gain and pregnancy has proved to correspond to the onset of symptoms. Very often, not the pregnancy itself but the effect of carrying an infant or toddler was identified with the onset of symptoms. Similarly, a change in job or increased work load may also justify further investigation, since eventually this may provoke conditions that will need to be addressed and corrected.

Ninety percent of all TIS patients complain of pain, paresthesia, and paresis. Frequently, the patient will have pain or paresthesia as the primary complaint. If so, the patient should be asked to sketch on a body diagram the exact

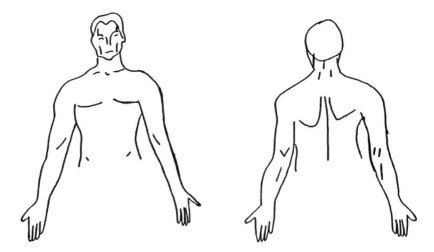

Fig. 7-6.　Patient sketches location of symptoms on body diagram.

location of the pain/numbness and to highlight the areas that are the worst (Fig. 7-6). Roos found that patients with nerve involvement of the upper plexus (i.e., C5–C7) report pain on the side of the neck that may radiate to the face, cranium, and anterior chest, over the scapula, and along the lateral aspect of the forearm into the hand (Fig. 7-1). Headaches and numbness of these areas are also commonly associated with an upper plexus problem.[16] According to Roos, patients with nerve involvement of the lower plexus, i.e., C8 and T1, report that the distribution of pain and numbness includes the suprascapular region, posterior neck and shoulder, and medial aspect of the arm and forearm and ulnar digits of the hand. In addition, both upper and lower plexus patients complain that the upper extremity and hand feel weak, tired, heavy, and cold[16] (Fig. 7-1).

It is important that the therapist find out if the patient's symptoms are predictable, that is, what aggravates the symptoms and what relieves or lessens them. Usually, I have found that most patients, if guided, can relate a change in their symptoms to an activity or particular posture. Upper plexus involvement may be indicated if the patient states that certain movements of the head or lifting produces their symptoms.[16] Involvement of the lower nerves of the plexus should be considered if the patient lists activities that depress the shoulder girdle, such as lifting, elevating the arm to drive, or styling the hair.[16] I have found that information pertaining to activities that produce the symptoms (i.e., upper versus lower plexus) coupled with the body diagram of the symptom pattern are important clues in localizing the area of the upper quarter to be initially examined.

Any additional questions related to past medical history such as previous cervical, thoracic, shoulder, or hand problems that display similar symptoms should be explored. Carpal tunnel syndrome and cervical disc and nerve root involvement can have the same pattern of involvement as TIS.

Physical Examination

Because multiple systems may be involved in TIS, the therapist must establish a systematic plan for evaluation. I have found it effective to organize the physical examination into two sections. The first section, a general upper quarter screen, should be done to rule out cervical disc and nerve root compression, shoulder dysfunction, and peripheral neuropathies. If this information is negative, the following six-part format should be used to localize the patient's problem (Fig. 7-7).

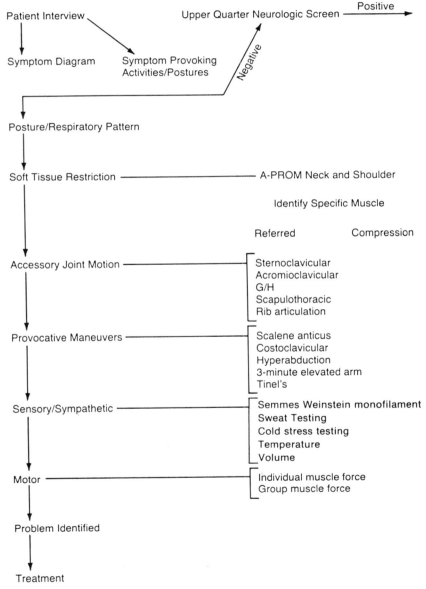

Fig. 7-7.   Scheme for physical therapy evaluation of TIS.

1. Upper quarter posture and respiratory pattern should be noted.
2. Active and passive motions of the head and shoulder should be observed to identify any restrictions, particularly those movements that reproduce the patient's symptoms. Based on these findings, individual muscles should then be checked for changes in length that might contribute to compression of the neurovascular structures or that might be the source of referred pain.
3. The amount of bony restriction should be assessed by accessory motion testing of the shoulder girdle, the cervical and thoracic spine, and the thoracic rib articulations.
4. The patient's response to the provocative maneuvers for TIS as classically described should be checked and a permanent record kept of these responses.
5. If the patient complains of pain and paresthesias, the extent of sensory and sympathetic involvement of the upper extremity and hand should be evaluated and documented.
6. If the patient complains of muscle weakness and fatigue, the amount of force that individual muscles and groups of muscles can generate should be measured by manual muscle testing or dynamometer analysis.

Postural Examination

Classically, faulty posture has been implicated as the cause for TIS. If posture is truly at fault, then evaluation of the patient's posture is required. The patient should be observed from all views, and any postural deviations and accessory breathing patterns noted. It is not uncommon to find insignificant postural deviations coexisting with those that are pertinent to the patient's problem. To determine which postural observations take priority, the examiner should compare the postural information with the patient's list of symptom-provoking posture/activities and the symptoms sketched by the patient on the body diagram. For example, if the patient listed postures/activities that required movement of the head or lifting, and the symptom diagram resembled an upper plexus symptom pattern (Fig. 7-1), I would focus first on those postural faults found in the cervical region. There is much documentation to show that many of the symptoms reported by these patients are a result of a shortened anterior scalene, which creates compression on the neurovascular bundle.[14,22,38,40] Often, the first clue to a unilaterally shortened anterior scalene can be found through postural examination. From the anterior view, involvement of this muscle is evidenced by the position of the head in lateral flexion toward the affected side and rotation toward the contralateral side. From the lateral perspective, shortening of the anterior scalene is noted by an increase in cervical lordosis.

Depending on the severity of the patient's symptoms, the ipsilateral sternocleidomastoid and upper trapezius may also contribute to these postural deviations. Generally, involvement of these muscles is in response to the scalene dysfunction. Spasm of the sternocleidomastoid is most notable and readily seen from the anterior view of the patient. If the upper trapezius is involved, the slope of the shoulder will be affected and the height of the scapula will be elevated. These patients may also breathe using the accessory muscle rather than diaphragmatic respiratory patterns.

Postural deviations involving the shoulder, chest, and scapulothoracic regions should be considered if the patient's body diagram resembles the pattern for lower plexus involvement (Fig. 7-1) and elevation of the arm is listed as a symptom-provoking activity. Narrowing of the costoclavicular space and shortening of the pectoralis minor have frequently been implicated in compression of the plexus and subclavian vessels in cases of TIS.[25,39] Common postural deviations are forwardly placed and abducted shoulders and accentuation of the thoracic curvature, which is suggestive of shortened pectoral and medial shoulder rotator muscles.[42] The affected shoulder may also be depressed, increasing the slope of the shoulder, as observed from anterior or posterior views of the patient.

If the patient's body diagram sketch does not match the upper and lower symptoms pattern of Roos[16] and/or the activities that aggravate the symptoms do not correspond, the patient may possibly have components of both upper and lower plexus involvement. Total involvement of both cervical and anterior chest and scapulothoracic musculature is not uncommon. Under these circumstances, the examiner should evaluate possible causes of the observed postural deviations (see Ch. 4 for further discussion of posture and the shoulder).

Evaluation of Soft Tissue Restrictions

The next step of examination is to locate the muscle(s) that may be responsible for producing the patient's symptoms, a task made easier because the list of contributing postural deviations has already been narrowed during the postural examination. For example, if the postural examination provided evidence that the scalene anticus and medius were shortened, the next steps should be (1) to measure the amount of active motion these muscles will permit without provoking symptoms and (2) to note whether the addition of a passive stretch at the end of range aggravated the patient's symptoms. Because these scalene anticus and medius muscles affect three planes of cervical motion, goniometric measurements should be taken of (1) cervical extension, (2) lateral flexion of the head toward the contralateral side, and (3) rotation of the head toward the affected side.

The postural examination may provide the only clue that the pectoralis minor is shortened. In such cases, shoulder range of motion (ROM) is generally not affected by a shortened pectoralis minor. The muscle's length should be assessed by having the patient lie supine on a firm surface. If the muscle is of normal length, the posterior aspect of the shoulder will lie in contact with the surface of the table. However, if the muscle is shortened, the shoulder will be in a forward position because the coracoid process of the scapula is being pulled downward anteriorly.[40] Once again, the assumption should not be made that this soft tissue restriction is responsible for the patient's symptoms unless the patient's symptoms are reproduced. Frequently, a passive stretch to the muscle will be necessary to elicit the symptoms. Passive stretching of the pectoralis minor can be done by pushing the posterior aspect of the shoulder against the surface of the table while the patient is supine.

It is important that the reader understand how the previous examples were used to illustrate the importance of the first steps of the TIS evaluation scheme (Fig. 7-7). Knowledge of where and when the patient hurts is established during the initial interview. Next, general postural deviations and how the patient moved were observed and recorded. Based on the information from the postural examination, the length of individual muscles was evaluated and reproduction of the patient's symptoms was attempted. Whenever possible, active and passive ROM measurements should be obtained for later assessment of treatment effectiveness.

The importance of evaluating for soft tissue restriction is twofold: first, to locate the muscle that restricts the motion and, second, to identify whether the muscle is responsible for compression of the neurovascular structures or referral of the pain. Reproducing the symptoms by compression of the brachial plexus and subclavian vessels is well established and falls under the traditional classification of TIS. Similar upper extremity symptoms have also been documented in shortened skeletal muscle and fascia containing myofascial trigger points. This phenomenon has been called referred pain or myofascial dysfunction.[41–43] Travell and Simons,[41] Cyriax,[42] and Gorrell[43] have found that the pain that results from compression of myofascial trigger points located in the upper quarter is referred to the thorax, upper extremity, and hand in predictable patterns. Although several investigators have reported points of muscle tenderness or irritability in TIS and cervicobrachial syndrome patients,[8,16] the theory of myofascial pain has not been adequately explored in TIS patients. It has been my experience that many symptoms of TIS patients are not always the result of direct compression of the plexus and subclavian vessels. Instead, careful examination of a specific muscle reveals irritable points within it and, if the points are compressed by fingertip pressure, forceful contraction, or a passive stretch, the patient will experience the "symptoms of TIS." I have found muscles that regularly contain myofascial trigger points in some patients with upper plexus symptom patterns to be the scalenes, levator scapula, subclavius, and the clavicular portion of the pectoralis major. Other muscles found with less frequency include the sternocleidomastoid, infraspinatus, and multifidus (Table 7-3). In some patients with typical lower plexus symptom patterns, I have found myofascial trigger points in the pectoralis minor and the intermediate portion of the pectoralis major. Muscles that produce referral of the lower plexus symptom pattern, but which I have found with less frequency, include the upper trapezius, medial head of the triceps, and subscapularis (Table 7-3).

Reproduction of the patient's pain by way of muscular compression of the neurovascular structures may only require the patient to actively stretch the muscle from its origin to insertion. However, the patient often will be limited by pain and therefore will not be able to stretch the involved muscle adequately or maintain the stretch long enough to reproduce the symptoms. For this rea-

Table 7-3. Muscles That Refer Myofascial Pain to Mimic Thoracic Inlet Syndrome Upper and Lower PLexus Symptom Patterns

Upper Plexus	Lower Plexus
Scalene anticus	Pectoralis minor
Subclavius	Sternal fibers pectoralis major
Levator scapulae	Upper trapezius
Clavicular section pectoralis major	Triceps medial head
Sternocleidomastoid	Subscapularis
Infraspinatus	Pectoralis minor[a]
Multifidus	
Scalene anticus[a]	
Scalene medius[a]	
Subclavius[a]	

[a] Muscles classically implicated in compression of the brachial plexus and subclavian vessels, which results in upper and lower plexus symptom patterns.

son, the examiner may need to passively stretch and maintain the muscle in a lengthened position to elicit the patient's complaints (Table 7-3). If this does not produce the symptoms, the muscle should then be checked for myofascial trigger points. First, the examiner should palpate over the muscle to localize an area within the muscle or its fascia. Generally, all that the examiner need do to reproduce the symptoms (if this is a myofascial trigger point) is to apply and maintain a compressive force by fingertip pressure over the hyperirritable point. If palpation is not successful, an alternative method of trigger point localization is to have the patient forcefully contract the muscle (i.e., shorten it and maintain it until the symptoms are elicited).[41] Further discussion of trigger point evaluation may be found in Chapter 12.

Because I have seen TIS patients whose symptoms were secondary to neurovascular compression by a shortened muscle as well as referred pain from myofascial trigger points, the reader may want to become familiar with both methods of evaluation and treatment.

Muscles to Examine for Shortening and Myofascial Trigger Points in TIS Patients with Upper Plexus Involvement (Table 7-3)

Anterior Scalene

Shortening of the scalene musculature can entrap the brachial plexus and subclavian vessel or refer pain from trigger points within the muscle itself and, depending on the severity of muscle involvement, both situations can occur.[41] Pain referred from a trigger point within the scalene will be experienced on the anterior and posterior aspects of the shoulder, lateral arm, and forearm, and distally into the radial side of the hand (Fig. 7-8). Pain resulting from nerve entrapment has been reported to follow a medial distribution or the C8–T1 dermatomal pattern as well as a lateral distribution or the C5–C6 dermatomal distribution.[41] To determine whether the pain is a result of active trigger points within the muscle, Travell and Simons suggest using the scalene cramp test. For this test, the subject rotates the head toward the side of pain and actively

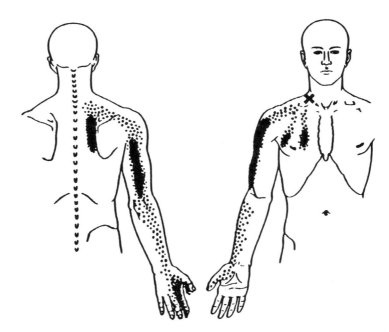

Fig. 7-8. Referred pain pattern for the right anterior scalene. (From Travell and Simons,[41] with permission.)

pulls the chin down toward the clavicle by flexion of the head. The trigger points will be aggravated by forced contraction of the muscle, and the pain will be referred.[41] If the subject is experiencing too much pain to perceive a change in pain with this test, these investigators suggest using the scalene-relief test to reduce the pressure of the clavicle against the muscle. To perform this test, the patient places the forearm against the forehead while raising and pulling the shoulder forward. If this position is held for several minutes, relief from the pain should occur.[41] The evaluation for compression of the plexus and subclavian vessels by the anterior scalene has been previously described in this chapter in the discussion of Adson's test.

Subclavius

I have found that the subclavius muscle is a frequent offender in this syndrome. This muscle can be stretched to compress the neurovascular structures when the examiner passively lifts the affected shoulder girdle cephalad while the subject forcefully exhales to lower the first rib.[44] The reader should note that this technique is different from the costoclavicular maneuver, which narrows the space between the first thoracic rib and the clavicle. The pattern of referred pain for the subclavius muscle includes the anterolateral aspect of the

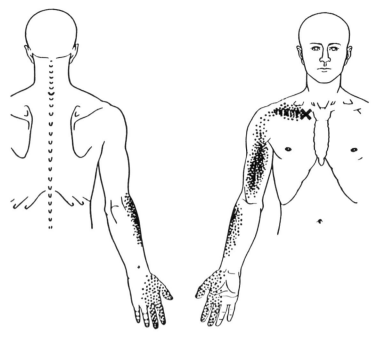

Fig. 7-9.   Referred pain pattern for the right subclavius. (From Travell and Simons,[41] with permission.)

shoulder, arm, and forearm, and both the dorsal and volar aspects of the thumb, index, and middle fingers[41] (Fig. 7-9). Myofascial trigger points within this muscle can be found by palpation of the muscle between its origin and insertion.

Levator Scapula

The neurovascular structures of the thoracic inlet cannot be compressed by the levator scapula, but I have found that it is likely to refer pain similar to a partial upper plexus pattern in TIS. The pattern of referral includes the posterior neck, shoulder, and the area between the scapulae (Fig. 7-10). This muscle, when shortened, will restrict rotation toward the affected side, neck flexion, and full abduction of the scapula.[41] Travell and Simons suggest that two trigger points may be found in this muscle by palpation along the lateral edge of the upper trapezius and the superior angle of the scapula.[41]

I have found that the clavicular portions of the pectoralis major, sterno-cleidomastoid, infraspinatus, and multifidus refer pain in a manner similar to upper plexus compression patterns. The reader may wish to consult reference 41, on myofascial pain.

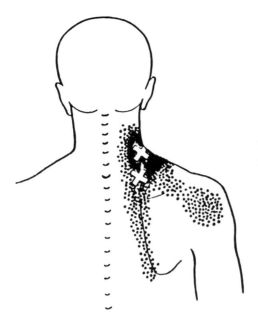

Fig. 7-10.   Referred pain pattern for the right levator scapulae. (From Travell and Simons,[41] with permission.)

Muscles to Examine for Shortening and Myofascial Trigger Points in TIS Patients with Lower Plexus Involvement (Table 7-3)

Pectoralis Minor

Stretching of the pectoralis minor to evaluate its role in compression of the neurovascular structures can be done in the following manner. The patient should be positioned supine with the affected arm supported and with the shoulder in adduction and medial rotation. The examiner should await the onset of symptoms while simultaneously flexing the adducted and medially rotated shoulder (to rotate the coracoid process upwardly) and while the subject forcefully exhales (to lower the ribs).

To locate myofascial trigger points within this muscle, the opposite procedure is described by Travell and Simons for compression of the pectoralis minor. The supine subject forcefully raises the affected shoulder off the table, keeping the arm relaxed and inhales. During this procedure, the examiner should palpate for irritable points within the now-exposed muscle. The pattern of referral from this muscle includes the anterior chest, medial aspect of the arm and forearm, and volar aspects of the ulnar three digits[41] (Fig. 7-11). These investigators believe that it is not uncommon to find associated trigger points in the pectoralis major, and I acknowledge this finding in TIS patients. The intermediate sternal fibers of the pectoralis major refer pain in the pattern that includes the anterior chest wall and typical C8–T1 dermatomal distribution noted by Roos.[16] To locate the trigger points, Travell and Simons suggest a pinching type of palpation of the muscle with the arm abducted to 90°.[41]

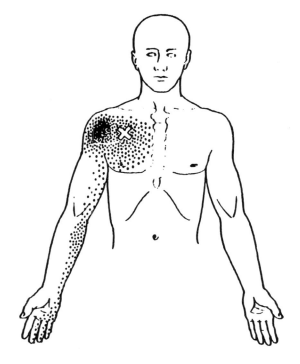

Fig. 7-11. Referred pain pattern for pectoralis minor muscle. (From Travell and Simons,[41] with permission.)

Additional muscles that may refer pain mimicking a lower plexus compression pattern in part include the upper trapezius, the medial head of the triceps, and the subscapularis.

Motion Testing for TIS

I refer the reader to a manual therapy treatment protocol described by Smith explicitly for management of the TIS patient.[45] Smith describes a seven-step protocol for increasing the mobility of the shoulder girdle and the first and second thoracic ribs. The protocol involves joint mobilization of the sternoclavicular and acromioclavicular joints, scapula, and thoracic ribs, and soft tissue stretching. The results of treatment are reported and support the effectiveness of this method of management. I have used some of Smith's treatment suggestions and have found that not all TIS patients require mobilization since they have only soft tissue restrictions; other patients are initially in such pain that mobilization is not tolerated. The fact that not all patients respond similarly emphasizes the point that a single standard treatment protocol for all patients is not always successful, and that treatment should be based on the findings of the physical examination and tailored accordingly.

Provocation Maneuver Examination

Review of the procedures and purposes of the scalene anticus, costoclav-icular, and hyperabduction tests can be found in the first sections of this chapter. Although the validity of these maneuvers is unknown, these tests continue to be frequently used in the diagnosis of TIS. I propose that provocative maneuvers remain a part of the physical therapist's examination scheme, not for the purpose of diagnosis, but as a means of establishing validity of these maneuvers. I suggest the following protocol:

1. Each maneuver is performed bilaterally in accordance with the classic description.
2. The patient's pulse is monitored and the response is defined as positive if there is a reduction in the quality of the pulse or cessation of the pulse, as negative if there has been no change in the pulse.
3. If symptoms are elicited, a record is made of the length of time required to reproduce these symptoms.
4. The above information is gathered on initial evaluation, during the course of therapy, and prior to discharge.

With this systematic approach, the examiner may be able to establish provocative maneuver validity and whether there is a relationship between the patient's clinical status and the patient's response to provocative maneuver testing (predictive validity).

Another provocative test described by several researchers is percussion or tapping along the pathway of the plexus from the superior thoracic outlet toward to axilla (Fig. 7-12). These researchers have found that percussion reveals areas of local tenderness in TIS patients.[13]

According to Kaplan's translation of the classic Tinel's sign, local pain produced by pressure applied to a nerve is a sign of nerve irritation. However, pressure on the nerve resulting in a tingling felt in the distribution of the nerve is a sign of axon regeneration.[46] In several TIS patients, I have noted that percussion of the nerve initially produces localized pain; however, as the patient's clinical status improves, the local pain response changes to the "radiating tingling" of nerve regeneration. The therapist may want to take note of the response to nerve percussion during the course of treatment in order to document whether a relationship between the nerve sign and the patient's clinical status exists.

Sensory and Sympathetic Evaluation

Paresthesia is a common complaint of the TIS patient. This symptom suggests sensory involvement, and should be documented so that the extent of involvement is known and the effectiveness of treatment recorded. Therapists can evaluate cutaneous sensation of the upper extremity with pressure-sensitive

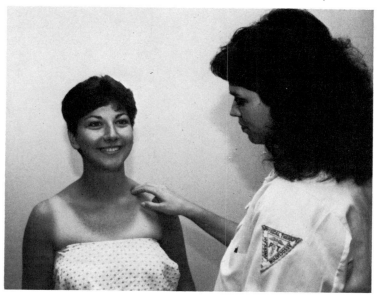

Fig. 7-12.　Percussion at the superior opening of the thorax for Tinel's sign.

monofilaments, known as Semmes Weinstein monofilaments (Fig. 7-13). These nylon filaments are calibrated so that when a specific amount of pressure is applied to the tip, it will bend, indicating that the filament's threshold has been reached. Twenty filaments ranging from 0.0045 to 447 g can be used to map out sensory threshold.[47] The scale of interpretation for this test has been developed for the palm of the hand, but it is possible to map out sensory thresholds for the entire upper extremity.

Gelberman and colleagues have investigated the value of using threshold and innervation density tests for sensibility testing of peripheral nerve compression syndromes. They have found the threshold tests, such as vibration and Semmes Weinstein monofilaments, to consistently reflect subtle and gradual decreases in nerve function before innervation density tests, such as static and moving two-point discrimination. In fact, the innervation density tests remained normal until sensory conduction had nearly ceased.[48]

Because 90 percent of all TIS patients complain of paresthesias of the upper extremity, I have started to use the monofilaments for TIS patients; the cutaneous sensation is mapped out for the involved extremity based on the area sketched by the patient on the body diagram. The threshold value obtained from testing the patient's uninvolved extremity is used as the norm (Fig. 7-12). Because these patients' complaints are more often sensory than motor, this easily administered noninvasive test may reveal more information than tests for motor nerve involvement. Another bonus of this test is that the patient may be tested in the symptom-producing posture.

If the patient reports swelling, blotchy skin, increased or decreased sweat-

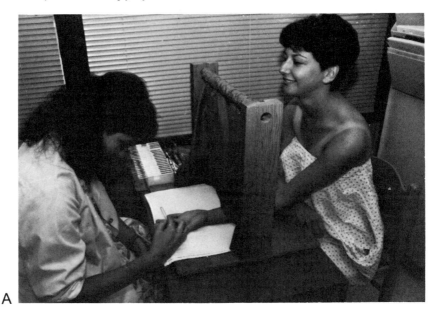

A

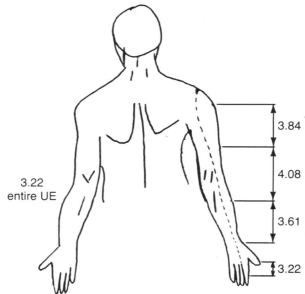

B

Fig. 7-13. (A) Evaluation of cutaneous sensibility with Semmes Weinstein monofilaments. (B) Monofilament mapping of upper extremity paresthesia. Right upper extremity, patient's affected side; left upper extremity, uninvolved side.

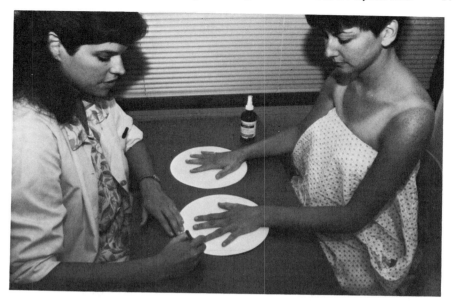

Fig. 7-14. Evaluation of sympathetic function with Ninhydrin sweat test.

ing of the hand, or a difference in hand temperature, involvement of the sympathetic nervous system is indicated. Because sweating and the diameter of blood vessels are controlled by the very thin sympathetic fibers that innervate them, these, too, can be involved in compression and myofascial dysfunction. Ninhydrin sweat testing[49] (Fig. 7-14), skin temperature mapping, volumetric and circumferential measurements, and cold recovery time[50] (Fig. 7-15) can all be used to evaluate sympathetic nervous system response.

PHYSICAL THERAPY TREATMENT OF THE TIS PATIENT

Treatment of the TIS patient is based solely on the information collected from the patient interview and physical examination. The purpose of this section is not to describe a "cookbook" protocol for the therapist to follow, but to illustrate how very different the physical therapy management of these patients can be. The traditional philosophy of conservative management of the TIS patient has been to correct the faulty posture. This philosophy appears to hold true whether the patient's pain is secondary to neurovascular compression or myofascial dysfunction.

To achieve improvement in the patient's situation, I have found that the patient must successfully complete three phases of treatment (Fig. 7-16). In the first phase, both the therapist and the patient must be able to demonstrate the ability to control the intensity of the symptoms. If the symptom is pain,

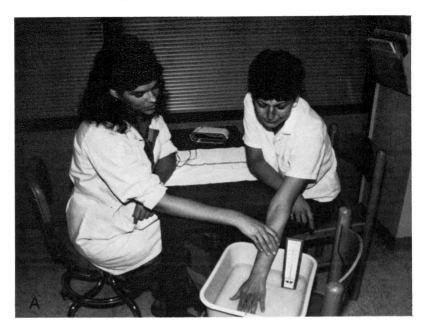

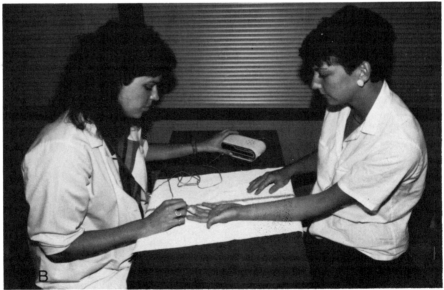

Fig. 7-15. Evaluation of cold recovery after (**A**) submerging hand in cold water bath and (**B**) monitoring of hand temperature before and after submersion with temperature thermistor.

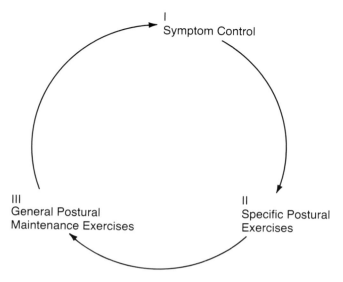

Fig. 7-16.   The three phases of physical therapy treatment for TIS.

there must be an understanding of *how* the intensity of the pain can be affected, and *what activity/posture* provokes the symptoms. Treatment in the symptom control phase may simply be management of trigger points in the muscle, use of heat/ice, or avoidance of symptom-producing tasks. Once the patient recognizes and understands that he has control over the symptoms, treatment can advance to the next phase. In the second phase, treatment is directed at specific exercises to change the symptom-producing musculoskeletal faults. Both the therapist and the patient must understand that the symptoms may be exacerbated during this phase of treatment. If both understand their limitations in control of the symptoms, as established in the first phase of treatment, exacerbation of symptoms should not be a problem. Once the symptoms are controlled and postural corrections are attained, the final phase of treatment is a postural maintenance program. This final phase consists of general postural exercises to maintain the patient in the asymptomatic status, which is extremely difficult considering the frequency of recurrence in this patient population.

There are no distinct dividing lines between the three phases of treatment. It is not at all uncommon for a patient in the second or third phase of treatment to report back to therapy with the original symptoms. In most cases, symptom recurrence is only temporary; however, to bring the symptoms back under control requires a return to the initial phase of treatment. The key to success in TIS is educating the patient so that he or she understands what is occurring and what intervention should be taken, and how to decide when to seek therapist assistance.

Throughout the remainder of this section, two clinical case studies will be used to illustrate key points of treatment. These cases are used only as examples and are by no means used to suggest that this is the only method of management. The first case illustrates management of myofascial dysfunction, and the second case describes management of neurovascular compression.

Case Study 1

J.K., a 39-year-old office manager/keypunch operator complained of pain between the scapulae radiating to the shoulder and down the lateral aspect of the arm, hypersensitivity along the lateral border of the forearm, and cold and numbness of the thumb and index finger (Fig. 7-17). She said that the forearm and hands symptoms were always present, but that the arm and scapular symptoms were dull aches in the morning that intensified to constant pain by the end of a full day of typing and desk work. Her self-rating of pain on examination was 3 on a scale of 10, but would reach as high as a 7 on bad days.

Pertinent clinical findings included reproduction of J.K.'s symptoms when fingertip pressure was applied to the right levator scapula, as well as with passive flexion of the head, stretching the levator scapulae. Reduction in the symptoms was achieved by the combination of passive extension and right rotation of the head. Semmes Weinstein monofilament testing along the lateral aspect of the upper extremity and hand demonstrated significant loss of sensation as compared with the contralateral extremity. Increased sympathetic function in the right hand in comparison to the left hand was also noted on sweat testing.

J.K. reported a pain rating of 0 and normalization of sensation after 10 treatments over a period of 20 days.

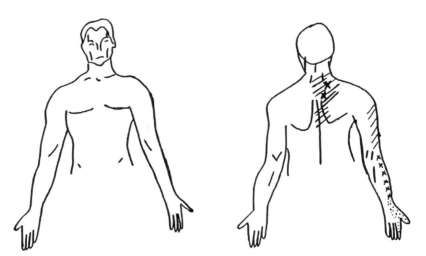

Fig. 7-17. Symptom pattern as described by J.K. in case study 1 (x, trigger point; ///, pain; **, hypersensitive; and :::, cold).

Case Study 2

L.M., a 28-year-old laborer, claimed that his symptoms were the result of operating a jackhammer 1½ years previously. His complaints included pain and swelling of the right anterior chest and right-sided neck pain that radiated across the shoulder and the lateral aspect of the arm and proximal third of the forearm (Fig. 7-18). At rest, L.M. rated his pain as 1 on a scale of 10; however, any use of the upper extremity or hand would elevate the pain to a rating of 7. This patient related that his symptoms were not any better following bilateral carpal tunnel releases, bilateral first thoracic rib resection, resection of the proximal one-third of the right clavicle, and a dozen right stellate ganglion blocks.

Pertinent physical findings included palpation tenderness of the right scalenes, sternocleidomastoid, upper trapezius, medial end of the clavicle, and clavectomy scars. Forced or deep inspiration was painful and lying supine was impossible. Cervical motion was restricted to 15° each of left lateral flexion, rotation, and extension. All planes of right shoulder active motion were restricted by two-thirds of the arc of full motion. Postural examination revealed abnormal forward flexion, right lateral flexion, right rotation of the head, and an elevated and abducted right shoulder.

Initial Phase of Treatment

Modalities have traditionally been used to provide pain relief and reduce muscle spasm during the initial phase of treatment of TIS. As early as 1919, Stopford and Telford described the successful use of faradic stimulation and

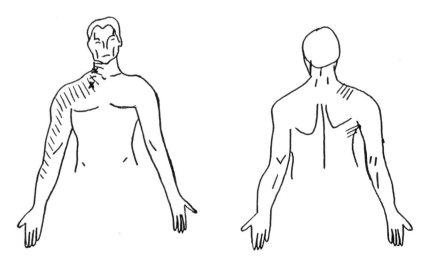

Fig. 7-18. Symptom pattern as described by L.M. in case study 2 (///, pain).

massage to relieve the symptoms caused by spasm of the upper trapezius.[34] To manage pain in this patient population, other therapists have included moist heat, infrared, ice, and massage as their first line of treatment.[1,13,35,38] I prefer the analgesia obtained after application of ice over an area of muscle tenderness. For example, the use of ice in myofascial dysfunction as in case study 1 anesthetized the levator scapula. This was crucial to the success of the first phase of treatment, because J.K. then felt that the pain was controllable. Once in control of the pain, she permitted the treatment that was necessary to begin deactivation of the myofascial trigger point.

In severely involved cases, such as that of L.M. in case study 2, the immediate treatment goal may be only to show the patient that the amount of pain he or she is experiencing can be temporarily reduced. The patient must have the feeling of being able to control the intensity of the symptoms experienced; adding passive stretch or vigorous massage may interfere with this objective.

During the initial phase when pain control is the priority, most investigators suggest that the patient avoid any activity or posture that will aggravate the symptoms.[1,13,24] The examiner should be well aware of these postures/activities, having obtained this information from the patient's initial interview and from reproduction of the patient's pain during physical examination. Because the objective of this phase of treatment is to control pain, part of the control will come from understanding what postures/activities elicit the pain. Therefore, to complete this phase, it is imperative that the therapist guide the patient so that he or she understands what postures/activities evoke their symptoms in order to avoid them. Unfortunately, many patients find that job-related activities produce their symptoms. In most cases, avoidance of work is not an acceptable solution; however, task modification is a feasible option. For example, in case study 1, typing from copy placed on the right side of the typewriter aggravated this patient's symptoms by compression of an active trigger point in the right levator scapula. Instead of avoiding all typing, the position of the copy was changed to one directly at eye level and in front of the patient. This position eliminated the need for the constant contraction of the right levator scapula, which contributed to this patient's symptoms.

For L.M., case study 2, merely the unsupported weight of the upper extremity depressed the shoulder girdle. Depression was then the stimulus for the right scalenes, sternocleidomastoid, and upper trapezius to contract continuously to elevate the shoulder girdle. To avoid continuous contraction of these muscles, which in turn compressed the upper plexus, L.M. made a conscious effort 24 hours a day to support the extremity passively. When seated, he placed the arm on a tabletop, chair armrest, or pillow. When standing, he found that the right arm could be cradled either by the left arm or by placing his hand in his pocket. Spurling and Grantham describe a position in which the hand is passively placed behind the head to relax the anterior scalene. According to these researchers, 300 of the 400 patients who avoided tension on the scalene were successfully managed.[35] Hansson used other passive methods of support, such as a sling, a figure eight wrap around the shoulders similar

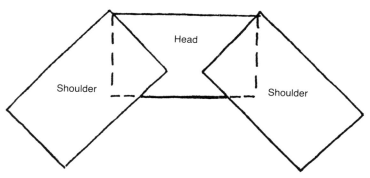

Fig. 7-19. Supine pillow arrangement for flexion of cervical spine, abduction of scapulae, and support of shoulders to relieve scalene anticus spasm. (From Reichert,[36] with permission.)

to a clavicular sling, or an airplane splint, to support the weight of the upper extremity.[51] For women with pendulous breasts, extra padding to increase the surface area of the shoulder straps or an underwire support brassiere to distribute the weight against the trunk rather than across the shoulders have been described.[13,24] Reichert suggested that these patients also required a change in their sleep habits, as positions assumed during sleep would continue to aggravate the anterior scalene. To prevent this, Reichert recommended strategic placement of three pillows, one pillow to support and slightly flex the cervical spine and the others to abduct the scapulae and provide support for each shoulder (Fig. 7-19). The combination of this resting posture and shoulder-shrugging exercises resulted in successful treatment in 60 of 74 patients.[36]

In the initial phase, the patient should learn that the symptoms can be controlled by therapeutic modalities and by avoidance of postures and activities that provoke the symptoms. It is not practical to advance to the second phase of care without this understanding and a conscious effort to control the symptoms. Success in the final phases of treatment will be less than optimal if this principle is not followed.

Second Phase of Treatment

Once the patient understands that it is possible to change the intensity of the symptoms and that he or she can demonstrate this control, treatment phase two should be initiated. The primary objective during this phase of management is correction of the previously identified musculoskeletal faults. In myofascial dysfunction, the muscle learns to avoid pain by shortening.[41] The levator scapula of J.K. in case study 1 was shortened, as evidenced by restricted forward flexion and left rotation of the head. Ice and stretch will quiet an active myofascial trigger point, but active exercise is necessary to maintain a full painfree

ROM of the muscle. To obtain full motion of the head, J.K. actively stretched the muscle to the point of discomfort, maintaining this position for 10 seconds. Initially, all planes of motion were stretched independently of one another; as she progressed, shoulder depression was combined with full forward flexion and left rotation of the head. Eventually, these exercises could be performed without the assistance of ice or heat.

During this phase of treatment, it is important that both the therapist and the patient realize that treatment will reproduce the patient's symptoms. This symptom reproduction will be the result of either compression of the active trigger point or compression of the shortened muscle against the neurovascular structures. I have found that it is beneficial for both the therapist and the patient to agree on the maximum level of discomfort that will be allowed during the course of each day's treatment. Thus, the patient maintains the feeling of control over the intensity of the pain. This concept worked well during L.M.'s second phase of care. Once he learned that the pain could be reduced to a level of 1 or 2 on a scale of 10 after treatment with application of heat, he began to tolerate a pain rating ranging from 4 to 6 during treatment.

When the number of musculoskeletal faults seem overwhelming, the examiner should approach treatment in a stepwise fashion and should not try to correct all postural deviations at once. Often, when one area is corrected, the other faults are self-correcting. Although L.M. had extensive shoulder, chest, and neck soft tissue restrictions, the initial treatment was directed only toward the limitations of cervical movement and then toward the shoulder. Because head movement was so restricted, active neck ROM exercises were pursued first in a progressive fashion. The first treatment objective of this phase was to move the head only to the point of discomfort. Several sessions later, movement was taken further into the range of discomfort; the final step was tolerance of more vigorous contract–relax techniques. During this phase, ice continued to precede active exercise, and heat or ultrasound for muscle relaxation followed exercise at the patient's request.

During this phase of treatment, the patient will begin to experience relief and will quite naturally want to pursue long-neglected tasks and activities. To avoid unnecessary setbacks caused by the overzealous patient who carries in a sack of groceries, rakes leaves, shovels snow, vacuums, or tackles a desk full of paper work, it is the therapist's task to frequently remind the patient to remain conscious of symptom-producing postures/activities. These reminders should also include guidelines for progressively increasing the patient's level of activity or to teach the patient how to modify the task altogether.

Final Phase of Treatment

The final phase of treatment should proceed once the patient demonstrates continued control of symptom intensity and the ability to correct the specific musculoskeletal faults without difficulty. The patient may not necessarily enter this final phase of treatment symptom free. It is not at all uncommon for residual

Table 7-4. General Postural Maintenance Exercises for TIS

Do each exercise ___ times each day.

1. Stand erect with the arms at the sides. (A) Bending the neck to the left, attempt to touch the left ear to the left shoulder without shrugging shoulder. (B) Bending the neck to the right, attempt to touch the right ear to the right shoulder without shrugging the shoulder. (C) Relax and repeat.

2. Stand facing the corner of the room with one hand on each wall, arms at shoulder level, palms forward, elbows bent, and abdominal muscles contracted. (A) Slowly let the upper part of the trunk lean forward and press the chest into the corner. Inhale as the body leans forward. Return to the original position by pushing out with the hands. Exhale with this movement.

3. Stand erect with the arms at the sides, holding in each hand a ___ pound weight. (A) Shrug the shoulders forward and upward. (B) Relax. (C) Shrug the shoulders backward and upward. (D) Relax. (E) Shrug the shoulders upward. (F) Relax and repeat.

4. Stand erect with the arms out straight from the sides at shoulder level; hold a ___ pound weight in each hand (palms should be down). (A) Raise the arms sideways and up until the backs of the hands meet above the head (keep elbows straight). (B) Relax and repeat.

5. Lie face down with right arm outstretched overhead with the head turned toward the left. (A) Raise the arm off the supporting surface. Hold this position for a count of three. Inhale as the arm is raised. (B) Exhale and return to original position. (C) Repeat. Do the same with the left arm with the head turned toward the right.

6. Lie on the back with arms at the sides, with a rolled towel or small pillow under the upper part of the back between the shoulder blades and no pillow under the head. (A) Inhale slowly and raise the arms upward and backward overhead. (B) Exhale and lower the arms to the sides. Repeat 5 to 20 times.

Clinician should add further exercise specific for patient's needs.

(Adapted from Peet et al.,[1] with permission.)

low-grade symptoms to persist. In some cases, these symptoms will gradually subside; other patients may have to learn to accommodate themselves to some residual symptoms.

Failure of conservative management to provide long-lasting relief for TIS patients is secondary to unsatisfactory completion of this phase of treatment. To maintain postural correction, the patient must not only continue to recognize activities/postures that will aggravate symptoms, but must also continue to perform generalized postural exercises to maintain symptom-free status.

The exercises outlined by Peet et al.[1] and later adapted by others[2,33] as the prescribed protocol for the treatment of TIS are quite satisfactory for the purpose of postural maintenance (Table 7-4). Exercises specific to the patient's particular needs should also supplement this program.

Occasionally, patients will not obtain relief from physical therapy management or will still have severe functional restrictions secondary to their symptoms. In those cases, if all means of conservative management have been exhausted, the patient's problem may not be one for the physical therapist to manage. If examination provided evidence of neurovascular compression, the therapist should not feel that all was lost, as the report of McGough et al. showed improved surgical success if the patient had exhausted long-term physical therapy management before a different type of treatment was considered.[13]

Summary of Physical Therapy Evaluation and Treatment

The traditional philosophy of those who conservatively manage the TIS patient is that postural faults are responsible for the symptoms. I suggest that development of a successful plan for management of the TIS patient is dependent on a carefully guided patient interview and a thorough physical examination. Physical examination for TIS should proceed only if the upper quarter neurologic screen yields negative information for cervical disc and nerve root compression, shoulder dysfunction, and peripheral neuropathies. I suggest a six-part format for examination of the TIS patient, to be supplemented with information obtained from the patient interview and symptom diagram. Included in this multipart evaluation format are (1) a generalized postural examination with attention to the pattern of respiration, (2) evaluation of soft tissue restriction with emphasis on evaluation for shortened muscles that might either compress the neurovascular structures or refer pain by myofascial dysfunction, (3) accessory motion testing, (4) a guideline for use of the classic TIS provocative maneuvers, (5) evaluation of upper extremity and hand sensation and sympathetic nervous system involvement, and (6) testing the force generated by individual muscles or groups of muscles.

Once the patient's problem is localized, treatment should follow in three phases. Two case studies have been provided to serve as examples of a method of management of TIS patients. The purpose of the first phase is to teach the patient how to bring the symptoms into control and to assist the patient in gaining awareness in avoiding postures/activities that evoke the symptoms. The second phase of treatment is directed at correction of specific symptom-producing postural faults; continued attention is paid to the goals of the initial phase. The primary purpose of the final phase of care is to prevent symptom recurrence by instructing the patient in generalized postural maintenance exercises to be carried out in addition to the exercises specific to the patient's musculoskeletal needs. I believe that this final phase of care is often neglected, which may account for the number of patients who do not achieve long-lasting relief following conservative management of TIS.

REFERENCES

1. Peet RM, Henriksen JD, Anderson TP, Martin GM: Thoracic outlet syndrome: evaluation of a therapeutic exercise program. Staff meetings, Mayo Clin 31:281, 1956
2. Kelly TR: Thoracic outlet syndrome: current concepts of treatment. Ann Surg 190:657, 1979
3. Roos DB: New concepts of thoracic outlet syndrome that explains etiology, symptoms, diagnosis and treatment. Vasc Surg 13:313, 1979
4. Crawford FA: Thoracic outlet syndrome. Surg Clin North Am 60:947, 1980
5. Dale WA: Thoracic outlet compression syndrome. Arch Surg 117:1437, 1982
6. Warwick R, Williams PL (eds): Gray's Anatomy. 35th British Ed. WB Saunders, Philadelphia, 1973

7. Gardner E, Gray DJ, O'Rahilly R: Anatomy: A Regional Study of Human Structure. 4th Ed. WB Saunders, Philadelphia, 1975
8. Johnson DA: Posture and cervicobrachial pain syndromes. JAMA 159:1507, 1955
9. Hadler NA: Medical Management of the Regional Musculoskeletal Diseases. Grune & Stratton, Orlando, FL, 1984
10. Williams HT, Carpenter NH: Surgical treatment of the thoracic outlet compression syndrome. Arch Surg 113:850, 1978
11. Urschel HC, Razzuk MA, Albers JE, et al: Reoperation for recurrent thoracic outlet syndrome. Ann Thorac Surg 21:19, 1979
12. Caldwell JW, Crane CR, Krusen EM: Nerve conduction studies: an aid in the diagnosis of thoracic outlet syndrome. South Med J 64:210, 1971
13. McGough EC, Pearce MB, Byrne JP: Management of thoracic outlet syndrome. J Thorac Cardiovasc Surg 77:169, 1979
14. Raff J: Surgery for cervical rib and scalenus anticus syndrome. JAMA 157:219, 1955
15. Judy KL, Heymann RL: Vascular complications of thoracic outlet syndrome. Am J Surg 123:521, 1972
16. Roos DB: The place for scalenectomy and first-rib resection in thoracic outlet syndrome. Surgery 92:1077, 1982
17. Urschel HC, Razzuk MA: Management of thoracic outlet syndrome. N Engl J Med 285:1140, 1972
18. Pisko-Dubienski ZA, Hollingsworth J: Clinical application of Doppler ultrasonography in the thoracic outlet syndrome. Can J Surg 21:145, 1978
19. Geroudis R, Barnes RW: Thoracic outlet arterial compression: prevalence in normal persons. Angiography 31:538, 1980
20. Coote H: Pressure on the axillary vessels and nerve by an exostosis from a cervical rib interference with the circulation of the arm. Removal of the rib and exostosis recovery. Med Times Gaz 11:108, 1861
21. Falconer MA, Weddell G: Costoclavicular compression of the subclavian artery and vein. Lancet 2:539, 1943
22. Adson AW, Coffey JR: Cervical rib. Ann Surg 85:839, 1927
23. Roos B: Congenital anomalies associated with thoracic outlet syndrome. Am J Surg 132:771, 1976
24. Jaeger SH, Read R, Smullens S, Breme P: Thoracic outlet syndrome: diagnosis and treatment. p. 378. In Hunter J, Mackin E, Bell J, Callahan A (eds): Rehabilitation of the Hand. CV Mosby, St. Louis, 1984
25. Wright IS: The neurovascular syndrome produced by hyperabduction of the arms. Am Heart J 29:1, 1945
26. Sanders RJ, Monsour JW, Gerber WF, et al: Scalenectomy versus first rib resection for the treatment of thoracic outlet syndrome. Surgery 85:109, 1978
27. Stanton PE, McClusky DA, Richardson HD, Lamis PA: Thoracic outlet syndrome: a comprehensive evaluation. South Med J 71:1070, 1978
28. London GW: Normal ulnar nerve conduction velocity across the thoracic outlet: comparison of two measuring techniques. J Neurol Neurosurg Psychol 38:756, 1975
29. Jebsen RH: Motor conduction velocities in the median and ulnar nerves. Arch Phys Med Rehabil 48:185, 1967
30. Honet JC, Jebsen RH, Perrin EB: Variability of nerve conduction velocity determinations in normal persons. Arch Phys Med Rehabil 49:650, 1968
31. Glover JL, Worth MD, Bendick PJ, et al: Evoked responses in the diagnosis of thoracic outlet syndrome. Surgery 89:86, 1980

32. Dale WA, Lewis MR: Management of thoracic outlet syndrome. Ann Surg 181:575, 1975
33. Roos DB: Experience with first rib resection for thoracic outlet syndrome. Ann Surg 173:429, 1971
34. Stopford JS, Telford ED: Compression of the lower trunk of the brachial plexus by a first dorsal rib. Br J Surg 7:168, 1919
35. Spurling RG, Grantham EG: The painful arm and shoulder with especial reference to the problem of scalene neurocirculatory compression. J Miss Med Assoc 38:340, 1941
36. Reichert FL: Compression of the brachial plexus: the scalene anticus syndrome. JAMA 118:294, 1942
37. Haggart GE: Value of conservative management of cervicobrachial pain. JAMA 137:508, 1948
38. McGowen JM, Velinsky M: Costoclavicular compression. Arch Surg 59:62, 1949
39. Raff J: Surgery for cervical rib and scalenus anticuus syndrome. JAMA 157:219, 1955
40. Kendall FP, McCreary EK: Muscle Testing and Function. 3rd Ed. Williams & Wilkins, Baltimore, 1983
41. Travell JG, Simons DG: Myofascial Pain and Dysfunction. Waverly Press, Baltimore, 1983
42. Cyriax J: Rheumatic headache. Br Med J 2:1367, 1938
43. Gorrell RL: Musculofascial pain. JAMA 142:557, 1950
44. Evjenth O, Hamberg J: The spinal column and the temporomandibular joint. Ch. 3. In Muscle Stretching in Manual Therapy. Vol. 2. Alfta Rehab Forlag, Sweden, 1984
45. Smith KF: The thoracic outlet syndrome: a protocol of treatment. J Orthop Sport Phys Ther 1:89, 1979
46. Kaplan EB: The "tingling" sign in peripheral nerve lesions. p. 8. In Spinner M (ed): Injuries to the Major Branches of Peripheral Nerves of the Forearm. 2nd Ed. WB Saunders, Philadelphia, 1978
47. von Frey M, Kiesow F: Uber die Function der Tastkorperchen Yeit. Psychol Physiol Sinnesory 20:126, 1899
48. Gelberman RH, Szabo RM, Williamson RV, Dimick M: Sensibility testing in peripheral-nerve compression syndromes. J Bone Joint Surg 65A:632, 1983
49. Moberg E: Objective methods for determining the functional value of sensibility in the hand. J Bone Joint Surg 40:454, 1958
50. Porter J, Snider R, Bardana E, et al: The diagnosis and treatment of Raynaud's phenomenon. Surgery 77:11, 1975
51. Hansson KG: Scalene anticus syndrome. Surg Clin North Am 22:611, 1942
52. Cherington M: Ulnar nerve conduction velocity in thoracic outlet syndrome. N Engl J Med 294:1185, 1976
53. Daube JR: Nerve conduction studies in thoracic outlet syndrome. Neurology 25:347, 1975 (abstr)

8 | Evaluation and Treatment of Brachial Plexus Lesions

Bruce H. Greenfield
Dorie B. Syen

The brachial plexus supplies both motor and sensory innervation to the upper extremities and related shoulder girdle structures. Lesions to the brachial plexus compromise the neurologic integrity and, hence, the function of the shoulder and related upper extremity. Evaluation of shoulder dysfunction should include an assessment of the integrity and functional status of the brachial plexus. The complex structure of the brachial plexus requires a thorough understanding of the multiple innervation patterns to the various muscles. An understanding of the mechanisms of injuries to the brachial plexus, pathophysiologic changes of nerve fibers and nerve roots, and potential for recovery is essential for proper and effective clinical management. Therefore, the following chapter provides a review of the anatomy of the brachial plexus, classification of brachial plexus injuries, description of pathomechanical and pathologic changes to the specific nerve fibers and nerve roots, and a review of a clarifying evaluation to assess the nature and extent of brachial plexus lesions. A clinical case study offers a combined physical and occupational therapy management of a patient with a brachial plexus injury.

ANATOMY OF THE BRACHIAL PLEXUS

The anatomy of the brachial plexus is divided into a review of the gross anatomy of the plexus and its relationship to surrounding structures, as well as a review of the microscopic anatomy of the nerve and nerve trunks.

191

Superficial Anatomy

The brachial plexus comprises the anterior primary divisions of spinal segments C5, C6, C7, C8, and T1, as shown in Figure 8-1. The components of the brachial plexus include the following:

1. Undivided anterior primary rami
2. Trunks—upper, middle, lower
3. Divisions of the trunks—anterior and posterior
4. Cords—lateral, posterior, and medial
5. Branches—peripheral nerves derived from the cords

The segmental motor innervation of the brachial plexus to the muscles of the shoulder is shown in Figure 8-2. The anatomy of the plexus has been pre-

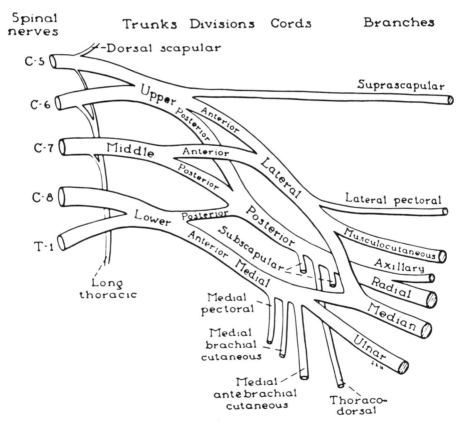

Fig. 8-1. Segmental motor innervation of the muscles of the shoulder. (From Hollinshead WH: Functional Anatomy of the Limbs and Back. 4th Ed. WB Saunders, Philadelphia, 1976, with permission.)

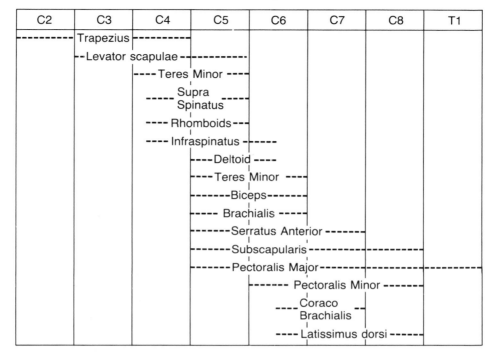

C2	C3	C4	C5	C6	C7	C8	T1

Fig. 8-2.   Additional segmental motor innervation of the muscles of the shoulder.

viously described.[1] The fourth cervical nerve usually gives a branch to the fifth cervical, and the first thoracic nerve frequently receives one from the second thoracic. When the branch from C4 is large, the branch from T2 is frequently absent and the branch from T1 is reduced in size. This constitutes the prefixed type of plexus. Conversely, when the branch from C4 is small or absent, the contribution of C5 is reduced in size, that of T1 is larger, and the branch from T2 is always present. This arrangement constitutes the post-fixed type of plexus.

The most typical arrangement of the brachial plexus is as follows: the fifth and sixth cervical nerves unite at the lateral border of the scalenus medius muscles to form the upper trunk of the plexus. The eighth cervical and first thoracic nerves unite behind the scalenus anterior to form the lower trunk of the plexus, while the seventh cervical nerve itself constitutes the middle trunk. These three trunks course downward and laterally and just above or behind the clavicle, each splitting into an anterior and a posterior division. The anterior division of the upper and middle trunks unite to form a cord, which is situated on the lateral side of the axillary artery and is called the lateral cord. The anterior division of the lower trunk passes downward, first behind and then on the medial side of the axillary artery, and forms the medial cord; this cord frequently receives fibers from the seventh cervical nerve. The posterior divisions of all three trunks unite to form the posterior cord, which is situated at first above and then behind the axillary artery.[1]

Autonomic sympathetic nerve fibers are present in all parts of the brachial plexus, consisting mostly of postganglionic fibers derived from the sympathetic ganglionated chain. The only preganglionic fibers in the brachial plexus are those of primary ramus T1.[1] Because the sympathetic supply to the eye travels through the T1 nerve root, the occurrence of Horner's syndrome, characterized by constriction of the pupil and ptosis of the eyelid on the involved side, in a patient who has sustained a traction injury is presumptive evidence of avulsion to that root.[2] Further discussion of Horner's syndrome follows in the section under Clarifying Evaluation.

Anatomic Relationships to the Brachial Plexus

The clinician should understand the relationship of the brachial plexus to the anatomic structures about the neck, shoulder girdle, and arms. To effectively isolate a plexus lesion, especially in the presence of open trauma, the clinician must identify the plexus and its relationship to the anatomic structures. For example, knowledge of the portion of plexus that lies between the clavicle and the first rib, in the presence of clavicular fracture, can help the clinician isolate the affected nerve and predict the affected muscles. Topographic relationships of the plexus are delineated in *Gray's Anatomy*.[1]

In the neck, the brachial plexus is situated in the posterior triangle, which is the angle between the clavicle and the lower posterior border of the sternocleidomastoid muscle. The plexus in this area is covered by skin, platysma, and deep fascia.

The plexus emerges between the scalenus anterior and scalenus medius muscles, passes behind the anterior convexity of the medial two-thirds of the clavicle, and lies on the first digitation of the serratus anterior and subscapularis muscles. In the axilla, the lateral and posterior cords of the plexus are on the lateral side of the axillary artery and the medial cord is behind the axillary artery. The cords surround the middle part of the axillary artery on three sides, the medial cord lying on the medial side, the posterior cord behind, and the lateral cord on the lateral side of the axillary artery. In the lower part of the axilla, the cord split into the nerves for the upper limb.

Anatomy of the Nerve Trunks

The nerve trunks and their branches are composed of parallel bundles of nerve fibers comprising the efferent and afferent axons and their ensheathing Schwann cells, which, in some cases, contain myelin sheaths.[1] The fibers are grouped together within trunks in a number of fasciculi, each of which contains from a few to many hundreds of nerve fibers. The architecture of the nerve trunk is shown in Figure 8-3. A dense irregular connective tissue sheath, the

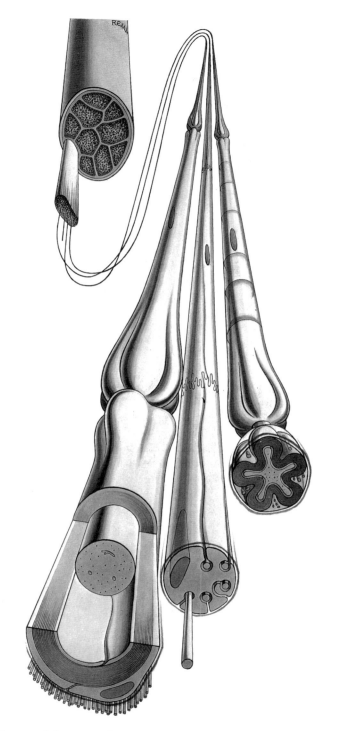

Fig. 8-3. Structural features of peripheral nerve fibers and a nerve trunk cut away, showing a large number of fasciculi, which each contain a large number of nerve fibers. (From Williams and Warwick,[1] with permission.)

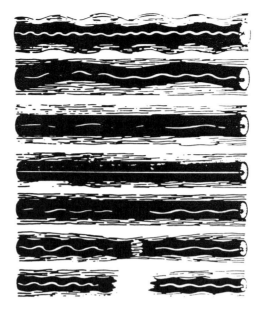

Fig. 8-4. Example of the undulating structure of the funiculi, which contains nerve fibers of a nerve trunk to the point of failure. (From Sunderland,[3] with permission.)

epineurium, surrounds the whole trunk, and a similar but less fibrous perineurium encloses each fasciculus of nerve fibers. The spaces between nerve fibers are penetrated by a loose delicate connective tissue network, the endoneurium. These connective tissue sheaths serve as planes of access for the vasculature of peripheral nerves, as well as protective cushions for the nerve fibers.

Features of Nerve Trunks Providing Protection from Physical Deformation

Several factors protect the brachial plexus and related nerve trunks from both traction and deformation injuries. First, with two notable exceptions, the ulnar nerve at the elbow and the sciatic nerve at the hip, the nerve trunks cross the flexor aspect of joints. Because extension is more limited in range than flexion, the nerves are subjected to less tension during limb movements.

Second, the nerve trunk runs an undulating course in its bed, the funiculi run an undulating course in the epineurium, and the nerve fibers run an undulating course inside the funiculi, as shown in Figure 8-4. This means that the length of nerve fibers between any two fixed points on the limb is considerably greater than the distance between those points.

Third, during traction, the perineurium, by virtue of a relatively large amount of elastic fibers compared with the endoneurium and epineurium, imparts a degree of elasticity in the nerve trunk. Fourth, each peripheral nerve contains, within the nerve trunk, a large amount of epineurial connective tissue that separates the fasciculi. According to Sunderland,[3] values of epineurial connective tissue of various peripheral nerves range in the body from 30 to 75 percent of the cross-sectional area of the total number of nerve fibers contained in each nerve trunk. Therefore, the epineurium, by providing a loose matrix for the contained fasciculi, cushions the nerve fibers against deforming forces.

Features of the Nerve Roots Providing Protection from Injury

The nerve roots at the intervertebral foramen possess several mechanisms that protect them from traction injury.[3] Repetitive strains are placed on the nerve roots forming the brachial plexus during normal cervical spine, shoulder girdle, and shoulder motions. Overstretching of nerve roots by transmitted forces generated in this manner is normally prevented by the following factors.

First, the dura is adherent to and part of the nerve complex at the level of the intervertebral foramen so that when traction pulls the entire system outward, a dural funnel is drawn laterally into the foramen. The dura, at a junction of the intervertebral foramen, being cone-shaped, plugs the foramen in such a way as to resist further displacement of the nerve, as shown in Figure 8-5. Second, the fourth, fifth, sixth, and seventh cervical nerve roots are securely attached to the vertebral column. Each nerve root, on leaving the foramen, is lodged into the gutter of the corresponding transverse process, bound securely by reflections of the prevertebral fascia and by slips from the dura attachment to the transverse processes (Fig. 8-5). Sunderland suggests that the significance of this attachment emerges on examination of the relative susceptibility to avulsion injury of the several nerve roots contributing to the brachial plexus. Traction injuries, which do not avulse nerve roots, more commonly involve the upper spinal nerves where these attachments exist, whereas the

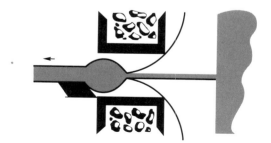

Fig. 8-5.   Displacement of the nerve complex laterally through the foramen is resisted by plugging the funnel-shaped dura, as well as the dural attachment to the transverse process. (From Sunderland,[3] with permission.)

Table 8-1. Etiologic Classification of Brachial Plexus Injuries as Related to the Shoulder

Traumatic
    Open injuries
    Closed injuries
        Obstetric
        Postnatal exogenous
Compression
    Exogenous (sometimes isolated branches)
    Anatomic predisposition (sometimes isolated branches)
    Genetically determined (sometimes isolated branches)
Tumors
    Primary tumors of brachial plexus
    Secondary involvement of plexus by tumors of surrounding tissues
Vascular
    Local vascular processes or lesions
    Participation in generalized vasculopathies (e.g., polyarteritis nodosa and lupus erythematosus)
Physical factors
    Radiotherapy
    Electric shock
Infectious, inflammatory, and toxic processes
    Involvement of local sepsis
    Viral or infectious
Cryptogenic (neuralgic amyotrophy)
    Parainfectious
    Related to serum therapy
    Genetic predisposition
    Cryptogenic

(Modified from Mumenthaler et al.,[7] with permission.)

incidence of avulsion injuries is much higher in the case of the lower nerve roots, which do not have these soft tissue attachments to the transverse processes.

CLASSIFICATION OF BRACHIAL PLEXUS INJURIES

Numerous types of classifications of brachial plexus injuries, illustrated in Table 8-1, have been proposed. The majority of brachial plexus lesions result from trauma, either direct, as if struck by an instrument, or indirect, as in a traction lesion to the cervical spine or upper extremity. Lesions may be described as preganglionic or post-ganglionic. Preganglionic avulsion injuries indicate that the nerve root has been torn from the spinal cord and preclude the possibility of recovery. Post-ganglionic lesions may be either in continuity (root and sheath intact) or ruptured (root intact and nerve sheath ruptured).[4] Spontaneous recovery may occur with the first injury, but, without surgical repair of the rupture, no recovery will occur in the second lesion.

Finally, the post-ganglionic avulsion is classified as either supraclavicular, which involves the trunks and divisions of the plexus, or infraclavicular, which involves the cords and branches.[5] In a series of 420 brachial plexus cases that underwent operations, Alnot reported that 75 percent were supraclavicular lesions and 25 percent were infraclavicular lesions.[5]

Supraclavicular Lesion

Isolated supraclavicular lesions affect either the upper, middle, or lower trunks of the brachial plexus. However, according to Alnot, in his series of patients, 15 percent of the supraclavicular lesions were double level, affecting two trunks, or combined supraclavicular and infraclavicular lesions. These lesions occur when the arm is forced violently into abduction and the middle part of the plexus is blocked temporarily in the coracoid region. Terminal branches are torn away and concomitant supraclavicular lesions occur when the head is jerked violently to the opposite side. Lower down in the plexus, the musculocutaneous nerve (which is tightly attached near the origin of the coracobrachialis muscle), the axillary nerve in the quadrilateral space behind the shoulder, or the suprascapular nerve in the suprascapular notch of the scapula is entrapped and torn.

Upper Trunk Lesion

Palsy of the C5 and C6 roots of the brachial plexus is known as Erb's palsy or Duchenne-Erb paralysis.[6] The muscles affected include the deltoid, biceps, brachialis, infraspinatus, supraspinatus, and serratus anterior. Also usually involved are the rhomboids, levator scapula, and supinator muscles. Therefore, this injury causes severe restriction of movement at the shoulder and elbow joints. The patient is unable to abduct or externally rotate his or her shoulder. The patient cannot supinate the forearm because of weakness of the supinator muscle. Sensory involvement is usually confined along the deltoid muscle and along the distribution of the musculocutaneous nerve. According to Comtet et al., partial or total spontaneous recovery of traumatic Duchenne-Erb paralysis is a frequent occurrence.[6] The delay between the injury and reinnervation of the corresponding muscle varies from 3 to 18 months, even to 24 months. Therefore, long-term rehabilitation with periods of reevaluations is imperative.

Middle Trunk Lesion

The middle trunk receives innervation from the C7 nerve root and courses distally to form a major portion of the posterior cord. The middle trunk offers a major neural contribution to the radial nerve. Therefore, a lesion affecting the middle trunk of the brachial plexus weakens the extensor muscles of the arm and forearm, excluding the brachioradialis, which receives primary innervation from the C6 nerve root. Sensory deficit occurs along the radial distribution of the posterior arm and forearm and along the dorsal radial aspect of the hand.

Lower Trunk Lesion

The lower trunk of the brachial plexus receives innervation from nerve roots C7 and T1. Therefore, injury to the lower trunk affects motor control in the fingers and wrist. The extent of disability is determined by whether the plexus is prefixed or post-fixed. The intrinsic muscles of the hand are only slightly affected in a lesion involving a prefixed plexus, whereas paralysis of the flexors of the hand and forearm occur in a lesion to a post-fixed plexus.[7] Sensory deficit is present along the ulnar border of the arm, forearm, and hand. The presence of Horner's syndrome, characterized by ptosis of the eyelid and constriction of the pupil on the side of the lesion, occurs if the sympathetic fibers contained within the anterior primary ramus of T1 are injured.[2] The sympathetic fibers of T1 provide motor control to the eye.

Infraclavicular Lesion

Infraclavicular lesions include injuries to the cords or the individual peripheral nerves of the brachial plexus. In Alnot's series of 105 patients with infraclavicular brachial plexus injuries, 90 percent of the cases were seen in young people (15 to 30 years of age) after car or motorcycle accidents.[5] The causes included (1) anteromedial shoulder dislocation, which caused most of the isolated lesions of the axillary nerve and the posterior cord; (2) violent downward and backward movement of the shoulder, which caused stretching of the plexus; and (3) complex trauma with multiple fractures of the clavicle, the scapula, or the upper extremity of the humerus, which caused more diffused lesions affecting multiple cords and terminal branches.

Lateral Cord Lesion

According to Alnot, injury to the lateral cord is rare.[5] Because the musculocutaneous nerve and the lateral head of the median nerve are affected, motor deficit consists of palsy of elbow flexion, associated with a deficit of muscle pronators of the forearm and wrist and finger flexors. When the lesion is proximal, the lateral pectoral nerve is injured, resulting in partial or total palsy of the upper portion of the pectoralis major muscle. Sensory deficit is localized at the forearm and at the thumb level.

Medial Cord Lesion

Isolated injury to the medial cord is also rare. Upper medio-ulnar palsy results in injury that is total in the distribution of the ulnar nerve and only partial in the distribution of the median nerve, the flexor pollicis longus muscle, and the flexor digitorum profundus muscle of the index finger. Partial palsy of the lower portion of the pectoralis muscle results in injury to the medial pectoral nerve.[5]

Posterior Cord Lesion

A posterior cord lesion involves the areas of distribution of the radial, axillary, subscapular, and thoracodorsal nerves. The lesion results in weakness of the extensors in the arm, with impairment of medial rotation and elevation of the arm at the shoulder.

Peripheral Nerve Lesion

Common peripheral nerve or branch injuries include, but are not limited to lesions of the long thoracic nerve, axillary nerve, dorsal scapular nerve, and suprascapular nerve. Injuries to the dorsal scapular and suprascapular nerves are reviewed in Chapter 4.

Long Thoracic Nerve Lesion

The long thoracic nerve originates from the individual primary rami C5, C6, and C7 after these nerves emerge from their respective intervertebral foramen. The nerve reaches the serratus anterior muscle by traversing the neck behind the brachial plexus cords, entering the medial aspect of the axilla, and continuing downward along the lateral wall of the thorax.[1] Although isolated injuries to the long thoracic nerve are rare, traumatic wounds or traction injuries to the neck that result in isolated weakness of the serratus anterior muscle with winging of the medial border of the scapula are presumptive evidence of a long thoracic nerve lesion.[2] Normal shoulder abduction and flexion results from a synchronized pattern of movements between scapula rotation and humeral bone elevation. Variations in the scapulohumeral rhythm in the literature have been reported.[8-10] For every 15° of abduction of the arm, 10° occurs at the glenohumeral joint and 5° occurs from rotation of the scapula along the posterior thoracic wall.[8] The rotation of the scapula results from a force couple mechanism combining the upward pull of the upper trapezius muscle, the downward pull of the lower trapezius muscle, and the outward pull of the serratus anterior muscle.[11] Therefore, palsy of the serratus anterior muscle in the presence of a long thoracic nerve injury, during abduction or flexion of the arm, results in partial loss of scapular rotation. The ability of the upper and lower trapezius muscles to temporarily compensate the loss of the serratus anterior muscle to externally rotate the scapula allows for close to full range (180°) flexion and abduction of the arm.[12] However, these muscles quickly fatigue after four or five repetitions, resulting in significant loss of full active shoulder flexion and abduction range of motion.

Axillary Nerve Lesion

The axillary nerve originates from spinal segments C5 and C6, courses to the distal aspect of the posterior cord of the brachial plexus, and advances laterally through the axilla.[1] The nerve bends around the posterior aspect of the surgical neck of the humerus to innervate the deltoid muscle and the overlying skin, as well as the teres minor muscle.

The most frequent cause of isolated axillary nerve lesion is anteromedial shoulder dislocation.[5] In 80 percent of cases, anteromedial dislocation results in a neuropraxia of the axillary nerve, with total recovery in 4 to 6 months' time.[5]

Complete lesion to the axillary nerve results in loss of active shoulder abduction. Sensory changes include an area of anesthesia along the deltoid muscle. However, even in the presence of a total axillary nerve lesion, some active shoulder abduction and external rotation is possible. Residual shoulder abduction results from the actions of the supraspinatus and infraspinatus muscles, as well as the biceps muscle. The stabilization of the humeral head by the supraspinatus muscle combined with the action of the long head of the biceps muscle allows, in some cases, full overhead abduction. Specifically, by externally rotating the arm, the patient places the long head of the biceps muscle in the line of abduction pull. However, the strength of abduction under these conditions is poor, and loss of muscle power occurs quickly with repetitive movements.

PATHOMECHANICS OF TRAUMATIC INJURIES TO THE NERVES

According to Stevens, the majority of traumatic injuries to the brachial plexus results in traction or tensile strains.[13] The brachial plexus is stretched between two firm points of attachment, the transverse processes proximally and the clavopectoral fascial junction distally, in the upper axilla. Stevens compares the cords of the plexus as a traction apparatus with a neutral axis at the C7 vertebra, when the arm is at the horizontal position. Specifically, he compares the brachial plexus as a single cord with five separate points of attachment firmly snubbed at the transverse processes, as shown in Figure 8-6. According to Stevens, a traction apparatus must have a neutral axis and a line of resistance. When the force of traction falls through this neutral center of axis at the C7 vertebra, the traction is equally borne by all parts of the apparatus, represented by nerve roots C5 through T1. A slight deviation from this neutral axis creates an unequal pull to one side or the other of the apparatus. That is, if the line of traction falls outside the neutral axis of C7, the entire force is transmitted from the neutral axis and all tension is released on the cords on the other side. Therefore, if tension is imparted to an arm elevated above the horizontal, stress is increased to the lower roots of the brachial plexus. Conversely, if tension is imparted to an arm depressed below the horizontal, stress is increased to

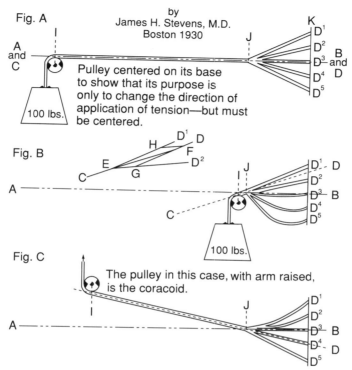

Fig. 8-6. Traction apparatus representing brachial plexus. (From Stevens,[13] with permission.)

the upper roots of the brachial plexus (Fig. 8-6).[13] Therefore, the relative position of the shoulder and neck at the time of injury, as well as the magnitude of the forces, dictates the area and extent of injury to the brachial plexus.

PATHOPHYSIOLOGY OF INJURY

The extent of injury to the nerve trunk, ranging from a nondegenerative neuropraxia to a severance of the nerve or plexus (neurotmesis), will dictate the course of treatment (surgical versus nonsurgical) and the prognosis and relative time frames for full recovery.

Five major degrees of injury are described by Sunderland[14]:

1. *First-degree nerve injury.* This injury is characterized by interruption of conduction at the site of injury with preservation of the anatomic continuity

of all components comprising the nerve trunk, including the axon. Clinical features include temporary loss of motor function to the affected muscles, but the presence of electric potential due to axonal continuity is retained. Cutaneous sensory loss may occur, but will recover in advance of motor function. Most patients recover spontaneously within 6 weeks after injury.

2. *Second-degree nerve injury.* In this injury, the axon is severed and fails to survive below the level of injury and, for a variable but short distance, the axon degenerates proximal to the point of the lesion. However, the endoneurium is preserved within the endoneurial tube. Histologic changes to the nerve include breakdown of the myelin sheath, Schwann cell degeneration, and phagocytic activity with eventual fibrosis. Clinical features include temporary complete loss of motor, sensory, and sympathetic functions in the autonomous distribution of the injured nerve. Several months will pass before recovery begins, with proximal reinnervation occurring before distal reinnervation to the involved muscles.

3. *Third-degree nerve injury.* This condition is characterized by axonal disintegration, Wallerian degeneration both distal and proximal to the site of the lesion, and disorganization of the internal structure of the endoneural fasciculi. The general fascicular pattern of the nerve trunk is retained with minimal damage to both the perineurium and epineurium. Because the endoneural tube is destroyed, intrafascicular fibrosis may obviate axonal regeneration. Many axons fail to reach their original or functionally related endoneurial tubes, and are instead misdirected into foreign endoneurial tubes. Clinically, motor, sensory, and sympathetic functions of the related nerves are lost. The recovery is long, up to 2 to 3 years, with a chance of significant residual dysfunction.

4. *Fourth-degree nerve injury.* This type of injury is similar to third-degree nerve injury, but the perineurium is disrupted. Therefore, the chance for a residual dysfunction due to fibrosis and mixing of regenerating fibers at the site of injury, which may distort the normal pattern of innervation, is high.

5. *Fifth-degree nerve injury.* In this injury, the entire nerve trunk is severed, with resultant complete loss of function to the affected structures. Obviously, without surgical grafting, recovery is negligible.

CLARIFYING EVALUATION

A thorough and systematic clarifying evaluation is essential for the clinician to assess accurately the nature and extent of the brachial plexus lesion and to develop an appropriate and effective treatment plan. Because most brachial plexus lesions slowly improve over a long period of time, the clinician must maintain and update accurate records concerning the progress of the patient. The clinician should use any one of a number of charts for recording results of the physical examination, as shown in Figure 8-7. Evaluation and

BRACHIAL PLEXUS

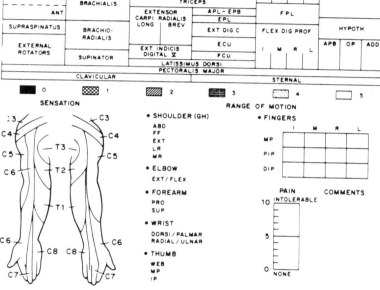

Fig. 8-7. Chart for recording results of physical examination for brachial plexus injury. (From Leffert RD: Rehabilitation of the patient with an injury to the brachial plexus. In Hunter JM, Schneider LH, Mackin EJ, Callahan AD (eds): Rehabilitation of the Hand. 3rd Ed. CV Mosby, St. Louis, 1990, with permission.)

treatment is a conjoint effort by a physical and an occupational therapist who specializes in the treatment of hand and upper extremity injuries. Knowledge of hand management and rehabilitation is particularly important in lower trunk injuries to the brachial plexus. Additionally, in the presence of fourth- and fifth-degree nerve injuries to the brachial plexus, occupational therapy offers strategies for splinting as well as equipment modification or assurance to assist permanently dysfunctional individuals.

HISTORY

Mechanisms of Injury

Because most brachial plexus injuries result from trauma, a thorough history should include questions concerning the nature and mechanisms of injury. According to Stevens, the different varieties of stress, and the relative position of the arm and head at the time of the stress, make tremendous differences in the kinds of lesions suffered, in the locality of the lesion, and in prognosis.[13] The magnitude of forces, that is, high-speed versus slow-speed injuries, is important to ascertain. According to Frampton, high-speed, large-impact accidents are commonly associated with preganglionic plexus injuries, while slow-speed, small-impact accidents are commonly associated with postganglionic injuries.[4] Examples of high-velocity injuries are those resulting from falls from speeding motorcycles, while examples of low-velocity injuries are those resulting from a fall down a stairway.

Pain

The area and nature of pain should be documented. Pain, described as a constant burning, crushing pain with sudden shoots of paroxysms of pain, is central in nature. This pain occurs as a result of deafferentation of the spinal cord at the damaged root level, leading to undampened excitation of the cells in the dorsal horn of the spinal cord. The confused barrage of abnormal firings is received and interpreted centrally as pain and is eventually felt in the dermatomes of the nerve root that is avulsed.[15] In a series of 188 patients with post-traumatic brachial plexus lesions, Bruxelle et al. found that 91 percent experienced pain at least 3 years after injury.[15] Pain may also result from secondary injuries to bones or related soft tissues. The report of any anesthesias or paresthesias should be noted and documented. The presence of Horner's syndrome, which is characterized by enophthalmos, myosis, and ptosis, along with a deficit of facial sweating on the affected side, reflects damage to the T1 nerve root. Questions concerning the course of events since injury or a change in the severity of the symptoms establish an indication of an improving or worsening lesion. A condition that is resolving spontaneously may indicate first- or second-degree nerve injuries, while a condition that has not changed across the course of 6 weeks may indicate at least a third-degree nerve injury, according to Sunderland's classification of nerve injuries.

Finally, the clinician should document the patient's occupation, handedness, and previous state of health to assist in establishing feasible goals for the patient's return to his or her premorbid activity level.

Physical Evaluation

The components of the physical evaluation include (1) posture; (2) passive range of motion of the cervical spine, shoulder, and upper extremity; (3) motor strength; (4) sensation; (5) palpation; and (6) special tests. The occupational therapy evaluation includes assessment for (1) edema, (2) coordination, (3) activities of daily living, and (4) vocational and avocational pursuits. The physical evaluation should be repeated frequently during the process of rehabilitation to carefully assess subtle signs of nerve reinnervation.

Posture

The patient is observed from the front, side, and behind. From behind, the clinician observes for muscle atrophy along the upper quarter muscles, as well as winging of the scapula. Winging of the scapula signifies weakness of the serratus anterior muscle, which may indicate a lesion of the long thoracic nerve. Ipsilateral atrophy of the supraspinatus or infraspinatus muscles can signify suprascapular nerve entrapment. Atrophy of the deltoid muscle, in addition to the supraspinatus and infraspinatus muscles, can indicate an upper trunk plexus lesion, such as Duchenne-Erb Paralysis of the C5 and C6 nerve trunks. Isolated atrophy of the deltoid muscle indicates an isolated axillary nerve lesion. From the side, the clinician should observe for changes consistent with a forward head posture: accentuated upper thoracic spine kyphosis, protraction and elevation of the scapulae, increased cervical spine inclination, and backward bending at the atlanto-occipital junction. The forward head posture results in muscle imbalances that can further result in entrapment of various nerves of the brachial plexus in the area of the thoracic outlet.[16] Thoracic outlet syndrome is discussed in detail in Chapter 7. From the front, the clinician should observe the attitude or position of the upper extremity and hand. An arm position of adduction and internal rotation can result from Duchenne-Erb paralysis. Pronation of the forearm with flexion at the wrist and metacarpophalangeal and proximal interphalangeal joints can result from injury to the lower trunk of the brachial plexus.[6] External deformities along the clavicle, which may indicate fracture, should be noted. Both nonunions and malunions of the clavicle can result in significant compression of the brachial plexus. The supraclavicular fossa is inspected for the presence of swelling or ecchymosis in those patients with recent injury and for nodularity and induration in the brachial plexus where the injury is old.[4] The eyes are observed for constriction of the pupils or ptosis of the eyelids, which can indicate the presence of Horner's syndrome.[2]

Passive Range of Motion

The passive range of motion of all joints of the shoulder girdle and upper limb must be assessed and recorded using a standard goniometer. Deficits of joint motion from immobility result in contractures of joint capsule, adhesions in the joints, and shortening of both muscle and tendons above the affected joints. The classic studies of Akeson et al. demonstrated the deleterious affects of 9 weeks of immobilization on periarticular structures, including the loss of water and glycoaminoglycans, randomization and abnormal cross-linking of newly synthesized collagen, and infiltration in the joint spaces of fatty fibrous materials.[17]

Motor Strength

Several manuals are available that review proper isolation, stabilization, and grading procedures for manual muscle testing.[18,19] Most grading systems grade muscle for 0 to 5, with 0 being a flaccid muscle and 5 representing normal muscle strength.[18] A complete upper extremity test should be performed initially to provide the clinician a data base from which to measure improvement. Therefore, retests should be performed periodically. A thorough manual muscle test assists the clinician in pinpointing the site and extent of the plexus lesion. Establishing an appropriate strengthening program is based on isolating and grading involved muscles. Isokinetic testing can also assist clinicians in measuring muscle strength deficits, usually for peak torque, power, and work, compared with the uninvolved upper extremity. Refer to Chapter 3 for a review of isokinetic testing protocols in the shoulder.

Sensation

Assessment of sensory loss assists in the diagnosis of the level and extent of the plexus lesion. Total avulsion of the plexus results in total anesthesia of the related areas. However, in a mixed lesion, and when recovery is occurring, the sensory pattern may vary in the arm. The sensory evaluation may include deep pressure, light touch, temperature, stereognosis, and two-point discrimination, depending on the patient's status.[4] Sensory changes are documented along dermatomes, as illustrated in Figure 8-7.

Coordination

Loss of sensation and muscle control in the presence of a brachial plexus injury results in a loss of gross and fine motor coordination in the affected upper extremity. There are numerous tests on the market designed to assess an individual's coordination. Each requires varying amounts of fine and/or gross motor coordination. The Purdue pegboard (Lafayette Instructional Co., Lafayette, Ind.), for example, assists the clinician in assessing the patient's manual dexterity. Patients are requested to place pegs with both the right and left hands, singularly and in tandem, and to perform a specific assembly task using pins, collars and washers. These tests are timed and compared with normative values.[20] It is up to the therapist to determine the most appropriate tests based on the patient's level of functioning.

Vascular

In the presence of severe brachial plexus injuries, particularly with associated fractures of the clavicle, disruption of the subclavian or axillary arteries may occur. Additionally, all patients who have had a significant nerve injury will have evidence of vasomotor changes.[2] Assessment of the brachial and radial pulses and inspection for dusky, cool skin indicating venous insufficiency should be performed by the clinician.

Edema

Edema must be assessed and treated to prevent stiffness in the joints. The concept of volumetrics to measure upper extremity edema is well established. The patient's hand is submerged in a lucite container (Volumeter, Volumeters Unlimited, Idyllwild, CA), and the amount of water displaced is measured using a 500-ml graduated cylinder. Both extremities should be measured and the results recorded. Circumferential measurements of the hand and forearm are another method of measuring edema. However, this technique is best suited for individual digit swelling or in the case of open wounds, which may preclude the patient getting the extremity wet. Manual palpation is also used to measure edema. The severity of the edema is usually rated from 1 to 3, with 1 being minimal and 3 being severe or pitting edema.

Palpation

Manual palpation is used to assess for myofascial trigger points about the affected shoulder girdle and upper extremity musculature. Trigger points result from tight and contracted muscles or from partially denervated muscles exhibiting poor muscle control and altered movement patterns. Active trigger points refer pain into the affected upper extremity, as well as the shoulder girdle, neck, and head.[21,22]

Special Tests

The presence of Tinel's sign, demonstrated by tapping over the brachial plexus above the clavicle, can be quite useful in distinguishing rupture from a lesion in continuity.[2,4] A distal Tinel's sign indicates a lesion in continuity where the axonal connections within the nerve trunk are intact. This may correspond to a first-degree nerve injury or a regenerating second- or third-degree nerve injury, as described by Sunderland. Conversely, the presence of a localized tenderness to tapping above the clavicle indicates a possible neuroma resulting from disruption of part of the plexus. This type of injury would correspond to a fourth- or fifth-degree nerve injury.

Activities of Daily Living

The patient is questioned regarding all aspects of self-care to identify those specific tasks he or she is not able to perform owing to the extent of the brachial plexus injury. Such areas include self-care skills such as feeding, bathing, grooming, and dressing. Based on the specific limitations of the patient, the occupational therapist then determines whether to provide the patient with specific adaptive equipment or to instruct the patient in one-handed techniques.

Assessment for Splinting

In the case of a complete brachial plexus injury, the patient is fitted with a flail arm splint that allows the patient to use the extremity at home and at work. The splint is fitted early, to prevent the patient from relying on one-handed methods as a means of performing specific activities.[4] In the case of a C5–C6–C7 injury, the patient might require a long wrist and finger extension assist splint (Fig. 8-8). The patient may also be fitted with a resting hand splint

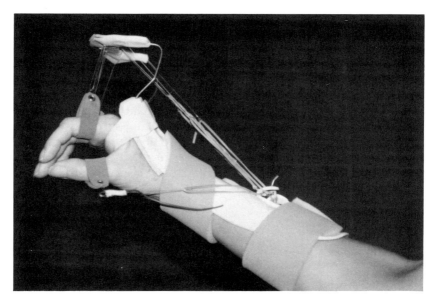

Fig. 8-8. A long metacarpophalangeal extension splint used with a patient who has weak wrist extension and trace finger extension.

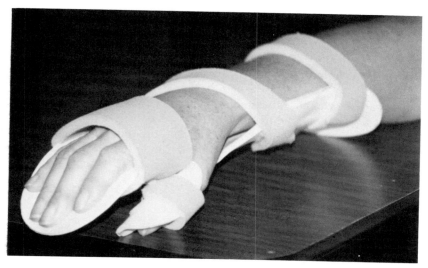

Fig. 8-9. A resting hand splint used following a brachial plexus lesion to prevent overstretching of weak and finger extensor muscles by maintaining the wrist in approximately 20° of dorsiflexion.

(Fig. 8-9) to wear at night to help maintain the wrist and fingers in a balanced position.

Vocational

A detailed job description is obtained to assess the patient's potential to return to work. In addition, a functional capacity evaluation can be performed later in the rehabilitation process to assess the patient's physical demand level.

Avocational

Becaue the brachial plexus-injured patient is unable to work, avocational pursuits are often an important source of much-needed diversional activity. The occupational therapist questions the patient closely as to premorbid hobbies or potential areas of interests. Activities of interest are developed that encourage use of the affected extremity.

Laboratory Evaluations of Brachial Plexus Lesions

Also included in the overall evaluation of a patient with a brachial plexus injury are laboratory evaluations involving electrodiagnostic testing, myelography, and radiographic assessment. These evaluations help the clinician diagnose the area and extent of the lesion and provide baseline measurements to help evaluate progress.

Radiographic Assessment

Every patient who has sustained a significant injury to the brachial plexus should have a complete radiographic series done of the cervical spine and involved shoulder gridle, including the clavicle.[2] Fractures of the clavicle with callus, which can impinge on the nerve trunks along the costoclavicular juncture, or fractures of the cervical transverse processes, which can indicate a root avulsion, must be ruled out.[2,4]

Myelography

Myelography is used to indicate the status of the nerve roots in the presence of traction injuries to the brachial plexus. According to Leffert, root avulsion can occur in the presence of a normal myelogram.[2] However, a well-documented study by Yeoman indicates the efficacy of myelography as a valuable adjunct to the diagnosis of brachial plexus root lesions.[23]

Electromyography

Because the loss of axonal continuity results in predictable, time-related electric charges, knowledge and assessment of these electric charges can be used to provide information concerning muscle denervation and reinnervation.[2]

For example, while normally innervated muscle exhibits no spontaneous electric activity at rest when examined with needle electrodes, denervated muscle produces readily recognizable small potentials (fibrillations) or large potentials (sharp waves), which are the hallmark of denervation. These electric discharges usually appear 3 weeks following injury to the plexus and signal the onset of Wallerian degeneration of a specific nerve. The clinician is able to localize the lesion by sampling muscles innervated by different nerves and root levels.

Additionally, when a root avulsion is suspected in a patient who has sustained a traction injury of the brachial plexus, the clinician should also peform an electromyographic evaluation of the posterior cervical musculature. The posterior cervical muscles are segmentally innervated by the posterior primary rami of the spinal nerves that provide the anterior primary rami to form the plexus. Denervation of the deep posterior cervical muscles is highly correlated with root avulsion. Conversely, if the electromyogram is positive for the muscles innervated by the anterior primary rami but not for the posterior cervical muscles, whatever possible damage exists is presumed to be infraganglionic in nature.[24]

Nerve Conduction Studies

Nerve conduction velocity tests may be used to help distinguish muscular weakness in the affected upper extremity from cervical intervertebral disc protrusion, anterior horn cell disease, or a brachial plexus lesion. Because anterior horn cell diseases and intervertebral disc protrusions do not influence nerve conduction latency, the clinician can be certain that a proximal nerve conduction delay is a result of a brachial plexus lesion.[25]

Another type of electrodiagnostic testing is the F response, an outgrowth of the measurement of velocity of conduction; this is a late reaction that potentially results from the backfiring of antidromically activated anterior horn cells. Electrical stimulation of motor points assesses the strength–duration curves of affected muscles.[26] A denervated or partially denervated muscle requires more time and current than a normally innervated muscle. Serial strength–duration testing, therefore, allows the clinician to assess neuromuscular recovery.[26]

REHABILITATION GOALS AND TREATMENT

The approach to rehabilitation for brachial plexus lesions is directed at maintaining or improving soft tissue mobility, muscle strength and function within the constraint of the nerve injury, and function. Because regeneration is excruciatingly slow, rehabilitation, in severe cases, is a long-term process, lasting as long as 3 years. Therefore, patient and family education, as well as home exercise programs, are an integral component of treatment.

Surgical grafting in the presence of fourth- and fifth-degree nerve injuries necessitates, on the part of the therapist, knowledge of soft tissue healing constraints. The relatively high chance of residual upper extremity dysfunction in some cases requires vocational and avocational retraining, as well as occupational therapy intervention for assistance-providing devices and splints.

According to Frampton,[4] rehabilitation falls into three stages: the early stage, consisting of diagnosis, neurovascular repair, and education concerning passive movement and self-care of the affected extremity; the middle stage, when recovery is occurring and intensive reeducation may be indicated; and the late stage, when no future recovery is expected and assessment for reconstructive surgery can take place. The time frames and extent of each phase are predicted based on the extent of the lesion and the individual's own motivation and recuperative capabilities. Goals, treatments, and rationales for the treatments for each stage of rehabilitation are exemplified in the case study presented below.

CLINICAL CASE STUDY

The following case study presents a typical brachial plexus injury affecting the shoulder and upper extremity function. Initial findings are delineated in the clarifying evaluation. The goals and phases of treatment are presented as a combined physical and occupational therapy approach. Rationales for specific treatments are presented, when relevant.

History.   A 25-year-old right-handed man was involved in a motor vehicle accident and suffered a traction lesion to his brachial plexus. Electrodiagnostic testing indicated an infraganglionic lesion to his left brachial plexus at Erb's joint, that portion of the brachial plexus where C5 and C6 unite to join the upper trunk. Radiologic studies indicated no fractures at the cervical spine or clavicle. The patient was referred to physical and occupational therapy 4 weeks after the initial injury.

The patient reported numbness and tingling along the lateral aspect of his left shoulder, in the area of the deltoid muscle, and weakness in his left shoulder, elbow, wrist, and hand. He reports intermittent pain in his left shoulder and neck made worse with attempted elevation of his left arm. He reported less numbness and increased strength in his left arm since the initial injury.

Vocation.   The patient works as a carpenter.

Postural/visual inspection.   Atrophy was observed in the deltoid, supraspinatus, and infraspinatus muscles on the left compared with the right side. His left arm was held in internal rotation along his lateral trunk, with his forearm pronated and his wrist and fingers in slight flexion.

Passive range of motion.   Elevation in the plane of scapula measured 120°, external rotation in adduction measured 30°, external rotation in 45° abduction measured 60°, and external rotation in 90° abduction measured 70°. His elbow, forearm, wrist, and hand passive range of motion were all within normal limits.

Active range of motion.   Elevation in the plane of scapula measured 60°, external rotation in adduction from full internal rotation measured 20°, elbow flexion measured 30°, and supination measured 50°. The patient had full pronation and wrist and finger flexion and extension.

Motor strength.   Motor strength was graded as follows:

Grade 0 = no contraction
Grade 1 = trace
Grade 2 = poor
Grade 3 = fair
Grade 4 = good
Grade 5 = normal

The patient's muscles were graded as follows: deltoid = 2, supraspinatus = 3, infraspinatus = 3, teres minor = 2, biceps brachii = 2, brachialis = 2, serratus anterior = 5, subscapularis = 3, extensor carpi radialis longus and brevis = 3, and supinator = 3. His grip strength was 88 lb on the right and 10 lb on the left.

Sensation.   Sensation was impaired to light touch and to sharp/dull along the lateral aspect of the left shoulder, in the area of the deltoid muscle, and along the radial side of the forearm.

Coordination.   Coordination was assessed using the Purdue pegboard and rated as follows: right hand, 14; left hand, 2; both hands, 4; assembly task, 6.

Edema. The patient had 2+ edema palpated along the dorsum of the left fingers at the proximal interphalangeal joints and metacarpal joints and along the dorsum of the left hand. His volumetric measurements were 482 cc on the right and 525 cc on the left.

Palpation. Trigger points were palpated in muscle bellies of the left upper trapezius, left rhomboid, and left subscapularis muscles.

Activities of daily living (ADL). The patient was unable to perform the following self-care activities:

Feeding—unable to cut his food.
Bathing—unable to wash his right shoulder and upper arm.
Grooming—unable to apply deodorant to his right underarm.
Dressing—unable to tie shoes, button shirt, zip pants or jacket, and buckle belt.

Assessment. This is a patient whose history revealed a traction injury to the upper trunk of the brachial plexus involving nerve trunks C5 and C6. Because he demonstrated at least poor muscle control of the affected muscles, which is spontaneously improving since the initial injury, the extent of the injury is classified as between a first-degree and second-degree injury, according to Sunderland's classification.[14] Therefore, one can expect combined resolution of nerve function, with full return of function of the left upper extremity.

Passive range of motion is moderately limited in the affected shoulder with restrictions of the related joint capsule, fascia, tendon, and muscle. Soft tissue limitations are consistent with the findings of Akeson et al.,[17] Tabary et al.,[27] and Cooper,[28] who studied the affects of immobilization on periarticular capsule, tendon, and muscle, respectively. The loss of motor control results in altered scapulohumeral rhythm. The rotator cuff muscles, particularly the supraspinatus, infraspinatus, and teres minor muscles, are unable to adequately control gliding of the humeral head during elevation of the shoulder. The resultant weakness, even in the presence of a weak deltoid muscle, results in impingement of the suprahumeral soft tissues underneath the unyielding coroocoacromial ligament. Chronic impingement results in inflammation and degeneration of the rotator cuff tendons.

Compensation of the scapula muscles to elevate the arm in the presence of weakness of the rotator cuff and deltoid muscles results in irritation and trigger points in both the left upper trapezius and left rhomboid muscles. A trigger point palpated in the subscapularis muscle is the result of the shoulder and arm positioned in internal rotation and along the lateral trunk wall, which maintained the subscapularis muscle in a shortened position. The contracted subscapularis muscle resulted in the greater limitation of passive external rotation with the arm adducted along the lateral trunk wall, as opposed to external rotation with the arm abducted to 45° or 90°. (R. Donatelli, personal communication, 1989).

The weakness in the left upper extremity and hand result in a loss of normal muscle pumping activity to remove interstitial fluid. In addition, the patient tended to keep his arm down at his side. These two factors result in increased edema in the left upper extremity, especially the left fingers and hand, compared with the right. The weakness in the left upper extremity, as well as the patient's decreased manual dexterity, interfered with some self-care activities. Fortunately, the patient is right-handed, which will expedite his return to employment as a carpenter.

Rehabilitation Goals and Treatment

Early Stage

First goal.   The first goal is to reduce pain.

Treatment: Heat, low-voltage surge stimulation, and spray and stretch (see Ch 12) were applied to the active trigger points in the left upper trapezius and left rhomboid muscles in our patient. Transcutaneous neuromuscular stimulation, using a high-rate, low-intensity conventional setting with dual channels and four electrodes, was applied around the left shoulder. The transcutaneous neuromuscular stimulation device was worn 8 hours per day.

Rationale: According to Travell and Simons, myofascial trigger points in the shoulder girdle muscles refer pain into the left shoulder and arm in a consistent pattern.[21] Therefore, reduction of trigger point tenderness in the left upper trapezius and left rhomboid muscles will alleviate part of this patient's pain. The conventional transcutaneous neuromuscular stimulation setting stimulates large A-beta sensory fibers that modulate impulses from the small A-delta and C fibers in the dorsal horn of the spinal cord.[29,30] Pain impulses along the A-delta and C fibers in this patient resulted from irritation of nociceptor endings in the connective tissue sheaths surrounding the nerve fibers and trunks, due to the traction injury.[30]

Second Goal.   The second goal is to restore full passive range of motion and soft tissue mobility.

Treatment: In our patient, low-voltage surge stimulation followed by spray and stretch techniques were applied to the active trigger points in the muscle belly of the subscapularis. Mobilization techniques, in the grades III and IV range according to Maitland's classification, were applied to the various joints in the left upper extremity.[31] Special attention was directed at manual distraction of the specific details concerning mobilization techniques at the shoulder complex.

Patients with this condition are given a program of range of motion self-exercises in order to preserve the range of motion at those joints where there is no, or only limited, active range of motion. Each patient is given an active range of motion exercise program for the uninvolved joints so that these joints do not become restricted due to disuse of the extremity in general. The patient's family should be familiar with the exercise program so that they can encourage the patient to follow through and become active participants in the patient's rehabilitation.

Rationale: In our patient, the painful limitation of external rotation with the shoulder adducted along the lateral trunk wall results from a contracted subscapularis muscle. Therefore, spray and stretch, followed by distraction of the medial scapula border, elongates the subscapularis muscle and improves external rotation with the shoulder in the adducted position. Mobilization techniques at the shoulder are directed at the inferior and anterior capsules, respectively, to promote abduction and external rotation movements, respectively. The scientific literature indicates no optimum time frames for applying grade IV manual stretching to the periarticular capsule. Clinically, we use three sets of 1-minute grade IV oscillations into the restricted tissue preceded by heat and followed by ice.

Third Goal. The third goal is to avoid neural dissociation to the reinnervating muscles.

Treatment: High-frequency muscle stimulation was applied to the partially denervated muscles. The preferred duty cycle was 10 seconds on and 20 seconds off, for a period of 30 minutes. The patient was instructed to use a home stimulator, three to four times daily.

Rationale: According to strength–duration studies, muscle stimulation to a partially denervated muscle requires a higher current and longer pulse duration than does stimulation to a normally innervated muscle.[26] In addition to maintaining reinnervating muscle tissue viability, electrically induced muscle contractions facilitate normal circulation, decrease edema, and present potential nutritional or tropic skin changes.[32,33]

Fourth Goal. Reducing edema is the fourth goal.

Treatment: Retrograde massage was applied to the hand from a distal to proximal direction, with the patient's hand and forearm elevated above his heart.[34] In addition, the patient and his wife were provided with written instructions regarding elevation of the arm, retrograde massage, and fist pumping to activate muscle pumping action in the hand and forearm.

Coban (3M Medical-Surgical, St Paul, MN) is a gentle elastic wrap used for edema control. It is wrapped diagonally from the fingertips proximally and should overlap approximately ¼ in. The advantages of Coban are that it is reusable (thus reducing costs), may be worn for prolonged periods, and allows for full range of motion.[35]

Rationale: Retrograde massage, in a gravity-assisted position, facilitates the reabsorption of interstitial fluids into the lymphatic system. First pumping, resulting in alternate contraction and relaxation of the musculature in the hand and forearm, promotes venous blood return to the heart.

Fifth Goal. The fifth goal is to increase the patient's ADL independence.

Treatment: The patient was issued adaptive equipment to increase his self-care independence until he exhibited a greater degree of motor control. For example, he was issued a rocker knife to help him cut his meat and a button hook to help him button his shirt. In addition, he was instructed in specific one-handed methods of performing certain tasks, such as tying his shoe laces.

Sixth Goal. Providing emotional support education is the sixth goal.

Treatment: Patient and family education and psychological referral were used to accomplish the sixth goal.

In certain instances, the therapist must help the patient through the initial stages of denial, anger, and depression associated with a severe brachial plexus injury. A patient's emotional state will affect his or her performance in therapy. The therapist should be an active listener and recognize the normal process of emotional recovery in patients with severe disability. Fear is a major component and compounds a patient's anxiety. This anxiety can often be reduced if the patient is educated as to the nature and extent of the injury, the course of recovery, the course of therapy, and the prognosis for recovery. One cannot stress enough the importance of involving the patient's family in the rehabilitation process. Family relationships often become strained as a result of serious injury. Financial issues may become a source of worry and concern for all involved. The family members may need as much support as the patient and will also benefit from the education process.

Middle Stage

First Goal.   The first goal in the middle stage is to reeducate reinnervating muscles.

Treatment: Manual proprioceptive neuromuscular facilitation techniques emphasizing diagonal patterns, with the patient supine, were begun at approximately 3 weeks after the initial evaluation. Light-weight isotonic strengthening was added to the program, using adjustable-weight cuffs. Initial isotonic strengthening emphasized external rotation movement patterns at the shoulder, as well as flexion and extension movements at the elbow and pronation and supination at the forearm. As strength improved, the patient was progressed to isokinetic strengthening at slow speeds of approximately 60°/s, emphasizing rotational movement patterns in the shoulder. The patient was progressed to isokinetic diagonal movement patterns in the supine position when isokinetic testing indicated a difference of left to right external rotation strength, as measured in peak torque, and power was within 30 percent. Refer to Chapter 3 for isokinetic testing and strengthening strategies for the shoulder.

Modalities such as vibration and tapping are used while the patient is exercising or performing functional activities. Appropriate sensory stimuli can evoke desired muscular responses, and this stimulation must be followed by purposeful activities if motor learning is to take place.[36]

Rationale: Manual proprioceptive neuromuscular facilitation diagonals allow the clinician to assess early subtle strength changes across treatments. Early isotonic strengthening is directed at restoring strength in the shoulder rotator cuff muscles, specifically the supraspinatus, infraspinatus, and teres minor muscles. The goal is to restore, during elevation of the shoulder, the dynamic steering mechanism of the rotator cuff muscles on the humeral head.[37] The restoration of rotator cuff muscle strength reestablishes the normal balance between these muscles and the upward pull of the deltoid muscle. Elevation of the shoulder in the presence of weak rotator cuff muscles results in abutment and impingement of the suprahumeral soft tissues against a relatively unyielding corocoacromial ligament. Isokinetic strengthening is instituted as soon as the patient is actively exercising with 1- or 2-lb weights. Isokinetic contraction offers the advantage of accommodating resistance to maximally load a contracting muscle throughout the range of motion.[38] The patient exercises at preselected speeds, beginning with slower speeds, so that he or she can consistently "catch" and maintain the speed of the dynamometer. External rotational strengthening is emphasized early, as previously mentioned, to restore the dynamic glide of the humeral head along the glenoid fossa by reestablishing strength in the supraspinatus, infraspinatus, and teres minor muscles. Isokinetic testing is performed every 2 to 3 weeks to assess peak torque and power values of the involved compared with the uninvolved upper extremity. Isokinetic diagonal strengthening patterns are performed initially supine, to eliminate the affect of the muscles working directly against gravity. Diagonal patterns are eventually performed with the patient sitting or standing, after bilateral strength deficits between the left and right shoulder rotators are within 30 percent. Although not scientifically substantiated, we have observed that when bilateral shoulder rotational strength deficits are greater than 30 percent, impingement of the suprahumeral soft tissues and pain, during active shoulder elevation, occurs.

Occupational therapy: In occupational therapy, our patient worked on tabletop activities with his left upper extremity supported. The activities were directed toward strengthening his elbow, forearm, and wrist musculature. For example, he transferred pegs from one bucket placed in front of him to a bucket placed to his far left. This activity required active elbow flexion and extension in a gravity-eliminated position. As his shoulder strength improved, he was able to perform this same activity unsupported. Additionally, he was able to stack cones, which required active shoulder abduction against gravity. He used light weights to strengthen wrist flexion and extension, supination, and pronation. Elastic rubber tubing, such as Theraband (Hygenic, Akron, OH), was used at home to improve elbow and wrist strength. He was issued Theraputty and instructed in hand-strengthening exercises.

Second Goal. The second goal is to continue mobilization to the restricted joints.

Treatment: Low-load–prolonged stretching using surgical tubing was applied to the restricted periarticular capsules, especially the anterior aspect of the glenohumeral capsule, to promote external rotation. The patient was positioned with his shoulder in 45° of abduction and his elbow in 90° flexion. Surgical tubing attached to his wrist provided a 30-minute low-load stretch into external rotation.

Rationale: Using rat tail tendons, Lehman et al. demonstrated that the optimum method to stretch pericapsular tissue is to use low-load prolonged stretch.[39] According to Lehman et al., the prolonged stretching allows the viscoelastic materal in the capsular tissue, including the water and glycoaminoglycans, to creep or to elongate with the tissue.

Third Goal. If necessary, continue the third goal is to edema control techniques.

Fourth Goal. The fourth goal is to reevaluate the use of assistance-providing devices and to modify the use of these devices.

Fifth Goal. Increasing coordination is the fifth goal.

Treatment: As our patient's motor performance improved, coordination activities became an integral part of his treatment program. Initially, the activities focus on such gross motor skills as placing large pegs into a bucket while being timed and, later, placing those same pegs into a pegboard. As he continued to improve, the activities required more fine motor skills, such as manipulating nuts and bolts (graded from large to small), practicing on an ADL board, turning coins, etc. All activities were timed to document progress. Trombly and Scott state that in order to increase coordination, activities should be graded along a continuum from gross to fine and that as the patient's coordination improves, the activities should require faster speeds and more accuracy.[40]

Late Stage

First Goal. The first goal in the late stage is to optimize muscle strengthening within the constraints of reinnervation.

Treatment: Isokinetic strengthening is continued to all major affected muscle groups in the left upper extremity. Rotational and diagonal strengthening at the shoulder is continued. Fast-speed training, at 180°/s, is added when bilateral slow-speed deficits, at 60°/s, are within 25 percent. The patient is instructed in an aggressive home strengthening program using adjustable cuff weights. Functional training, including lifting, carrying various-size weights, hammering, and sawing activities, is instituted.

Rationale: Strengthening in the clinic is continued if the patient continues to exhibit strength gains with periodic isokinetic strength retests. Fast-speed training is instituted to improve muscular endurance. Fast-speed training is not instituted until slow-speed bilateral deficits are within 25 percent. We have observed clinically that, in the presence of slow-speed, bilateral deficits greater than 25 percent, the patient cannot consistently "catch" and maintain the faster speeds of the dynamometer. Functional training for this particular patient is designed to simulate the working conditions and motor requirements of carpentry.

Second Goal. Optimizing joint and soft tissue mobility is the second goal.

Third Goal. The third goal is to help the patient return to work.

Treatment: At 1 year postinjury, a job analysis was done to identify those tasks our patient would need to perform in order to be able to safely and accurately perform his job. At that time, the patient started on wood-working projects that required minimal fine motor tasks (i.e., sanding, staining, etc.). At 15 months, he progressed to working on more intricate projects and, at 18 months, he returned to work.

CONCLUSION

The case study illustrates the problem-solving approach to patient treatment. Signs and symptoms evaluated during the clarifying evaluation are prioritized in order of their clinical significance. Treatment is divided into three phases to allow the clinician to establish appropriate goals within the constraints of nerve reinnervation. The patient is progressed through each phase based on continued reeducation of signs and symptoms. The patient is discharged when clinical tests and evaluation indicate no further improvement in motor capabilities. The patient is discharged on a home program and is periodically reevaluated. Treatment is resumed if reevaluation confirms additional signs of motor reinnervation. A combined physical and occupational therapy approach recognizes the potential of significant long-term dysfunction of the patient's upper extremity.

REFERENCES

1. Williams PL, Warwick R: Gray's Anatomy. 36th British Ed. Churchill Livingstone, Edinburgh, 1980
2. Leffert RD: Clinical diagnosis, testing, and electromyographic study in brachial plexus traction injuries. Clin Orthop Rel Res 237:24, 1988
3. Sunderland S: Traumatized nerves, roots and ganglia: musculoskeletal factors and neuropathological consequences. p. 137. In Korr IM (ed): The Neurobiologic Mechanisms in Manipulative Therapy. Plenum, New York, 1978
4. Framptom VM: Management of brachial plexus lesions. J Hand Ther 115:120, 1988
5. Alnot JY: Traumatic brachial plexus palsy in the adult: retro- and infraclavicular lesions. Clin Orthop Rel Res 237:9, 1988
6. Comtet JJ, Sedel L, Fredenucci JF: Duchenne-Erb palsy: experience with direct surgery. Clin Orthop Rel Res 237:17, 1988
7. Mumenthaler M, Narakas A, Gilliat RW: Brachial plexus disorders. p. 1383. In Dyck PJ, Thomas PK, Lambert EH, Bunge R (eds): Peripheral Neuropathy. Vol. 2. WB Saunders, Philadelphia, 1984
8. Inman VT, Saunders M, Abbot LC: Observations on the function of the shoulder joint. J Bone Joint Surg 26A:1, 1944
9. Freedman L, Munro RR: Abduction of the arm in the scapular plane: scapular and glenohumeral movements. A roentgenographic study. J Bone Joint Surg 48A:1503, 1966
10. Poppen NK, Walker PS: Normal and abnormal motion of the shoulder. J Bone Joint Surg 58A:195, 1976
11. Inman VT, Ralston HJ, Saunders JB, et al: Relation of human electromyograms to muscular tension. Electroencephalogr Clin Neurophysiol 4:187, 1952
12. Kendall HO, Kendall FP, Wadsworth GE: Muscles: Testing and Function. 2nd Ed. Williams & Wilkins, Baltimore, 1971
13. Stevens JH: Brachial plexus paralysis. p. 344. In Codman EA (ed): The Shoulder. Krieger Publishing, Melbourne, 1937
14. Sunderland S: Nerves and Nerve Injuries. 2nd Ed. Churchill Livingstone, Edinburgh, 1978

15. Bruxelle J, Travers V, Thiebaut JB: Occurrence and treatment of pain after brachial plexus injury. Clin Orthop Rel Res 237:87, 1988
16. Janda V: Muscles, central nervous motor regulation and back problems. p. 29. In Korr IM (ed): The Neurobiologic Mechanisms in Manipulative Therapy. Plenum, New York, 1978
17. Akeson WH, Amiel D, Mechanis GI, et al: Collagen cross-linking alterations in joint contractures: changes in the reducible cross-links in periarticular connective tissue collagen after nine weeks of immobilization. Connect Tissue Res 5:15, 1977
18. Highet WB: Grading of motor and sensory recovery in nerve injuries. p. 356. In Seddon HJ (ed): Peripheral Nerve Injuries. Medical Research Council Report Series T2 282. Her Majesty's Stationery Office, London, 1954
19. Daniels L, Worthingham C: Muscle Testing. Techniques of Manual Examination. 4th Ed. WB Saunders, Philadelphia, 1980
20. Hamm NH, Curtis D: Normative data for the Purdue pegboard on a sample of adult senditates for vocational rehabilitation. Percept Mot Skills 50:309, 1980
21. Travell JG, Simons DG: Myofascial Pain and Dysfunction. The Trigger Point Manual. Williams & Wilkins, Baltimore, 1984
22. Janda V: Some aspects of extracranial causes of facial pain. J Prosthet Dent 56:4, 1986
23. Yeoman PM: Cervical myelography in traction injuries of the brachial plexus. J Bone Joint Surg 50B:25, 1968
24. Bufalini C, Pesatori G: Posterior cervical electromyography in the diagnosis and prognosis of brachial plexus injuries. J Bone Joint Surg 51B:627, 1969
25. Bonney G, Gilliat RW: Sensory nerve conduction after traction lesion of the brachial plexus. Proc R Soc Med 51:365, 1958
26. Scott PM: Clayton's Electrotherapy and Actinotherapy. 7th Ed. Balliere Tindall, London, 1975
27. Tabary JC, Tardieu C, Tardieu G, Tabary C: Experimental rapid sarcomere loss with concomitant hypoextensibility. Muscle Nerve 4:198, 1981
28. Cooper RR: Alterations during immobilization and regeneration of skeletal muscles in cats. J Bone Joint Surg 54:919, 1972
29. Lampe GN, Mannheimer JS: Stimulation Characteristics of T.E.N.S. FA Davis, Philadelphia, 1984
30. Guyton AC: Organ Physiology: Structure and Function of the Nervous System. 2nd Ed. WB Saunders, Philadelphia, 1976
31. Maitland GD: Peripheral Manipulation. 2nd Ed. Butterworths, London, 1977
32. Gutman E, Guttman L: Effects of electrotherapy on denervated muscles in rabbits. Lancet 1:169, 1942
33. Hatano E, et al: Electrical stimulation on denervated skeletal muscles. p. 469. In Goria A (ed): Posttraumatic Peripheral Nerve Regeneration: Experimental Basis and Clinical Implications. Raven Press, New York, 1981
34. Reynold C: The stiff hand. p. 95. In Malick H, Kasch M (eds): Manual on Management of Specific Hand Problems. AREN Publication, Pittsburgh, 1984
35. Enos L, Lane K, MacDougal B: Brief or new: the use of self-adherent wrap in hand rehabilitation. Am J Occup Ther 38:265, 1984
36. Trombly C, Scott A: Occupational Therapy for Physical Dysfunction. Williams & Wilkins, Baltimore, 1977, p. 71
37. Saha AK: Dynamic stability of the glenohumeral joint. Acta Orthop Scand 42:491, 1971

38. Hislop HJ, Perrine JJ: The isokinetic concept of exercise. Phys Ther 47:114, 1967
39. Lehman JF, Masock AJ, Warren CG, Koblanski JN: Effect of therapeutic temperature on tendon extensibility. Arch Phys Med Rehabil 51:48, 1970
40. Trombly C, Scott A: Occupational Therapy for Physical Dysfunction. Williams & Wilkins, Baltimore, 1984

9 | Common Shoulder Problems in the Athlete

David C. Reid
Linda Saboe
Robert Burnham

Shoulder Problems

Although many published series deal with isokinetic parameters in the lower extremity, few data relate to the upper limb.[1,2] The increasing interest in pericapsular problems in swimmers and the relationship of those pathologies to muscle imbalance have made it imperative to have a knowledge of the normal condition of the upper limb.[3-6] It is also becoming increasingly apparent that there is an overlap between the simple impingement problems of overuse and those related to varying degrees of instability in the shoulder. Furthermore, the role of immobilization after initial shoulder dislocation is open to review, along with the speed of progression of rehabilitation.[7-10] Discussion on the outcome of most shoulder surgery has been based largely on complication rates, redislocation rates, or the examiner's subjective opinions regarding functional improvement.[11-13] This has made it difficult to evaluate data regarding specific treatment regimens and rehabilitation protocols. This chapter discusses a series of studies that we have completed relating to these issues. All isokinetic tests were performed using a Cybex II isokinetic dynamometer (Cybex, Ronkonkoma, NY) and standard protocols.[1,14] Abduction and adduction were tested with the subject in a supported sitting position (Fig. 9-1), and external and internal rotation were tested with the subject in standing and lying positions with the arm at the side and abducted to 90°, respectively (Figs. 9-2 and 9-3). All data are reported for 60°/s using the best of three trials.

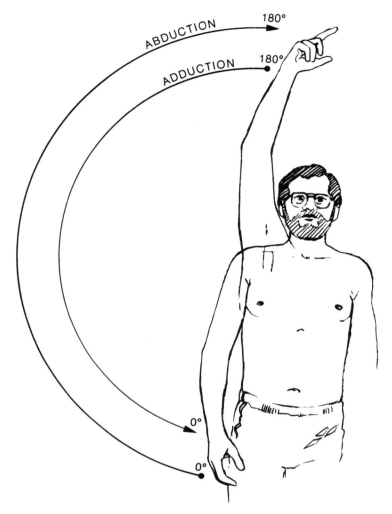

Fig. 9-1.   Abduction and adduction, both designated at 0° with the arm at the side.

Normal Subjects

The normal subjects were 40 moderately fit athletic individuals tested for a total of 80 shoulders. For all movements tested, men were approximately twice as strong as women (Fig. 9-4). There was no significant difference between dominant and nondominant arms. The strongest muscle group was the adductors, being about twice as strong as the abductors. If the adductors, being the strongest, are considered as 100 percent, the abductors are approximately 50 percent. The internal rotators were approximately 45 percent of the adductors and the external rotators were approximately 30 percent of the adductors

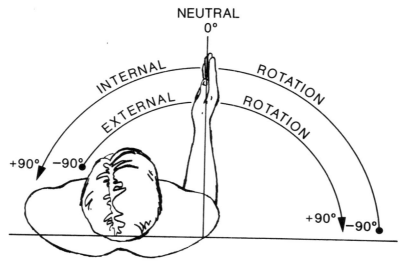

Fig. 9-2. Internal and external rotation with the upper arm held at the side. The neutral position is illustrated and positive and negative ranges are marked. ●——, Starting range; ——▶, finishing range.

when the arm was at 90° and 45 percent when the arm was in the neutral position. The external to internal rotation ratio was approximately 80 percent. A similar study was completed by Fowler, who agreed with the ratios for internal and external rotation at 90° abduction, but reported a ratio of 65 percent with the arm in the neutral position.[15] These ratios represent a normal healthy

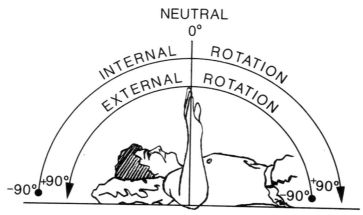

Fig. 9-3. Internal and external rotation with the arm abducted to 90°. The neutral position for each movement is marked. ●——, Starting range; ——▶, finishing range.

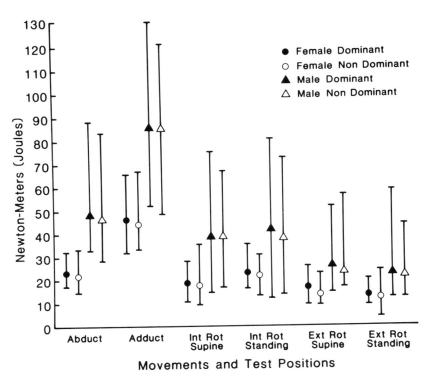

Fig. 9-4. Peak torques (Newton-meters) for each movement for the control or normal group are shown.

population and can be used as treatment goals for rehabilitation in much the same way as ratios are used for the quadriceps and hamstrings at the knee.

Swimmers

The incidence of shoulder pain is probably higher in swimmers than in those who participate in any other sport, constituting approximately 50 to 60 percent of all problems in highly competitive swimmers. This incidence is a marked increase over the 3 percent figure reported by Kennedy and Hawkins[5] in 1974 and Fowler[16] in 1979 and reflects the more intensive training at an increasingly young age.

The traditional concept of swimmer's shoulder is an anterior impingement syndrome involving mainly the supraspinatus or biceps tendon under the coracoacromial arch.[4] This is obviously an overuse syndrome. The contributing factors are anatomic impingement, impairment of the microcirculation, anatomic variations in the size of the bicipital groove, and muscle imbalance.[4,5,17,18] This last factor is significant in that it points to a potentially treatable entity by relatively simple means, namely, exercise. There is also a suggestion that a second constellation of signs and symptoms is present, particularly in swimmers who use the back and butterfly strokes, and involves a hypermobility syndrome with a tendency to painful subluxation. This, in turn, may generate a susceptibility to a painful impingement syndrome.[19–21]

We assessed 40 swimmers, 75 percent of whom had reached a national level of competition. Fifty percent of these swimmers had a past history of shoulder pain, reflecting the endurance or distance training of most swimmers with its repetitive abduction and circumduction maneuvers. Indeed, even swimming 10,000 meters a day, a nominal distance for many swimmers, would require that the athlete put each arm through at least 10,000 to 11,000 strokes a week.[1,6] It is important to recall that the upper extremities are the prime movers in swimming, with the lower extremities adding only a small percentage to speed, perhaps as little as 10 percent in the crawl stroke and a little more in the breast stroke.[1,22–24] Therefore, as training intensity increases, the stresses on the shoulder increase. Surprisingly, for the most part, the peak torques for swimmers were not significantly higher than for the fit athletic controls (Fig. 9-5). Female swimmers were the exception, having an upper limb strength of approximately 60 percent of that of males, reflecting the increased upper limb work of female swimmers over that of the general female athletic population. These findings have several implications.

First, isokinetic testing in stereotyped positions may not reflect the swimming stroke and, hence, may not provide a true assessment of the swimmer's power. Nevertheless, the importance of dry land training in strengthening the shoulder girdle area is sometimes neglected.

Second, swimming (even the so-called sprint events) is essentially an endurance sport when assessed from a metabolic viewpoint.[25,26] This concept is further supported by review of muscle biopsy specimens taken from the deltoid area of swimmers, which show a larger preponderance of type I fibers than do those taken from controls.[1] Dry land training should reflect this need, and high repetition work should form a large part of the strengthening program. Furthermore, future testing should include an endurance component so that a realistic assessment can be made of the swimmer's total power.

Last, the tests reported here were made at 60°/s, and testing at higher rates may be more sensitive to the differences among the swimming population.

In terms of practical advice, however, while conceding that dry land training is important, we believe that any swimmer with a history of shoulder pain, or one who is recovering from shoulder symptoms, should avoid resisted movements above shoulder level. Declined bench work and modified arm positions will give the desired strengthening effect without increasing the symptoms from impingement.

Because of the suggestion of muscle imbalance in the rotator group, special

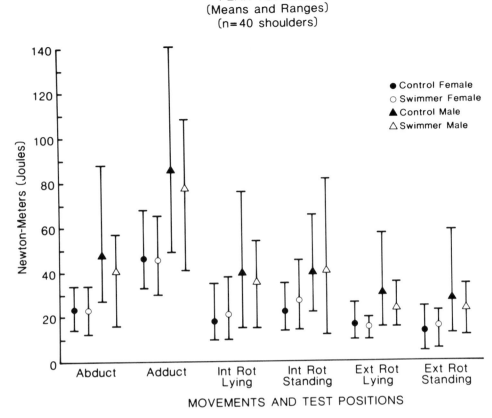

Fig. 9-5.   Peak torques of swimmers versus the control population.

emphasis was given to data relating to internal-external rotation ratios.[1] In our study, the internal rotators were stronger than the controls by approximately 10 percent; this is anticipated inasmuch as internal rotator strength correlates well with success in 100-meter freestyle swimming. Our results were not as dramatic as those of Fowler, who reported that external-internal rotation ratio in abduction was 62 percent in swimmers as opposed to 78 percent in control subjects.[15] In the neutral position, this difference was less remarkable, namely, 66 percent in controls and 53 percent in swimmers. Both of these studies reflect a slight proportionate weakness of the external rotation, and it is suggested that specific external rotator strengthening should form part of the treatment protocol for swimmers' shoulder. Naturally, muscle strengthening is combined with stroke modification. A swimmer in the acute phase of shoulder pain may have to discontinue swimming, or perhaps use only the breast stroke for several weeks, until the symptoms are resolved. Even then, the crawl or back stroke should be resumed cautiously.

Muscle tightness, particularly in the pectorals and anterior shoulder group, may be present in many young swimmers, and attention to this is mandatory for any treatment protocol.[27] However, stretching should be specific and directed at restoring normal range. Mobility of the swimmer's shoulder should be adequate to allow sufficient range of motion (ROM) for a comfortable stroke pattern. There is very little to be gained from excessive mobility. On the contrary, perverse stretching maneuvers may serve to produce functional instability. This is particularly true for those individuals with a tendency toward hypermobility. Preseason testing by team therapists should seek to identify swimmers with evidence of either local laxity of the shoulder or general ligament laxity and to protect them from excessive stretching. Often, the first clue to trouble is pain during turning or during the catch or entry phase of the back stroke. Although pain secondary to hypermobility or minor subluxation is difficult to treat, it responds to protection and slow, steady strengthening of the rotator groups. More dramatic hypermobility and frank subluxation rarely, if ever, respond to nonoperative treatment, and the swimmers may have to switch to the crawl or breast stroke.

Individuals with a history of bicipital tendinitis or supraspinatus tendinitis should also have the thoracic spine examined carefully. In some of these individuals, pre- and in-season mobilizations of the upper thoracic spine may allow easier achievement of full shoulder abduction and flexion. Thoracic mobility may destress the anterior structures under the coracoacromion arch during the extremes of range.

RECURRENT DISLOCATION

Recurrent anterior dislocation of the glenohumeral joint is a common phenomenon accounting for more than 80 percent of dislocations of the upper extremity.[13] In some individuals, the dislocation is predictable and can be avoided for the most part by modification of activity. In others, the unpredictability makes this an extremely disabling problem. The usual mechanism of dislocation, in day-to-day activities, is external rotation in the abducted position. However, in sporting activities, another situation is frequently described that involves simply abduction and adduction. For the volleyball player, it may occur during spiking or blocking; for the swimmer, during touching for the turn; and for the tennis player, during the serve. Little discussion has related to this particular mechanism. Furthermore, the role and efficacy of exercise in the prevention of dislocation is poorly understood.

By isokinetic testing, we evaluated 40 subjects who had dislocated a shoulder a minimum of three times. They all had symptoms sufficient to cause them to consider operative repairs. As would be anticipated, these subjects could not start to generate significant torque in the position of the apprehension test, namely, external rotation in abduction. However, surprisingly, the abductor and adductor groups reflected most weakness throughout the range, more so than the rotators.

Some individuals dislocated their shoulders during testing—not during rotation, but during forced adduction with the arm straight and externally rotated. In other words, as they contracted their adductors to bring their arm down, their shoulders dislocated. This may explain the mechanism of dislocation so frequently seen in sports. Furthermore, it emphasizes the concept that once someone has developed sufficient capsular laxity to allow recurrent dislocation, muscle strengthening will do little to alleviate the situation. Indeed, the very muscles that keep the humeral head securely in place, in the so-called safe positions of the joint, actively dislocate the head from the glenoid in the abducted position. That is, dislocation tends to be an active processs not simply a passive phenomenon accompanying abduction with external rotation.

These statements do not deny the usefulness of shoulder rehabilitation when muscle weakness exists but explain why muscle strengthening will not prevent redislocation if there is sufficient capsular laxity.

TREATMENT OF INITIAL DISLOCATION

The orthopedic literature reflects confusion as to the correct management of first dislocations.[7,8,13] The length of strict immobilization after reduction varies considerably, from 2 days to 8 weeks.[7-10] The result of these haphazard approaches is reflected in the subsequent redislocation rate, which is between 80 to 90 percent in persons less than 20 years of age at the time of their first dislocation,[13] approximately 60 percent for persons 20 to 30 years of age, and between 20 to 40 percent for those who are more than 40 years of age.[13] These figures have left most individuals with a feeling of inevitability; hence, many physicians and therapists feel that since there is a great chance of redislocation whatever the treatment, it is better to opt for early mobilization, early strengthening, and rapid return to sport, activity, or occupation—a rather fatalistic approach, based on poor control of early treatment, low patient compliance, and inadequate therapy.

A more careful review of the literature reveals an important underlying concept, first suggested by Watson-Jones in 1956,[28] that the initial period of immobilization is important in prevention of recurrences. This perspective has been recently adopted by several groups and is gaining momentum. In 50 individuals less than 30 years of age, the recurrence rate was reduced to less than 20 percent with treatment of 6 weeks of strict immobilization. Early isometric exercises are taught to the individual by the therapist while the arm is immobilized in a sling and swath, and are performed twice daily for the first 3 weeks. Axillary hygiene is performed with the arm strictly by the side, and the elbow is removed from the sling several times a day to allow flexion and extension, which assists comfort and prevents stiffness. Care is taken to avoid all external rotation. For the second 3-week period, gentle pendular exercises are given, mainly with the arm in a sling, and external rotation is allowed just short of neutral with the arm kept adducted against the body. External rotation is not permitted with the arm away from the side. Abduction with the arm internally rotated is permitted to 45°. Following this period, from 6 weeks on, the emphasis is on strengthening for about 4 weeks, allowing ROM to resume with gentle active motion. After this time, ROM can be actively pursued and becomes a major rehabilitation goal. Passive stretching should be avoided in the first 12 weeks after dislocation. In a few instances in which the shoulder appears particularly stiff, mobilization can be pursued more aggressively and slightly earlier, but only at 6 weeks after dislocation.

In 1984, Kuriyama et al. gave us a better insight as to the pathology of anterior dislocations by performing arthrograms on 143 first dislocations.[11] This group noticed that there were two main types of dislocations. Two-thirds of them were capsular tears, that is, the humeral head ripped out through the capsule. One-third were capsular detachments, that is, the glenoid labrum or adjacent capsule was detached from the glenoid margin. The importance of this observation is that capsular tears have a great propensity for healing, which is not so obvious with the labrum detachments. This concept is reinforced by the fact that of those shoulders that later redislocated, 90 percent were of the capsular detachment type—the danger group for redislocation. More important, those persons who were strictly immobilized for 3 weeks had a redislocation rate that was amazingly low: 3.4 percent versus 47.7 percent for those who were immobilized for a shorter period.[11]

Furthermore, Kuriyama et al. showed, with follow-up arthrograms, that capsular healing and rebuilding could be demonstrated at 3 weeks but not before.[11] This underlies the importance of early immobilization during this vulnerable 3-week period.

With these data as a background, every effort should be made to obtain patient compliance for early immobilization with a sling and swath, supplemented by carefully taught isometric exercises. The previously outlined regimen will provide excellent functional outcomes and reduce the devastatingly high redislocation rate that has come to be accepted as inevitable.

FUNCTIONAL OUTCOME OF SHOULDER REPAIRS

The three commonly used surgical techniques for stabilizing recurrent dislocating shoulders are the Magnuson-Stack, the Putti-Platt, and the Bristow repairs. These three repairs represent three different principles.

The Magnuson-Stack type of repair is a simple procedure, taking all layers, capsule, cuff, and subscapularis tendon, and overlapping all layers as one, and frequently fixing it with a staple, taking care to avoid the long head of biceps.[29,30]

The Putti-Platt repair is a more involved procedure, taking the capsule in one layer and the subscapularis tendon in another, and separately plicating each layer.[13] It tends to give a very tight repair, limiting external rotation; hence, it may be less than ideal for the treatment of athletes in some sports.

The Bristow repair is based around transfer of the tip of the coracoid process with the conjoint tendon of biceps and coracobrachialis to the neck of the scapula. As such, a dynamic sling is formed in the position of abduction and external rotation when these tendons tighten across the front of the neck of the scapula.[31,32] Although there is some debate as to whether the bone block forms a static impediment to dislocation, in many cases it is able to do so, sitting as it does in the fossa which may be occupied by a dislocating humeral head. It is the preferred type of operation for athletes because of the possibility of early restoration of nearly full ROM.

The decision for one operation over another has largely been based on complication and redislocation rates, and there is little information about functional outcomes.[13] Our data are incomplete but examine the functional endpoint of these three classes of operations. Our study so far includes 40 patients with Putti-Platt repairs and a preliminary series with the other procedures, with patients followed from 1 to 11 years (mean, 6 years).

Present information indicates that adequate rehabilitation provides normal strength on the operated side with all repairs. Furthermore, full ROM, or very minimally limited external rotation and abduction, is also possible. Occasionally, a person with a Putti-Platt repair may have an unacceptable range for a few selected sports. The incidence of this is very low. Full ROM is more rapidly achieved with the Bristow repair.

Based on this information, the type of operation should be selected based on the surgeon's skill and experience in performing that procedure and its known complication rates.

Awareness of multidirectional instability will prevent the pitfall of carrying out these traditional operations for dislocation unsuccessfully. It is imperative to consider the inferior capsular shift procedure whenever there is an element of inferior subluxation along with the anterior dislocation. One of the easiest clinical signs for detecting this is to put longitudinal traction along the relaxed arm while palpating beneath the tip of the acromion. A positive sign is present when a sulcus either appears or is palpable in response to this distracting maneuver.

Furthermore, all the procedures will be more compatible with early return to full function if coupled with an adequate rehabilitation protocol.

The known complications include redislocation, pain, vascular and neural compromise, loose or migrating internal fixation devices, interference with the biceps tendon, infection, and, in the Bristow repair, possible nonunion. Most of these complications are uncommon, with the exception of redislocation rates. A literature review reveals that after the Magnuson-Stack procedure, there is a redislocation rate of 0 to 17 percent, with an average of approximately 4 percent. The Putti-Platt procedure has a redislocation rate of between 0 to 8 percent, with an average of 4 percent, while the Bristow procedure is reported as having an average of slightly more than 2 percent redislocation, with a range of 0 to 3 percent.[10,13,31,32]

With care taken to obtain an adequate bone block and good screw fixation, and with well-planned therapy, the Bristow procedure is likely to give the earliest return to normal function and the lowest redislocation rate.

Rehabilitation includes isometric exercises for the first 3 weeks after surgery, with pendular and gentle active exercises for the next 3 weeks. No resistance is given; abduction is limited to 45° and external rotation to neutral. At 6 weeks, it is assumed that bone healing is well underway and that the capsular repair is sound. Subsequent rehabilitation is guided by pain. Heavy resisted work and forced external rotation are delayed until postoperative week 12.

SHOULDER SUBLUXATION

Shoulder subluxation with functional impairment is particularly difficult to assess and treat. Nevertheless, an understanding of the synergic role of both the internal and external rotators has opened a potentially exciting avenue of treatment. Our current work involves the use of biofeedback techniques to gain functional control of the external rotators. These muscles particularly prevent unwanted anterior glide in the glenoid fossa during overhead motions. The concept is not so much to strengthen but to evolve and reinforce functional engrams for controlling subtle intra-articular glides. We are currently carrying out several prospective studies on this treatment approach, and the early responses are promising.

SUMMARY

Isokinetic data has been presented in relation to several problems of the shoulder, after initial establishment of normal values. These normal values are offered as treatment goals for a healthy athletic population. There is still a need for normal values to be established for older persons as well as for children before and after their growth spurts.

Swimmers' shoulder, an anterior impingement syndrome, has its basis in overuse, but the disproportionate strength of internal over external rotators may be a contributing factor and should be corrected during therapy for this condition. It is conceded that adequate ROM is essential for good swimming, but overstretching can produce problems of its own. Particular care should be taken to identify those persons who have a basic tendency for loose joints and to protect them adequately from perverse overstretching. Once developed, functional instability of the shoulder is very difficult to treat in swimmers and may necessitate a change in stroke, with elimination of the butterfly and back strokes.

In a study of persons with recurrent dislocations, the role of the adductor muscle group in precipitating dislocation has been described, explaining the failure of muscle-strengthening routines to prevent redislocations. Nevertheless, the importance of restoring normal muscle power, where wasting is present, is undeniable.

The incidence of recurrent dislocation can be directly linked to inadequate immobilization and progressive rehabilitation of the first traumatic dislocation.

With correct treatment, an 80 percent redislocation rate is not inevitable, even in a young age group.

Of the frequently used surgical repairs for recurrent dislocation of the shoulder, the Bristow procedure appears to give the earliest return to activity and function as well as the potentially lowest redislocation rate, making it the preferred operation for most athletes.

An exciting new area of treatment is the use of biofeedback in the control of the deep rotators in patients with subluxations. The thrust of this therapy is not so much just strengthening but the development of muscle control.

With the glenohumeral joint having so little bony structural stability, dynamic mechanisms for movement and control are paramount. Much of the muscle action is indirect, through force couples. As such, small alterations in balance of power and neural control can profoundly affect function. It is little wonder then that rehabilitation plays a pivotal role in all of the common orthopaedic problems in the shoulder area. The data presented in this chapter emphasize this fact.

REFERENCES

1. Elsner RC, Pedegana LR, Lang J: Protocol for strength testing as rehabilitation of the upper extremity. J Orthop Sports Phys Ther 4:229, 1983
2. McMurray DL: Determination of the isokinetic peak torques of the external and internal rotator muscles of the shoulder in a normal adult female population. MSc Thesis. University of Alabama. Birmingham, Alabama, 1983
3. Marino M: Profiling swimmers. Clin Sports Med 3:211, 1984
4. Domingrez RH: Shoulder pain in swimmers. Phys Sports Med 8:37, 1980
5. Kennedy JD, Hawkins RJ: Swimmer's shoulder. Phys Sports Med 2:34, 1974
6. Foster CR: Multidirectional instability of the shoulder in the athlete. Clin Sports Med 2:355, 1983
7. Rowe CR: Factors related to recurrences of anterior dislocation of the shoulder. Clin Orthop 20:21, 1961
8. Hastings DE: Recurrent subluxation of the glenohumeral joint. Am J Sports Med 9:352, 1981
9. Aroneu JG: Decreasing the incidence of first time anterior shoulder dislocations with rehabilitation. Am J Sports Med 12:283, 1984
10. Simonet WT, Cofield RH: Prognosis in anterior shoulder dislocation. Am J Sports Med 12:19, 1984
11. Kuriyama S, Fujimaki E, Katagiri T, Uemura S: Anterior dislocation of the shoulder joint sustained through skiing. Am J Sports Med 12:339, 1984
12. Pappas AM: Symptomatic shoulder instability due to lesions of the glenoid labrum. Am J Sports Med 11:279, 1983
13. Rockwood CA: Dislocations about the shoulder. In Rockwood CA, Green DP (eds): Fractures. JB Lippincott, Philadelphia, 1975
14. Cybex, Division of Lumex Corp: Isolated Joint Testing and Exercise. A Handbook for Using the Cybex II and the UBXT. Bayshore, New York, 1980
15. Fowler P: Unpublished data. University of Western Ontario, London, Ontario, 1985
16. Fowler P: Swimmer problems. Am J Sports Med 7:141, 1979

17. O'Donoghue DH: Subluxing biceps tendon in the athlete. J Sports Med 13:28, 1973
18. Hitchcock HH, Bechtol CO: Painful shoulders. J Bone Joint Surg (Am) 30:267, 1948
19. Strauss MB, Wrobel LJ, Neft RS, Cady GW: The shrugged-off shoulder: a comparison of patients with recurrent subluxations and dislocations. Physician Sports Med 11:85, 1983
20. Hastings DE, Coughlin LP: Recurrent subluxation of the glenohumeral joint. Am J Sports Med 9:352, 1981
21. Mathews LS, Oueida SJ: Glenohumeral instability in athletes. Spectrum, diagnosis and treatment. Adv Orthop Surg 8:236, 1985
22. Jopke T: Training swimmers. How coaches get results. Physician Sports Med 10:161, 1982
23. Sharp RL, Troop JP, Costil DL: Relationship between power and sprint free style swimming. Med Sci Sports Exerc 14:53, 1982
24. Rodeo S: Swimming breast stroke: a kinesiological analysis and considerations for strength training. NSCA J 4–8 Aug. and Sept., 1984
25. Costill DL, Fink WJ, Hargreaves M, et al: Metabolic characteristics of skeletal muscle during detraining from competitive swimming. Med Sci Sports Exerc 17:339, 1985
26. Magel JR, Andersen KL: Pulmonary diffusing capacity and cardiac output in young trained Norwegian swimmers and undetermined subjects. Med Sci Sports 1:131, 1969
27. Hovelius L, Eriksson K, Fredin H: Recurrences after initial dislocation for the shoulder. J Bone Joint Surg 65A:343, 1983
28. Watson-Jones R: Fractures and Joint Injuries. E & S Livingstone, Edinburgh, 1976
29. Aamoth GM, O'Phalen EH: Recurrent anterior dislocation of the shoulder: a review of 40 athletes treated by subscapularis transfer. Am J Sports Med 8:188, 1977
30. Miller LS, Donahue JR, Good RP, Staerk AJ: The Magnuson-Stack procedure for treatment of recurrent glenohumeral dislocations. Am J Sports Med 12:133, 1984
31. Halley DK, Olix MD: A review of the Bristow operation for recurrent anterior shoulder dislocation in athletes. Clin Orthop 106:175, 1979
32. Braly WG, Tullos H: A modification of the Bristow procedure for recurrent anterior dislocation of the shoulder. Am J Sports Med 13:81, 1985

10 | Throwing Injuries to the Shoulder

Turner A. Blackburn, Jr.

Why has the understanding of the throwing act and the injuries associated with it lagged behind that of the study of the knee and ankle? After all, baseball is "America's pastime." Could it be that the overwhelming number of ankle and knee injuries predisposed more intensive study of these joints? Because knee and ankle injuries occur in almost all sports, but throwing injuries only occur in throwers, could the emphasis of research have ignored them? Has the small "clique-ish" world of professional baseball disallowed changes or research that may be of benefit?

Unless there is a dislocation, separation, complete rotator cuff tear, or fracture, it is difficult to diagnose a pitcher's or thrower's complaint about an ache, pain, or overuse injury involving the shoulder. Examination techniques, history taking with an *understanding* of throwing, and an actual ability to see the injury without disabling the athlete with surgery have only recently been developed.

The advent of the arthroscopic diagnostic examination of the shoulder has allowed the correlation of physical examination and history with pathology. Three puncture holes in the shoulder capsule do not preclude the athlete's throwing again. Open procedures on the shoulder almost always produced sufficient scar tissue to prevent full form and flexibility, therefore also preventing a return to full function.

Because the arthroscope is generating more interest in throwers, the biomechanist is now studying the pitching act with much more enthusiasm. An understanding of the pitching act means a better understanding of the pitching injury. Many times, an adjustment in the biomechanics of the form of the thrower will be all that is needed to treat an injury.

The addition of specific exercises applied to the pitching act to recreate concentric or eccentric contractions that occur in specific positions has greatly enhanced the progress the athlete can make in recovering from an injury.

The goals and objectives of this chapter are to familiarize readers with the mechanics of throwing and injuries that occur when overuse or poor mechanics occur, and to provide insight into diagnosis and treatment of injuries. Specific injuries will be discussed with emphasis on soft tissue problems. Arthroscopic surgery will be discussed as surgical intervention. Rehabilitation techniques will be explored extensively with emphasis on proper form for exercise and a return to throwing outline.

MECHANISMS OF THROWING

The act of overhead throwing is a series of rotational movements that include the thrower getting the hand and, thus, the ball moving at speeds up to 100 mph. This orchestrated and coordinated movement requires skill and athletic ability as well as strength and flexibility. It requires input from all areas of the body, including legs, abdomen, back, shoulder, elbow, and wrist. The rotational movements actually allow a "whipping" motion to occur throughout the chain from foot to hand, propelling the ball.

As injuries occur in the throwing act, it becomes apparent that the shoulder takes its fair share of the load. The overhead toss calls for the elevation of the humerus, which obviously calls for proximal stabilization at the glenohumeral joint and the scapulothoracic joint. Raising the arm overhead uses the much-discussed scapulohumeral rhythm described by Codman.[1] The coordinated movement has a ratio of glenohumeral movement to scapular movement of 3:2.[2] The scapula is controlled by a balance of forces of the various portions of the trapezius, levator scapulae, and serratus anterior. There are associated movements at the acromioclavicular joint and sternoclavicular joint.[3] There is rotation of the clavicle along with retraction and protraction of the shoulder complex occurring at the sternoclavicular joint during the pitching act.

Windup

The pitching act begins with the windup. This phase of pitching will vary with every pitcher and the condition of the game as far as base runners. No injuries occur during this phase, but it is a very important part of throwing because it begins a series of events that puts the body into motion. Windup occurs from the beginning movements to the point where the ball hand and gloved hand separate.

This phase gets the arms up overhead after a downward swing. Body weight is first shifted forward on the right foot (for right-handed pitchers; weight shifts first to the left foot for left-handed pitchers) and then back to the left foot. As in most sports that require propelling of an object, the shift of body weight begins the real power move. Rotation begins in this phase as the shoulder turns 90° to the plate. The left knee is lifted and pulled upward and to the right as the hips also turn nearly 90°. The weight is now shifted forward slightly to the right foot, but the center of balance does not yet shift over the middle of the body. The body is coiled in rotation of right leg, hips, and trunk. The "scapulothoracic rhythm" has the arm position up and away from the body. The individual may show many variations in this movement, especially with knee lift height and rotation.

Cocking

As in any whipping type of action, activities do not occur at the same time, but along a continuous "chain." The cocking phase describes the positioning of the glenohumeral joint. The point at which the hands break to maximal external rotation is described as the cocking phase. At the same time that the hands break, the center of balance of the body moves forward. The left leg extends forward and plants with the foot pointed toward the plate. Once the center of balance is forward, the right leg, with foot pointed perpendicular to the line of throw, drives the body weight forward. At about the time of left foot plant, the arm is at its fullest external rotation. The left hand and arm are propelled into extension and horizontal abduction to help speed the rotation of the trunk to the left.

The glenohumeral joint is brought to an external rotation of approximately 140° to 160°. Slow-motion analysis shows that this occurs at the glenohumeral joint and the scapulothoracic joint. The humerus is abducted to 90°. Indeed, the descriptions of a pitcher as throwing "overhand," "three-quarters," or "sidearm" are misnomers. Most of these pitchers have their glenohumeral joint at 90° but their body leaning to the right or left gives them the appearance of being in these various positions. Trunk rotation brings the humerus back behind the frontal plane. As the left foot plants and begins the first deceleration of the body's frontal motion, the "whipping" action begins, which puts the humerus into 30° of horizontal abduction. Thus, the glenohumeral joint leads the forward frontal horizontal adduction of the humerus. Anterior structures of the glenohumeral joint are under great stress at this point. The internal rotators of the humerus are put under maximum stress and stretch.

During the cocking phase, the posterior deltoid brings the humerus back into horizontal adduction. The supraspinatus, infraspinatus, and teres minor must aid in pulling the arm back as well as stabilizing the humeral head. The subscapularis, as well as other internal rotators such as the pectoralis major and latissimus dorsi, fires in late cocking to stop the posterior movement of the humerus. But, because of the whipping chain effect that occurs, the pectoralis major, latissimus dorsi, and subscapularis begin to contract and start pulling the arm forward before the humerus is at full external rotation. Because acceleration occurs once the ball moves forward, these activities have already occurred in the "acceleration" muscles.[4] During this movement, the proximal stabilizers near the scapula are firing to maintain a solid base for the movement of the humerus. The elbow is flexed at 90°, with cocontraction in the triceps and biceps. The forearm is at neutral, and the wrist is slightly extended.

Acceleration

The acceleration phase starts with the forward motion of the ball until it is released. We must not forget that the ball is the last thing to move forward. The thrower's left foot is already planted and the hips have rotated back to the left. The trunk is rotating to the left. The humerus moves in a horizontal adduction direction for 40 ms and the ball comes forward in internal rotation for approximately 40 ms.

The elbow moves from 90° flexion to 25° to 30° extension. There is tremendous force across the anterior shoulder and the medial side of the elbow. The humeral head has forces that are trying to pull it anteriorly out of the socket. In this brief 80 ms, very high forces occur.

The scapular stabilizers continue to function during this stage. The rotator cuff muscles are active as stabilizers of the humeral head but do not show a high degree of activity.[5] The pectoralis major and latissimus dorsi have done their job by now and, although active, are not doing as much as during the cocking phase. The triceps work extremely hard in accelerating the elbow into extension. The point of ball release is somewhere near the ear level. The hand is moving as fast as the ball (as much as 90 to 95 mph).

Ball Release

The ball release is a very nebulous event. The fastest cameras have a difficult time discerning exactly when the ball leaves the fingertips. Just prior to the 6- to 7-ms event, the pronators of the forearm are controlling the type of pitch. The pitcher applies force to the ball through the fingers. All pitchers go into a relative amount of pronation. The wrist may be slightly flexed at release.

Deceleration

Once the ball is released, the body must slow down the hand and, therefore, the arm. The foot strike of the left foot starts this deceleration of the body. At ball release, it has been estimated that there may be 300 lb of force trying to pull the arm forward out of the socket.

The forces that occur during the first 40 ms after the ball release are the highest and most difficult to control. The rotator cuff, posteriorly, must accomplish this deceleration. The cuff fires at extremely high levels of electromyographic activity.[5] Deceleration is accomplished through an eccentric contraction of the posterior cuff. Again, the scapular stabilizers must also do their job to allow the cuff to do its job. The bicep contracts violently, slowing the elbow extension. This force is transmitted across the humeral head for stabilization.

Follow-Through

After the first 40 ms of activity of deceleration, the follow-through phase allows the rest of the absorption of the throwing energy to occur. It also puts throwers in a position to protect themselves from balls that may be hit back toward them. There is a stretch of the posterior shoulder structure as well as a diminished activity in the posterior cuff muscle.

INJURY MECHANICS

The American Medical Association's Standard Nomenclature of Athletic Injuries[6] describes the classifications of musculotendinous injuries that occur at the shoulder in throwing.

Grade I muscle strain:
   a. Mild
   b. No tearing
   c. Minimal symptoms
   d. Heal quickly
Grade II muscle strain:
   a. Moderate
   b. Tearing fibers
   c. Swelling
   d. Functional disability
   e. May take 6 weeks to heal
Grade III muscle strain:
   a. Severe
   b. Complete tear or rupture
   c. Severe loss of function
   d. Much time loss

Overloading occurs at the shoulder joint during the pitching motion and elbow injury occurs. This overload may be intrinsic or extrinsic. It may come from forces produced by the body itself intrinsically through muscle contractions, such as in the acceleration phase when anterior muscles contract and pull the arm forward. It may occur when the ball is released and the arm must be slowed, which produces higher forces than are usually found with concentric contractions during the acceleration phase. This extrinsic force produced when the ball is released must be controlled through eccentric contractions of the posterior cuff. Because most injuries occur during the acceleration and deceleration phases, the intrinsic–extrinsic concept helps one correlate the pitching motion with the injury.

During acceleration, the movements of horizontal adduction and internal rotation produce a grinding force on the glenoid labrum. The acceleration muscles are trying to pull the humerus anteriorly over the labrum and out of the fossa. Movement of the humeral head may damage the labrum anteriorly and superiorly. If the posterior stabilizing muscles (i.e., posterior rotator cuff) are weaker, the anterior force may succeed in damaging the anterior labrum. The forces during acceleration are high, but the rate remains relatively constant, so muscles rarely tear. During deceleration, forces are high and the rate of deceleration is increasing, thereby producing much higher forces on the posterior cuff muscles. This extrinsic loading causes tissue tearing in the posterior rotator cuff.

Overuse causes an inflammatory response to microtrauma, leaving the athlete sore. Early mild injuries such as this respond quickly to rest, exercises, and modalities. When these overuse situations are pushed, they become chronic and severe. Usually, the overuse situation causes a change in throwing biomechanics, and insult is added to injury. As weakness occurs because of abnormal biomechanics, more stress is put on structures that, when damaged, cause more severe damage, such as the rotator cuff. Poor mechanics may even put stress on the suprascapular nerve, which is sometimes injured in the throwing athlete.

The force that the bicep produces when slowing the elbow during deceleration is also applied across the anterior humerus. The long head of the biceps has an intimate attachment to the glenoid labrum. These high forces may help tear the biceps partially. Biceps tendinitis occurs in many throwing overuse syndromes. Rarely is the biceps at fault, but it is representative of other problems about the shoulder.

Because the arm is only taken to 90° of abduction in throwing, impingement syndromes in the pure sense of the word do not occur as in swimming, when the arm is taken overhead more than 90°. Extrinsic overload at the posterior rotator cuff causes tissue tearing at the superior cuff area. If there is rotator cuff weakness, impingement may occur on elevation to 90°. This will present itself as an impingement pain on examination when the arm is brought up more than 90°.

Of course, poor pitching mechanics can cause undue stress (i.e., decreased external rotation, horizontal abduction, or full horizontal adduction) during throwing. The most common combination seen is weakness in the posterior cuff muscle and a lack of full external rotation.

Anterior pain can usually be associated with opening up too soon. This happens when pitchers try to whip the arm by rotating the body away from the pitching arm sooner and faster than they should to create more arm speed. Injuries resulting in this situation are mild and respond to conservative measures quickly. Proper instruction in pitching technique is important to prevent injury. Exercise strengthens the shoulder.

EXAMINATION

The usual history of a thrower with a partial rotator cuff tear or labrum tear is one of 12 to 18 months of symptoms that come and go. Symptoms usually improve with rest. Return to play usually exacerbates them. Many times, players are told to rest and not to throw, and are given no exercises. Then they are asked to pitch in a game after 10 days. Naturally, reinjury occurs.

Those throwers with an anterior–superior labrum tear have problems at ball release when they describe they cannot "let the ball go." The partial rotator cuff lesion athlete has pain on trying to increase the intensity of the pitching act, but may be able to throw with no pain at lesser intensity.

Many athletes go home during the off-season months and "rest" the injury, then come back to spring training and have a difficult time. Young pitchers who just make a club may come to spring camp trying to impress the coaches, throwing harder and more times than they ever have. They are injured and say nothing, afraid they will be cut from the team, and end up hurting their careers.

The physical examination must be systematic and precise so that nothing is omitted. With the athlete sitting up straight, a visual inspection will reveal atrophy in the upper quadrant in both anterior and posterior positions. This may occur in the supraspinatus, infraspinatus, teres minor, and deltoid, and sometimes in the pectoralis major. Chronic problems in the shoulder area will show deltoid atrophy much as the quadricep will demonstrate atrophy with a knee problem. Supraspinatus nerve lesions are demonstrated by posterior cuff weakness.

The coordination of scapulothoracic involvement can be observed when the arm is raised overhead. The throwing side of the athlete will be hyperatrophied and may show abnormal positioning of the scapula.

Palpation of the shoulder can also be accomplished with the athlete in the sitting position. The coracoid process, where the short head of the bicep attaches as well as the shoulder depressors, may be sore. The long head of the biceps can be palpated next. The sternoclavicular joint, acromioclavicular joint, deltoid, subdeltoid bursae, trapezius, and levator scapula insertion can all be palpated with the athlete in a sitting position.

With the athlete supine and the humerus in neutral position, the long head of the biceps can be examined. With the humerus externally rotated, the subscapular tendon can be checked. With the humerus internally rotated, the supraspinatus insertion can be palpated for tenderness. With the athlete prone and the arm hanging off the table, the examiner's fingers can work under the posterior deltoid and palpate the posterior cuff.

Passive flexibility of the shoulder is now ascertained. When the athlete is sitting, a passive horizontal adduction maneuver (Fig. 10-1) indicates the tightness of the posterior structures. This motion is important for follow through. When the athlete is supine, external rotation of the shoulder is checked at 90°, 135°, and full abduction (Fig. 10-2). Passively, it should reach well into the 140° to 160° range. There should be no pain. Internal rotation will be reduced to as much as 45°, which appears normal in baseball pitchers. Pure abduction

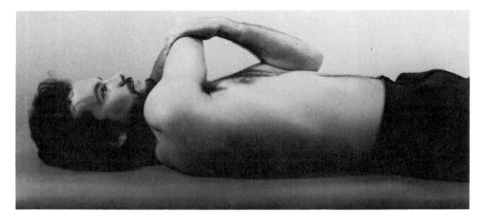

Fig. 10-1.   Horizontal adduction flexibility.

without winging of the scapula should be evident (Fig. 10-3). The shoulder should be able to reach 30° of horizontal abduction.

Several manual muscle tests give clues concerning specific injuries about the shoulder. Jobe and Moyers have taught us that the supraspinatus is best tested in the standing position with the arm abducted to 90° and horizontally abducted to 30°. The humerus is internally rotated fully[7] (Fig. 10-4). Pain and weakness here represent injury to the posterior rotator cuff and results from the impingement process. Baseball players with an otherwise normal shoulder will have pain in this test. The deltoid atrophies with injury and should be tested in flexion and abduction. External rotation is tested with the humerus at 90° abduction and 45° external rotation (Fig. 10-5). This represents the strength of the posterior cuff in the throwing position. The external rotation test at 0° of humeral abduction with the elbow at 90° tests the infraspinatus and teres minor (Fig. 10-6). The posterior musculature can be checked with the athlete prone and the arm horizontally abducted at 90°.

Joint testing involves several maneuvers. Laxity of the capsule can be elicited with the patient supine by manually trying to slide the humerus anteriorly (Fig. 10-7) and posteriorly (Fig. 10-8). During this maneuver, the popping of a torn labrum may be elicited (Fig. 10-9) by bringing the arm into full abduction and circumduction.

COMMON INJURIES

Deltoid

A deltoid strain can cause anterior pain. Grades I and II strains may slow the athlete down, but usually heal quickly. Conservative measures including ice, moist heat, ultrasound, and electric stimulation are of benefit. Exercises

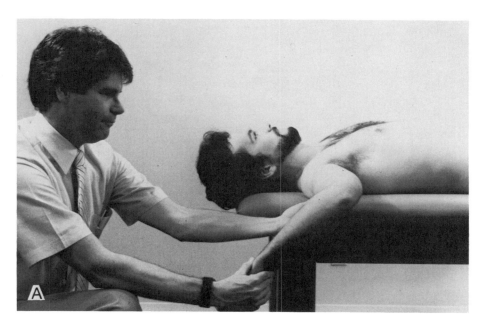

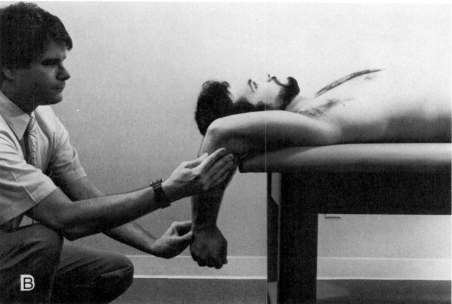

Fig. 10-2. **(A)** External rotation at 90° abduction. **(B)** External rotation at 135° abduction. (*Figure continues.*)

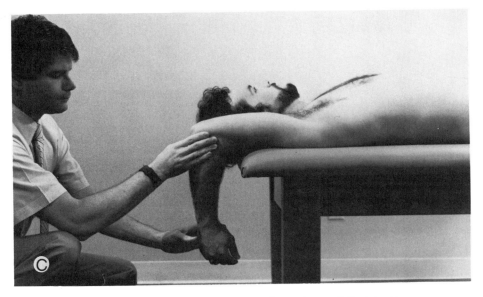

Fig. 10-2. *(Continued).* **(C)** External rotation at full abduction.

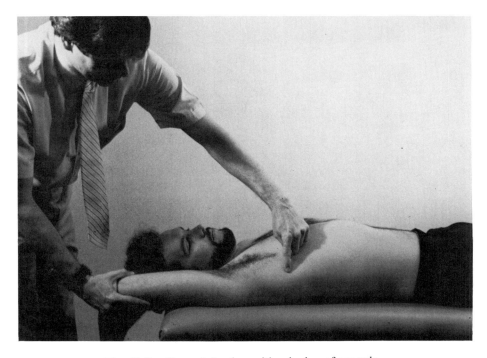

Fig. 10-3. Pure abduction with winging of scapula.

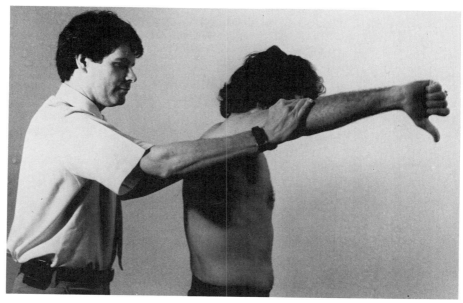

Fig. 10-4.   Supraspinatus position.

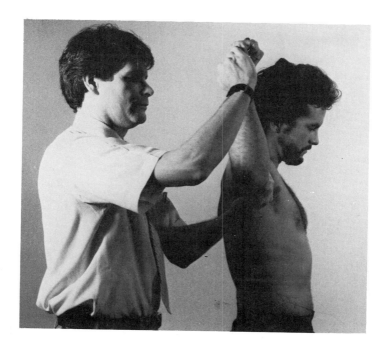

Fig. 10-5.   External rotation manual muscle test at 90°.

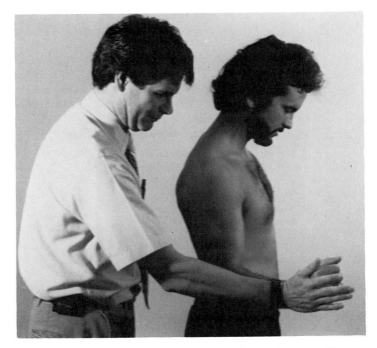

Fig. 10-6.   External rotation manual muscle test at 0°.

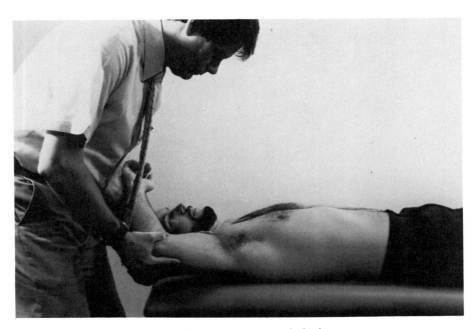

Fig. 10-7.   Anterior capsule laxity.

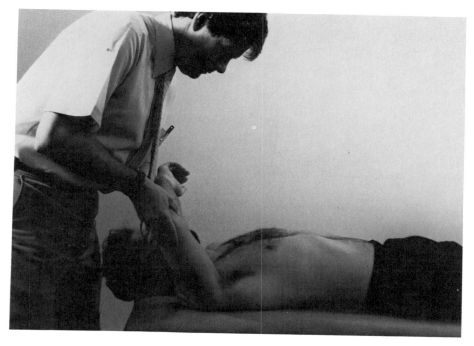

Fig. 10-8. Posterior capsule laxity.

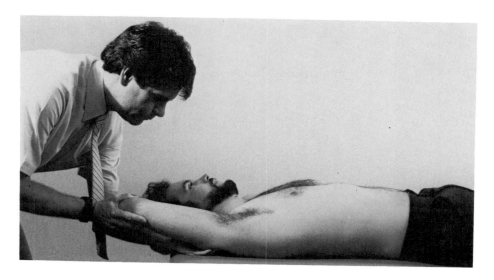

Fig. 10-9. Glenoid labrum grind test.

for the anterior deltoid are most important. In chronic shoulder problems, the anterior deltoid atrophies. It is a most important structure, especially in the acceleration phase of throwing.

Subdeltoid Bursitis

This inflammatory process can occur in the thrower. It is found by direct palpation of the bursa. It is usually associated with pain during the acceleration phase of throwing. Again, conservative measures apply. A steroid injection may be considered only in stubborn cases and only if there is no rotator cuff injury.

Subdeltoid Adhesions

If there are frequent repeated episodes of subdeltoid bursitis, a chronic inflammatory process will develop. This can lead to adhesions in the bursal sac. The player will have a reduction in range of motion (ROM), with a painful arc of movement. Other tests will prove negative for other problems. An injection of 0.5 percent bupivacaine and early light throwing can break up these adhesions. Chronic adhesions may have to be excised surgically.

Subscapular Tendonitis

During the acceleration phase, the subscapularis is very active in throwing. This muscle can develop tendonitis. Palpation will elicit this pain, and conservative measures and exercise should help the tendonitis heal.

Pectoralis Major Muscle Ruptures

A rare injury is the rupture of the pectoralis major. It is usually seen in the throwing of heavy objects, such as a javelin or discus. It also occurs in weight lifters. It occurs during the acceleration phase of throwing. Many times, it occurs at the sternal and clavicular origin of the pectoralis major. There may be a history of extrinsic overload and soreness locally. The pectoralis muscle belly can rupture by intrinsic overloading in the mid-phase of acceleration.

Latissimus Dorsi Muscle Rupture

Latissimus dorsi muscle ruptures are about as rare as pectoralis major ruptures. They occur when internal rotation forces are applied during the throwing act.

Biceps Tendonitis

Tendonitis of the long head of the biceps as it passes through the bicipital groove is overdiagnosed in the throwing athlete. Many times it is associated with other pathology. The biceps tendon long head has an important stabilization function in the throwing act. If other stabilizers (i.e., posterior rotator cuff) are weakened, the bicep must carry more of the load. The tendon is sore through excursion through the bicipital groove. Modalities and exercise remedy this problem. If there is rotator cuff weakness, the bicep carries more of a load supporting the glenohumeral joint, and injury occurs.

Recurrent Subluxation of the Long Head of the Biceps

The long head of the biceps can sublux during the cocking and early acceleration phase, especially in athletes who have shallow bicepital grooves. The long head has a 30° posterior angle where it attaches to the superior portion of the glenoid rim. This can cause subluxation when the humerus goes from external rotation to internal rotation. This subluxation can be produced by externally and internally rotating the humerus and palpating the subluxation with the fingertips.

Biceps Tendon Ruptures

The long head of the biceps may partially avulse at this insertion along the superior rim of the glenoid fossa. During acceleration and deceleration, the bicep is active and the high forces may partially tear the tendon and the glenoid labrum. This is an intra-articular problem and can be seen with arthroscope.

Glenoid Labrum Tears

The anterior glenoid labrum can tear by the shoulder grinding factor or by subluxation of the humeral head. The biceps long head can also pull a portion of it. The examiner can make it pop when checking for laxity of the anterior capsule. The thrower complains of a pain on acceleration of the arm. If the tear propagates anteriorly and inferiorly, the subluxation of the humeral head can be a problem. Arthroscopic surgery easily removes this joint irritant.

Subluxation of the Humerus

Most throwers have a loose-jointed shoulder. It is rare for a pitcher to dislocate a shoulder while throwing. The anterior and posterior capsules can be tested and found to be loose, but this is specific to the activity. If there is a subluxation problem, it is difficult to decide in what direction it occurs during the act of pitching because both directions can be affected during cocking, acceleration, and deceleration. An athlete with an anterior subluxation may have an anterior inferior labrum tear. Anterior instability may lead to rotator cuff injury as the cuff tries to stabilize the joint. An athlete with a posterior subluxation usually has a mid-posterior labrum tear. These can be treated arthroscopically, and the patient can be rehabilitated to full function.

Rotator Cuff Tears

Most throwers who injure the rotator cuff do not tear it completely. A partial tear develops in the thickness of the cuff. Deceleration of the throwing arm may cause this pathology. If the cuff becomes fatigued, microtrauma to the tendon begins to develop. Over time, an incomplete tear develops within the supraspinatus tendon insertion. This occurs on the undersurface of the cuff intra-articularly. Impingement syndromes do not tear the tendon, or the lesion would be external to the cuff. Anterior instability may also cause injury.

An athlete who has pain on deceleration of the throwing arm cannot get back to usual speed and ends up continuing to reinjure the arm. The athlete slowly develops weakness throughout the shoulder during this process.

Arthroscopic debridement can stimulate healing. With proper exercise, the athlete may return to full pitching in 6 months. Athletes with complete tears of the rotator cuff have a much smaller chance of returning to play.

SURGERY

A scar on the shoulder of a thrower usually spelled doom for the aspiring player. The advent of the arthroscope changed all this. Because very little scar tissue develops with arthroscopic puncture holes, the athlete achieves full ROM and can get into the throwing position. The arthroscope has allowed visualization of injuries that for so long have been hidden.

Three major problems can be handled with arthroscopic surgery. The torn glenoid labrum in the anterior–superior quadrant can be easily debrided. If the biceps tendon is frayed intra-articularly, debridement can reduce pain and instability. The necrotic tissue of a partial rotator cuff tear can be debrided and the "healing pump" started with increased blood supply caused by the surgery.

CONSERVATIVE CARE

Most injuries to the throwing shoulder do not result in surgery. Most are treated conservatively with modalities, anti-inflammatories, exercise, and a gradual return to throwing. These athletes usually do not have "frozen shoulders" or other shoulder conditions that make the evaluation difficult. The arthroscope has allowed a correlation of physical findings and history to actual injury.

Modality use can be beneficial. Use of moist heat before throwing and ice after throwing is the usual routine. Ultrasound with or without anti-inflammatory gel delivers its properties deep into the rotator cuff or other structures. High-voltage stimulators also aid in healing and pain relief. Transcutaneous electric nerve stimulation will help to control pain postoperatively. Iontophoresis may also be effective.

The most difficult situation is determining rotator cuff irritation. Early in the development of rotator cuff problems, the athlete can recover quickly from symptoms, but, because of continued high-pressure throwing, the injury is exacerbated. Rest and exercise and a graduated return to the throwing program allows the problem to heal without reinjury.

The glenoid labrum tear can be discovered on examination. The shoulder must be strengthened to prevent abnormal forces from causing further damage. As with a torn meniscus in the knee, the glenoid labrum tear is not an emergency situation. The athlete may continue to throw. The lesion will not heal; therefore, surgery will probably result.

Both the postoperative rotator cuff debridement and labrum excision follow the same rehabilitation program. Both are usually done as outpatient procedures. The patient usually uses a sling for 1 or 2 days for comfort. Postoperative dressings are removed at day 3, and bandages are used over the puncture holes until they heal.

At postoperative day 1, ROM and strengthening exercises begin. They are done to the patient's tolerance but are pushed along quickly, especially because of the need for full ROM. Codman exercises are effective early for mobilization of the glenohumeral joint. Supine flexion and abduction used with a wand allows the athlete to work these motions at least 25 times, three to five times daily. Often, the athlete develops a contracture between the scapula and humerus inferiorly at the glenohumeral joint. Manual stretching may be indicated by stabilizing the scapula and allowing for stretching of the humerus overhead. Putting a pad under the scapula raises the body and allows for more ROM work when the athlete must work alone and increase shoulder retraction.

External rotation stretching is by far one of the most important motions to perform. This motion applies graduated controlled stress to the healing and scarring area, allowing collagen to form in a much more organized fashion and keeping scar formation small and smooth so that impingement problems are prevented. The athlete performs the actively assisted external rotation stretch at 90°, 135°, and full abduction. The goal is development of more than normal external rotation and a pain-free ROM end.

Other ROMs must be exercised, including internal rotation. The follow-through phase requires good posterior flexibility and is accomplished by the horizontal adduction stretch.

For strengthening, a high-repetition, low-weight program appears to be the most therapeutic. Five sets of 10 repetitions and no weight, with progress up to 5 lb, is usually all that is required during the first 6 weeks. This program increases strength to the point at which the manual muscle test will be normal in all positions and not irritate the joint. All lifts require a dead stop at their extreme and are done at a measured pace. The athlete may work higher as this gets easier, but never with more than 10 lb. The athlete generally does not work with weight machines until capable of throwing normally.

Shoulder shrugs are done with scapular adduction and shoulder retraction. Forward flexion and pure abduction are done with the humerus externally rotated and the thumb up. The supraspinatus is exercised with the arm at 30° in forward flexion and the humerus internally rotated fully. The hand is lifted to eye level. The posterior shoulder structures are strengthened with prone horizontal abduction, with the glenohumeral joint at 100° and the arm externally rotated fully. Prone external rotation is done with the humerus supported on the exercise table. Side-lying external rotation is performed for infraspinatus and teres minor strengthening. The bicep curl and tricep extension or french curl increase strength in those important throwing muscles. The sitting push-up or dip strengthens the internal rotators, shoulder depressors, and triceps and is the only internal rotation strengthenig that is done. An imbalance of weaker posterior muscles versus anterior muscles may lead to injury. Appendix 10-1 is a shoulder exercise program that can be individualized for each patient.

At 4 weeks for the labrum tear and at 6 weeks for the partial rotator cuff tear, the athlete is expected to have full ROM with very little pain at extremes and a G+ to N manual muscle test for the shoulder. The interval throwing program (Appendix 10-2), another patient exercise program, should be started, allowing the athlete to condition the arm slowly. The original injury most likely occurred because of fatigue. The muscles of the arm are strong, but the tendon and joint structures are not ready for the high stresses of 90 mph fast balls. A thrower who now overworks the arm will reinjure the area.

The interval is 5 minutes of long toss and 5 minutes of short toss (Appendix 10-2). The athlete warms up with moist heat and stretching, then tosses the ball for several minutes at 30 ft, gradually building up to 90 ft. This is the long toss, which allows the pitcher to work on good form at low intensity. The pitcher then tosses the ball at 30 ft and throws at half speed or as tolerated. The thrower should rest for 30 minutes, do the prescribed exercises and then repeat the sequence. The thrower will have accomplished 20 minutes of throwing, but will not have fatigued the arm. The long toss progresses by 30 ft to 250 ft. The short toss progresses from 30 ft at half speed to 60 ft at half speed, then to three-quarter speed, three-quarter speed from mound, three-quarter speed from mound and curve balls, and finally works up to full speed. As athletes get stronger, they may reach plateaus that cannot be worked through; an additional few minutes or another interval may be of benefit. Athletes must listen to their body and not force progress too fast. It usually takes 3 months to recover from a labrum excision to full participation and 6 months for the partial rotator cuff tear. Speed gun testing will help the athlete determine progress. The athlete should continue the exercises vigorously. Because every athlete is different, progress will be individual.

PREVENTION

A player should not be sent home during the off season without a program, injured or not. A player who expects to throw the next season should have the arm conditioned all year by throwing a ball for 15 minutes three times weekly. A maintenance weight program centered around the supraspinatus lift, the prone horizontal abduction, prone external rotation, and external rotation stretching will help the shoulder stay strong. A pitcher never "rests."

Biomechanical analysis through high-speed video has become a reality. The coach and the athlete can observe biomechanical abnormalities and correct them.

The physician, therapist, trainer, and coach must work together in close harmony to assure the progress of the injured thrower. Exercise, rest, modalities, proper medication, and a graduated return to throwing program will enhance a player's return to throwing activity.

APPENDIX 10-1

SHOULDER EXERCISE PROGRAM

1. Circumduction

   Lean over with opposite arm on table. Let involved arm hang straight down. *Be relaxed.* Move body and let arm swing in circle clockwise, counterclockwise, forward and backward, and side to side. Do at least 1 minute every hour you are awake (Fig. 10-10).

2. Supine Flexion

   Lie on back. Grip hammer in both hands with elbow straight, take both arms over head as far as possible and hold for count of 5. Return to starting position. Repeat ____ times, ____ times per day (Fig. 10-11).

3. Supine External Rotation

   Lie on back with involved arm out to side at 90° and elbow at 90°. Use the hammer to push the arm straight back into external rotation. Hold for a count of 5. Relax and repeat ____ times, ____ times per day. Repeat this at 90°, 135°, and full abduction (Fig. 10-12).

4. Supine Internal Rotation

   Lie on back with involved arm out to side at 90° and elbow at 90°. Use hammer to push the arm straight into internal rotation. Hold for a count of 5. Relax and repeat ____ times, ____ times per day (Fig. 10-13).

5. Supine Abduction

   Lie on back with involved arm out to side as far as possible and arm externally rotated as far as possible. Slide arm *along floor* as close to ear as possible. Use hammer or hand to help pull. Hold for a count of 5. Relax and repeat ____ times, ____ times per day (Fig. 10-14).

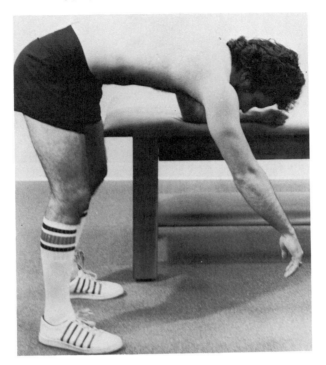

Fig. 10-10. Circumduction.

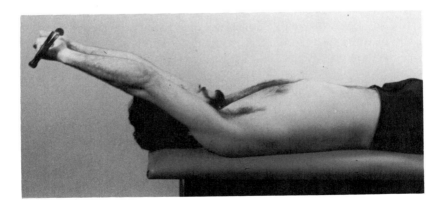

Fig. 10-11. Supine flexion.

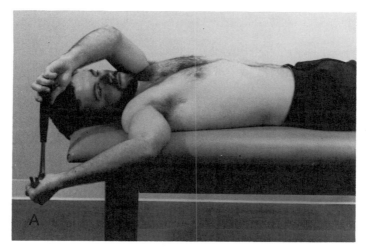

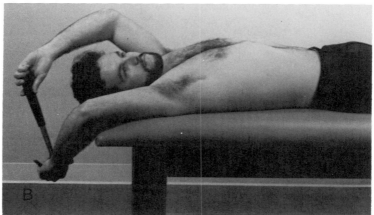

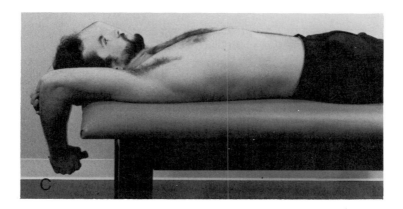

Fig. 10-12.   (**A & B**) Supine external rotation. (**C**) Supine external rotation.

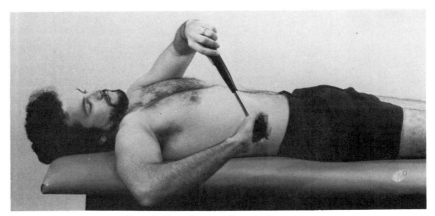

Fig. 10-13.   Supine internal rotation.

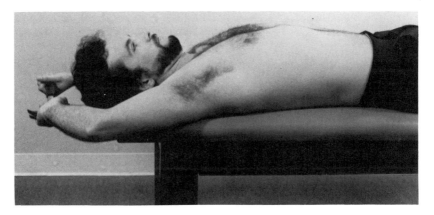

Fig. 10-14.   Supine abduction.

6. Rope and Pulley
    Rope and pulley should be in doorway, with pulley in one corner of the door jamb. Sit in a chair with back against door jamb under pulley. Clasp handles of pulley.
    A. With elbow straight, raise arm out to front using your muscle. When you have it as high as possible, then assist by pulling on the rope. Take arm as high as possible, hold for a count of 5, then lower the arm using as much muscle power as possible. Repeat ＿＿ times, ＿＿ times per day.
    B. With elbow straight, raise arm out to side, palm facing upward. Repeat ＿＿ times, ＿＿ times per day.
7. Shoulder Shrugs
    Stand with arms by your side. Lift shoulders straight up to your ear, hold for a count of 2, the pull shoulders back, pinch shoulder blades, and hold for a count of 2. Relax shoulder. Repeat ＿＿ times, ＿＿ times per day. Progress up to ＿＿ pounds held in your hands (Fig. 10-15).

8. Shoulder Flexion
    Stand. Raise arm out to front of body as high as possible. Hold this for a count of 2, then lower. Repeat ____ times, ____ times per day. Start with ____ pounds and progress to ____ pounds (Fig. 10-16).

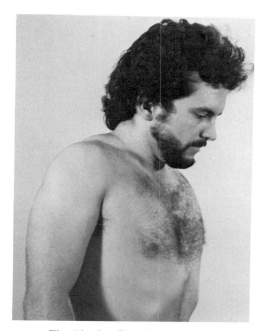

Fig. 10-15. Shoulder shrugs.

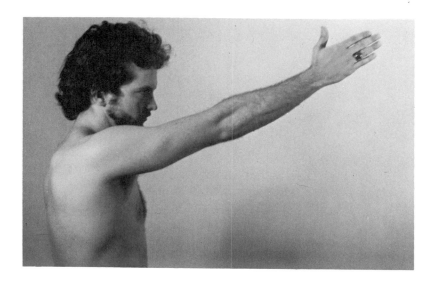

Fig. 10-16. Shoulder flexion.

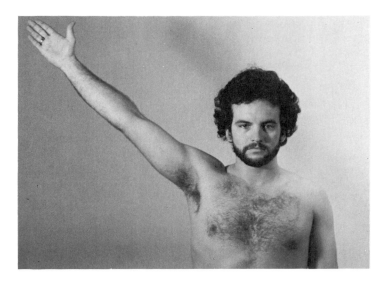

Fig. 10-17. Shoulder abduction.

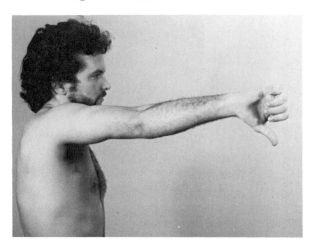

Fig. 10-18. Supraspinatus.

9A. Shoulder Abduction

Stand. Raise arm out to side of body as high as possible while rotating arm externally. Hold for a count of 2, then lower. Repeat ____ times, ____ times per day. Start with ____ pounds and progress to ____ pounds (Fig. 10-17).

9B. Supraspinatus

Raise the arm out to the side in front of body 30° with arm internally rotated. Hold thumb down. Lift to eye level (Fig. 10-18).

10. Prone Horizontal Abduction

Lie on table on stomach with involved arm hanging straight to the floor, thumb up. Hand should be at eye level. Raise arm out to side. Hold for a count of 2, lower and relax. Repeat _____ times, _____ times per day. Start with _____ pounds and work up to _____ pounds (Fig. 10-19).

11. Biceps Curl

Support arm on opposite hand. Bend elbow to full flexion, then straighten arm completely. Repeat _____ times, _____ times per day. Start with _____ pounds and work to _____ pounds (Fig. 10-20).

12. French Curl

Raise arm overhead. Take opposite hand and give support at elbow. Straighten arm overhead, hold for a count of 2. Relax. Repeat _____

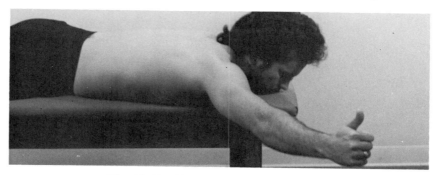

Fig. 10-19.   Prone horizontal abduction.

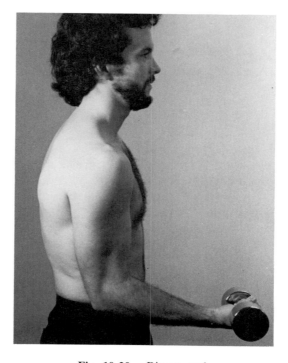

Fig. 10-20.   Biceps curl.

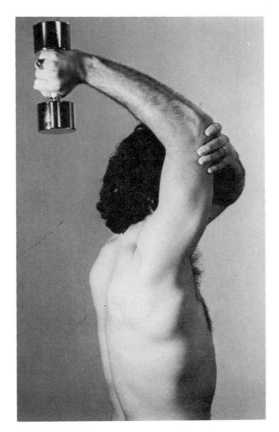

Fig. 10-21.   French curl.

times, _____ times per day. Start with _____ pounds and work to _____ pounds (Fig. 10-21).

13. Sitting Dip
    Sitting on edge of chair with hands by your side, lift buttocks off surface. Hold for a count of 2, then relax. Start with _____ times. Work up to _____ repetitions (Fig. 10-22).

14. Hanging
    Hang from chin-up bar; with feet on floor, bend knees and absorb a comfortable amount of weight. Perform for 1 minute, three times per day.

15A. External Rotation
    Lie prone with arm supported at the elbow. Lift weight into external rotation. Hold for a count of 2. Relax. Perform _____ times, _____ times per day. Start with _____ pounds and work up to _____ pounds (Fig. 10-23).

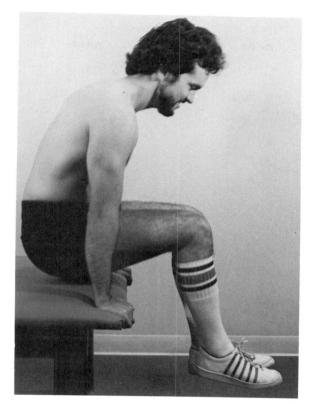

Fig. 10-22.   Sitting dip.

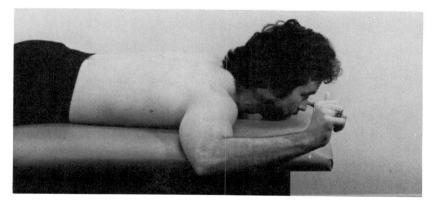

Fig. 10-23.   External rotation prone.

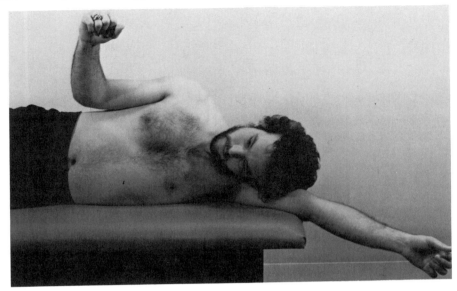

Fig. 10-24.   External rotation side-lying.

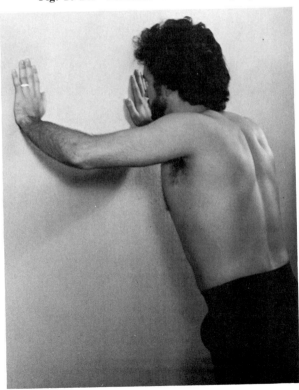

Fig. 10-25.   Progressive push-up.

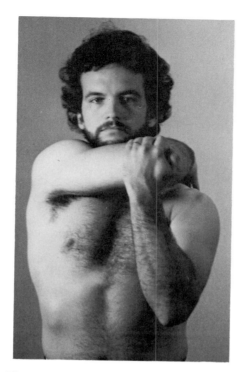

Fig. 10-26. Horizontal adduction stretch.

15B. External Rotation Side-Lying
Lie on opposite side, arm resting on side and elbow flexed at 90°. Rotate arm upward (Fig. 10-24).

16. Progressive Push-up
Start with push-up into the wall. Gradually progress to tabletop and eventually to floor. Do as tolerated (Fig. 10-25).

17. Horizontal Adduction Stretch
Grasp elbow of involved arm with opposite hand and pull arm across front of chest. Hold for a count of five. Relax. Repeat ____ times, ____ times per day (Fig. 10-26).

APPENDIX 10-2

INTERVAL THROWING PROGRAM

The interval throwing program is designed to allow you to work several times a day at a submaximal level, never trying to fatigue the arm, but to get a light workout. This will enable the arm to gradually become stronger and more conditioned to the throwing act. The program should begin with a thorough stretching of the throwing extremity and application of moist heat. It should be followed by ice, if appropriate. Even though you could throw at a more intense level, that is not the idea of this program. It is the slow buildup and conditioning of the arm that will allow you to progress and not reinjure yourself. Throw _____ (2) days and rest _____ (1) days. One interval equals one long toss and one short toss.

Begin each throwing session with several minutes of 30-ft tossing to get the arm warm for long toss. You may gradually work to your long-toss distance. You do not have to start at the set distance.

Your long toss may start with throws that will just roll to your partner and graduate to one hop and then the fly.

The long-toss and short-toss intervals may progress independently of each other.

Progress may not be in a straight line. There will be advances and regressions. Ease off when you hurt. Do not advance a phase until you are completely comfortable at your present phase. *Expect some soreness.*

PHASE I   _____ Interval/day (2)*
             _____ Rest between (15–30)

Long toss		*Short toss*	
Feet	_____ (90)	Feet	_____ (30)
Minutes	_____ (5)	Minutes	_____ (5)
Throws	_____ (25)	Throws	_____ (50)
Intensity	_____ (to tolerance)	Intensity	_____ (work to ½ speed)

PHASE II   _____ Interval/day (2)
              _____ Rest between (15–30)

Long toss		*Short toss*	
Feet	_____ (120)	Feet	_____ (60)
Minutes	_____ (5)	Minutes	_____ (5)
Throws	_____ (25)	Throws	_____ (50)
Intensity	_____ (to tolerance)	Intensity	_____ (work to ½ speed)

PHASE III   _____ Interval/day (2)
               _____ Rest between (15–30)

Long toss			Short toss		
Feet	—— (150)		Feet	—— (60)	
Minutes	—— (5)		Minutes	—— (5)	
Throws	—— (25)		Throw	—— (50)	
Intensity	—— (to tolerance)		Intensity	—— (work to ¾ speed)	

PHASE IV —— Interval/day (2)
—— Rest between (15–30)

Long toss			Short toss		
Feet	—— (180)		Feet	—— (60)	
Minutes	—— (5)		Minutes	—— (5)	
Throws	—— (25)		Throws	—— (50)	
Intensity	—— (to tolerance)		Intensity	—— (work to ¾ speed, mound)	

PHASE V —— Interval/day (2)
—— Rest between (15–30)

Long toss			Short toss		
Feet	—— (210)		Feet	—— (60)	
Minutes	—— (5)		Minutes	—— (5)	
Throws	—— (25)		Throws	—— (50)	
Intensity	—— (to tolerance)		Intensity	—— (½ to ¾ speed, mound breaking ball)	

PHASE VI —— Interval/day (20)
—— Rest between (15–30)

Long toss			Short toss		
Feet	—— (250)		Feet	—— (60+)	
Minutes	—— (5)		Minutes	—— (5)	
Throws	—— (25)		Throws	—— (50)	
Intensity	—— (to tolerance)		Intensity	—— (¾—full speed, mound, breaking ball)	

* Numbers in parentheses are suggestions.

REFERENCES

1. Codman EA: The Shoulder, Thomas Todd Co, Boston, 1934
2. Freedman L, Munro RR: Abduction of the arm in the scapular plane: scapular and glenohumeral movements. J Bone Joint Surg 48A:1503, 1966
3. Inman UT, Saunders JB, Abbott LC: Observations on the function of the shoulder joint. J Bone Joint Surg 26:1, 1944
4. Jobe FW, Moyers DR, Tibone JE, et al: AM EMG injury of the shoulder in pitching: a second report. Am J Sports Med 12:218, 1984

5. Jobe FW, Perry JB, Perry T, et al: An EMG analysis of the shoulder in throwing and pitching: a preliminary report. AMF Sports Med 11:3, 1983
6. American Medical Association. Standard Nomenclature of Athletic Injuries. p 99. American Medical Association, Chicago, 1975.
7. Jobe FW, Moyers DR: Delineation of diagnostic criteria and rehabilitation program for rotator cuff injuries. AMF Sports Med 10:336, 1982

11 | Mobilization of the Shoulder

Robert A. Donatelli

In the past decade, mobilization has been demonstrated clinically to be an important part of rehabilitation and assessment of restricted joint movement. Clinical application is based on an understanding of joint mechanics, connective tissue histology, and muscle function. Mobilization has developed into a clinical science, requiring the therapist to understand anatomic and histologic characteristics of synovial joints. Significant advancement have been made in describing the benefits of passive movement. Thanks to the hard work and dedication of such researchers as Akeson, Woo, Matthews, Amiel, and Peacock,[9,11,14] we have a better understanding of joint stiffness and wound healing. As clinicians, we can take this knowledge and apply our mobilization techniques during critical stages of wound healing to influence the extensibility of scar tissue and reduce the development of restrictive adhesions. We can also use this knowledge to prevent and treat joint stiffness by applying the appropriate stress to the muscles and connective tissue, promoting homeostasis.[1] It is through an understanding of normal tissue function, tissue changes during immobilization, and the structure of scar tissue that we can establish the criteria for mobilization.

This chapter will discuss mobilization from a basic science approach. The mobilization techniques for the shoulder will be described, with emphasis on the mechanical and neurophysiologic effects.

DEFINITION

Several terms must be defined when mobilization is discussed. Articulation, oscillation, distractions, manipulation, and mobilization all describe a specialized type of passive movement.

Articulatory techniques are derived from the osteopathic literature. They are defined as passive movement applied in a smooth rhythmic fashion to stretch contracted muscles, ligaments, and capsules gradually.[2] They include gentle techniques designed to stretch the joint in each of the planes of movement normal to it.[2] The force used during articulatory techniques is usually a prolonged stretch into the restriction or tissue limitation.

Oscillatory techniques are best defined by Maitland, who describes oscillations as passive movements to the joint, which can be of a small or large amplitude and applied anywhere in a range of movement, and which can be performed while the joint surfaces are held distracted or compressed.[3] There are four grades of oscillations: grade 1 is a small amplitude movement performed at the beginning of range; grade 2 is a large amplitude movement performed within the range, but not reaching the limit of the range; grade 3 is a large amplitude movement up to the limit of range; and grade 4 is a small amplitude movement performed at the limit of range.[3] Grades 1 and 2 are used for the neurophysiologic effects, and grades 3 and 4 are designed to initiate mechanical changes in the tissue.

Distraction is defined as "separation of surfaces of a joint by extension without injury or dislocation of the parts."[4] Distractive techniques are designed to separate the joint surface attempting to stress the capsule.

Manipulation is defined by *Dorland's Illustrated Medical Dictionary* as "skillful or dextrous treatment by the hand. In physical therapy, the forceful passive movement of a joint beyond its active limit of motion."[5] Maitland describes two manipulative procedures. Manipulation is a sudden movement or thrust, of small amplitude, performed at a speed that renders the patient powerless to prevent it.[3] Manipulation under anesthesia is a medical procedure used to restore normal joint movement by breaking adhesions.

Mobilization is defined as "the making of a fixed or ankylosed part movable. Restoration of motion to a joint."[4,5] To the clinician, mobilization is passive movement that is designed to improve soft tissue and joint mobility. It can include oscillations, articulations, distractions, or manipulations.

Mobilization, in this chapter, is defined as a specialized passive movement, attempting to restore the arthrokinematics and osteokinematics of joint movement. It includes articulations, oscillations, distractions, and thrust techniques. The techniques are built on active and passive joint mechanics. They are directed at the periarticular structures that have become restricted secondary to trauma and immobilization. These same techniques can be effective tools in the evaluation of joint movement.

ROLE OF MOBILIZATION

The major goal of the physical therapist is to restore normal function. The normal mechanics of synovial joints include a combination of arthrokinematics (the intimate mechanics of joint surfaces), osteokinematics (the movement of bones), and muscle function.[6]

Gray's Anatomy describes the intimate joint mechanics as roll, spin, and slide (as noted in Ch. 1). These movements occur during active movement between articular surfaces.[6] In addition to the active movements, there are accessory movements, two types of which are described in *Gray's Anatomy*. The first type occurs only when resistance is encountered during active movement; e.g., metacarpophalangeal joint rotation can only occur when a solid object is grasped by the hand.[6] The second type of accessory movement is purely a passive motion produced by an outside force[6]; e.g., if muscles surrounding the shoulder joint are relaxed, a distractive force can separate the head of the humerus from the glenoid cavity.

The combination of the active movements of roll, spin, and slide plus the accessory movements constitute joint mobility. For example, as the glenohumeral joint externally rotates in the adducted position, the humerus slides anteriorly, rolls posteriorly, and spins into external rotation. The activity of the rotator cuff muscles are largely responsible for this action. The muscle cannot produce the normal active range if joint mobility is limited. The goal of mobilization is to restore joint mobility.

EFFECTS OF PASSIVE MOVEMENT

Normal joint motion includes a dynamic combination of arthrokinematics, sufficient periarticular tissue extensibility, osteokinematics, and normal muscle function. Joint stiffness results from a loss or change in one or all of the components of joint mobility. Passive movement has its most therapeutic effect in the treatment of joint stiffness secondary to immobilization and trauma. Continuous passive movement has been demonstrated to be effective in reducing wound edema and joint effusion, eliminating joint restrictions following trauma.[1] Franks and associates found that continuous passive movement resulted in increased patient comfort and shorter hospital stays.[1] Passive movement has been shown to provide proprioceptive feedback to the central nervous system (CNS) by maintaining tension in the muscle.[1] It has also been hypothesized that stimulation of the proprioceptors interferes with transmission of pain through the CNS.[1] The nociceptive afferents (pain fibers) have a much higher threshold of excitation than do the mechanoreceptor afferents,[7,8] and there is evidence that the stimulation of peripheral mechanoreceptors blocks the transmission of pain to the brain.[7] Wyke explains this phenomenon as a direct release of inhibitory transmitters within the basal spinal nucleus, inhibiting the onward flow of incoming nociceptive afferent activity.[7] Mobilization is one method of enhancing the frequency of discharge from the mechanoreceptors, thereby diminishing the intensity of many types of pain. If the mechanoreceptor stimulation is of high enough frequency and is maintained long enough, the pain may be abolished.[7]

An important aspect of passive movement is in the prevention and treatment of the complications resulting from immobilization. The lack of stress to connective tissue results in changes in normal joint mobility. The periarticular tissue and muscles surrounding the joint demonstrate significant changes after periods of immobilization. Akeson et al. have substantiated a decrease in water and glycosaminoglycans (GAG, the fibrous tissue lubricant), an increase in fatty fibrous infiltrates (which may form adhesions as they mature into scar), an increase in abnormally placed collagen cross-links (which may contribute to the inhibition of collagen fiber gliding), and the loss of fiber orientation within ligaments (which significantly reduces their strength).[1,9] Passive movement or stress to the tissues can help to prevent these changes by maintaining tissue homeostasis.[1] The exact mechanisms of prevention are uncertain.

EFFECTS OF PASSIVE MOVEMENT ON SCAR TISSUE: INDICATIONS AND CONTRAINDICATIONS FOR MOBILIZATION

Research indicates that mobilization is most effective in reversing the changes that occur in connective tissue following immobilization.[1] Conversely, mobilization after trauma must be carefully analyzed. When is it safe to apply stress to scar tissue? How much stress should be applied to the scar in order to promote remodeling? In what direction should the stress be applied? These important questions must be answered before we can determine the indications for mobilization of scar tissue.

Research has demonstrated that stress applied early to healing wounds is important in establishing the characteristics of scar tissue. The production of scar tissue begins on the fourth day of wound healing and increases rapidly during the first 3 weeks.[10,11] Peacock has substantiated this peak production of scar by the increased quantities of hydroxyproline.[11] Hydroxyproline is a byproduct of collagen synthesis.[11,12] New collagen is deposited in the scar, at a rate higher than normal connective tissue, for up to 4 months. Research indicates that early stress to scar tissue influences the remodeling process. The collagen fibers are initially deposited within the scar in a random fashion. This random order changes as the tissue begins to remodel. The new collagen fibers align with the preexisting fibers, and the assimilation of the new fibers is part of the remodeling process. Scar tissue begins to resemble the previous normal tissues by the process of maturation.[10,11] Another important aspect of remodeling is the ability of the collagen fibers to glide. If this does not occur, the scar tissue can cause limitations in the mobility of the normal tissue.

The collagen fibril in its early stages is very weak. Intermolecular and intramolecular cross-linking of collagen molecules develop, designed to resist tensile forces.[11,12] The tensile strength of the collagen fibers continues to develop linearly for at least 3 months.[10,11] Arem and Madden demonstrated that after 14 weeks of scar maturation, elongation of the scar was no longer possible.[13] In contrast, the 3-week-old scar was significantly lengthened when subjected to tension.[13] It is evident that as scar tissue matures, it develops the capability to resist tensile forces. Peacock hypothesizes that the mechanism by which the length of the scar is increased becomes critical for the restoration of the gliding mechanism.[11] Stretching, or an increase in length of the scar, is a result of straightening or reorientation of the collagen fibers, without a change in their dimensions.[11] For this to occur, the collagen fibers must glide on each other. This gliding mechanism is hampered in unstressed scar tissue by the development of abnormally placed cross-links and a random orientation of the newly synthesized collagen fibrils.[9] Clinically, this can mean limited joint movement.

Joint stiffness results from immobilization and/or trauma. The limitations in movement result from the changes that occur in the periarticular tissues as described above. Mobilization is indicated when the lack of extensibility of the periartricular structures limits the arthrokinematic movement of joint surfaces. This limitation will produce compensations in normal motion and changes in muscle function. The patient experiences pain and limited movement of the involved joint. The therapeutic effects of mobilization on scar and immobilized tissue is important in reestablishing normal active range of motion (ROM). Mobilization of the immobilized tissue stimulates the production of GAGs, which is important for lubrication and maintaining a critical distance between collagen fibers to allow for the gliding mechanism to occur.[9,14] It also assures an orderly deposition of new collagen fibrils, thereby preventing abnormal cross-link formation.[9,14] Enneking and Horowitz[15] and Evans et al.[16] document that forceful manipulation breaks intracapsular fibrofatty adhesions that may have formed within the joint during immobilization.

As previously mentioned, early stress to scar tissue determines the tissue flexibility. Arem and Madden advocate stressing the tissue as early as the third week of scar tissue production.[13] Tissue flexibility is enhanced by passive movement of the young scar, and this is accomplished by promoting alignment of new collagen fibers with preexisting fibers, preventing the development of obstructive adhesions, and enhancing fiber glide. The direction, velocity, duration, and magnitude of the stress to scar tissue needs further investigation. The exact effects mobilization has on the remodeling process have not been determined. The forces applied during application of the mobilization techniques are controlled by the pain tolerance of the patient and tissue resistance. The direction of stress applied to connective tissues should be determined in the evaluation by the location of tissue resistance and assessment of joint mobility.

It is easier to understand the contraindications of mobilization by becoming aware of the common abuses of passive movement. The abuses of passive movement can be broken down into two categories: creation of excessive trauma to the tissues and the causing of "undesired" or abnormal mobility.[1]

Improper techniques, such as extreme force, poor direction of stress, and excessive velocity, may result in serious secondary injury or damage to the tissues surrounding the joint that is mobilized. In addition, mobilization to joints that are moving normally or that are hypermobile can create and/or increase joint instabilities.

Ultimately, selection of a specific technique will determine contraindications. For example, the very gentle grade 1 oscillations, as described by

Maitland, rarely have contraindications. These techniques are mainly used to block pain. They are of small amplitude and controlled velocity. In contrast, manipulative techniques have many contraindications. Haldeman describes the following conditions as major contraindications for thrust techniques: arthritides, dislocation, hypermobility, trauma or recent occurrence, bone weakness and destructive disease, circulatory disturbances, neurologic dysfunction, and infectious disease.[17]

In summary, connective tissue heals by formation of scar tissue. Peak production of scar occurs within the first 3 weeks of wound healing.[18] Between 3 weeks and 6 weeks, there is a decrease in fibroblast numbers. Controlled stress at this early stage is important in realignment of collagen fibers. At 14 weeks, scar length appears to be maximal. Influencing the mobility of the scar at this stage may be difficult, requiring a greater magnitude of force. The mechanical properties of untreated scar tissue were inferior to normal ligament tissue after 40 weeks of healing.[18] The ligament "scar" was found to be structurally abnormal chemically and mechanically at long-term follow-up.[18] Tipton et al.[19] clearly demonstrated that increased or decreased levels of systematic exercise will markedly influence the strength of ligaments. Exercise was found to increase the number of collagen fibrils and to alter their arrangement and thickness. In addition, ligaments from trained animals had a significantly higher hydroxyproline content than ligaments from immobilized animals.[19] Therefore, normal maturation of scar tissue is dependent on stress at early stages.

PRINCIPLES OF MOBILIZATION TECHNIQUES

The mobilization techniques are designed to restore intimate joint mechanics. Several general principles should be remembered during application of the techniques.

Hand Position

The mobilization hand should be placed as close as possible to the joint surfaces, and the forces applied should be directed at the periarticular tissues. The stabilization hand counteracts the movement of the mobilizing hand by applying an equal but opposite force or by preventing movement at surrounding joints.

Direction of Movement

The direction of forces to the joint should be away from pain and into resistance. The resistance represents the direction of capsular or joint limitation. Movement into the restriction is an attempt to make mechanical changes within the capsule and its surrounding tissue. The mechanical changes may include breaking up of adhesions, realignment of collagen, or increasing fiber glide. Certain movements stress specific parts of the capsule. It has been substantiated through arthrogram studies that external rotation of the glenohumeral joint stresses the anterior recess of the capsule.[20]

The direction of movement should not exceed the normal limits of the joint. When applying the mobilization techniques, the therapist must be aware of the joint's movement within the body planes (degrees of freedom) and the contour of the joint surfaces. The glenohumeral joint has three degrees of freedom, or it is capable of moving in all three body planes (frontal, sagittal, and transverse).[6] In addition, movement occurs at the joint surface. For example, Poppen and Walker have established that during the first 30° to 60° of shoulder elevation, the head of the humerus moves upward approximately 3 mm. Thereafter, it moves 1 or 2 mm upward and downward between each successive position.[21] The earlier works of Saha demonstrate the movements of roll, spin, and slide of the humeral head during elevation of the shoulder.[22] A more detailed analysis of shoulder joint movement is reviewed in Chapter 1. For the therapist to determine the direction of force, there must be an understanding of joint movement and the location and nature of the joint restriction.

Body Mechanics

It is important for the therapist to maintain good body mechanics during the application of mobilization techniques. The therapist should stand as close as possible to the patient. The therapist's hands and arms should be positioned to act as fulcrums and levers, and the therapist's position should allow for the most efficient application of techniques.

Duration and Amplitude

Several studies have been performed to determine the most effective technique for obtaining permanent elongation of collagenous tissue, using different loads and loading time. The studies used rat tendons to demonstrate the elongation of tissue under varied loads. The treatments included low-load and a long duration using 5 g and stretch for 15 minutes. High-load, short-duration treatment used 105 to 165 g for 5 minutes.[23,24] The results indicated that low-load long-duration stretch was more effective in obtaining a permanent elongation of the tissue. Several studies also indicated further improvement with the use of heat before or during the stretch and ice immediately afterward.[25,26]

GLENOHUMERAL JOINT TECHNIQUES

Figure 11-1: Inferior Glide of the Humerus

Patient position: supine, with the involved extremity close to the edge of the table. A strap stabilizes the scapula. The extremity is abducted to the desired range.

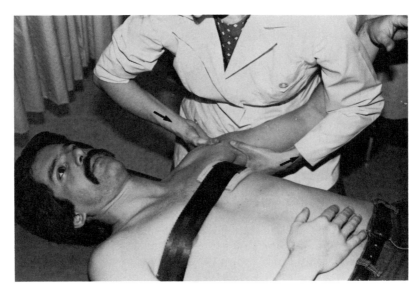

Fig. 11-1.

Therapist position: facing the lateral side of the upper arm. Left hand is into the axilla as close as possible to the joint line. The web space of the right hand is over the superior humeral head as close as possible to the acromion. The left hand maintains the abducted position while applying a distractive force. The right hand pushes the head of the humerus inferiorly, attempting to stress the axillary pouch or inferior portion of the glenohumeral capsule. Oscillatory techniques using grades 3 and 4 are effective. For more aggressive stretching to the inferior capsule, a prolonged stretch and manipulations are effective with the patient's arm held in 60° of abduction or less.

Figure 11-2: Longitudinal Distraction—Inferior Glide of the Humerus

Patient position: supine, with the involved extremity as close as possible to the edge of the table.

Therapist position: facing the joint, with the right hand into the axilla attempting to hold the glenoid. The left hand grips the epicondyles of the humerus, applying a downward traction on the humerus and stressing the inferior capsule. A prolonged stetch is effective with this technique.

Figure 11-3: Caudal Glide of the Humerus

Patient position: supine, with the involved extremity flexed to 90° at the shoulder.

Therapist position: as close as possible to the involved extremity, with

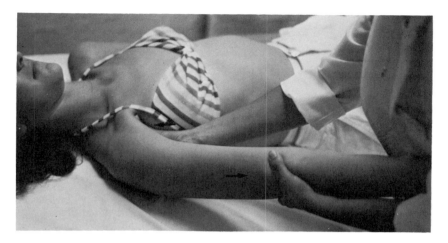

Fig. 11-2.

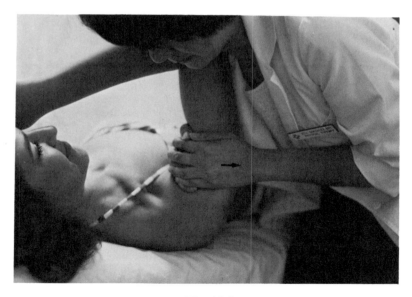

Fig. 11-3.

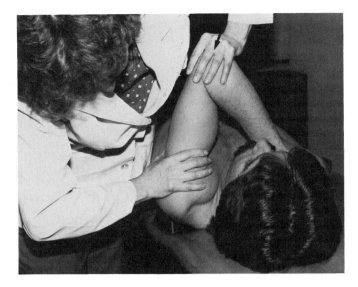

Fig. 11-4.

both hands grasping the humerus as close as possible to the head of the humerus. The hands pull the humerus inferiorly, stressing the inferior aspect of the glenohumeral capsule. A prolonged stretch is most effective.

Figure 11-4: Posterior Glide of the Humerus

Patient position: supine, with the involved extremity as close as possible to the edge of the table. A wedge is placed under the dorsal scapula. The extremity is flexed and horizontally adducted to the desired range. The elbow is flexed.

Therapist position: facing cranially, with the right hand maintaining the flexed and adducted position and the left hand over the elbow with the forearm parallel to the patient's forearm. The force is applied through the elbow, pushing the humerus posteriorly and stressing the posterior aspect of the glenohumeral capsule and the tendinous portion of the subscapularis. A prolonged stress or oscillatory techniques is useful.

Figure 11-5: Lateral Distraction of the Humerus

Patient position: as close as possible to the edge of the table, with the involved extremity flexed at the elbow and glenohumeral joint. The extremity rests on the therapist's shoulder. A strap stabilizes the scapula.

Therapist position: facing laterally, both hands grasp the humerus as close

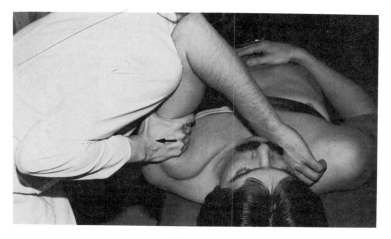

Fig. 11-5.

as possible to the joint. The force is a lateral pull to the humerus, stressing the anterior, posterior, superior, and inferior aspect of the capsule. A prolonged stretch is most effective.

Figure 11-6: Anterior Glide of the Humerus

Patient position: prone, with the involved extremity as close as possible to the edge of the table. The head of the humerus must be off the table. A wedge is placed just medial to the joint line under the coracoid process. The extremity is abducted in the plane of the scapula.

Therapist position: distal to the abducted part, facing cranially. The left hand applies an inferior pull to the humerus. The right hand moves the head of the humerus anteriorly, stressing the anterior recess and capsule. The tendinous portion of the subscapularis is also stressed with this technique. A prolonged stretch with oscillations at the end of the available range is very effective.

Figure 11-7: Anterior Glide of the Head of the Humerus

Patient position: supine, with the involved extremity as close as possible to the edge of the table. A strap may be used to stabilize the scapula (see Fig. 11-5).

Therapist position: facing cranially, with the right hand holding the head of the humerus as close as possible to the joint line. The left hand stabilizes the distal humerus, applying a slight distractive force. The force of the right hand moves the head of the humerus in an anterior direction, stretching the

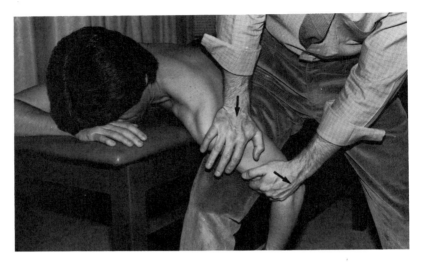

Fig. 11-6.

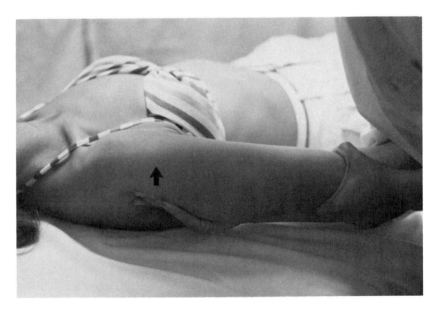

Fig. 11-7.

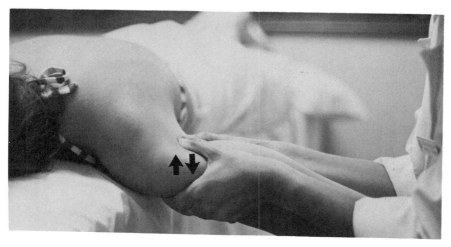

Fig. 11-8.

anterior capsular structures and the tendinous portion of the subscapularis. A prolonged stretch is most effective.

Figure 11-8: Anterior/Posterior Glide of the Head of the Humerus

Patient position: prone, with the involved extremity over the edge of the table abducted to the desired range. A strap may be used to stabilize the scapula.

Therapist position: facing laterally in a sitting position, with the forearm of the involved extremity held between the therapist's knees. Both hands grasp the head of the humerus and apply an up-and-down movement, oscillating the head of the humerus. Grades 1 and 2 are mainly used with this technique to stimulate mechanoreceptor activity.

Figure 11-9: Anterior/Posterior Glide of the Head of the Humerus

Patient position: supine, with the involved extremity supported by the table. A towel roll or wedge is placed under the elbow to hold the arm in the plane of the scapula (abduction anterior to the frontal plane).

Therapist position: facing laterally in a sitting position. The fingertips hold the head of the humerus while a gentle up-and-down movement is applied. This technique is used with grades 1 and 2 oscillations.

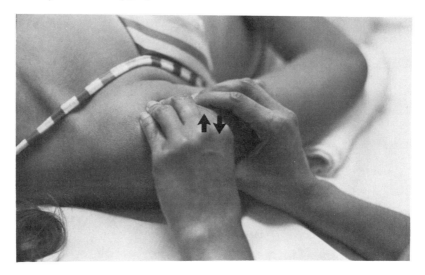

Fig. 11-9.

Figure 11-10: External Rotation of the Humerus

Patient position: supine, with the involved extremity supported by the table. The arm is held in the plane of the scapula.

Therapist position: facing laterally, with the right hand grasping the distal

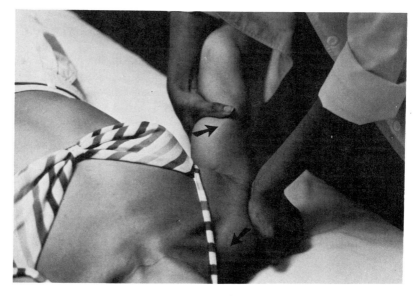

Fig. 11-10.

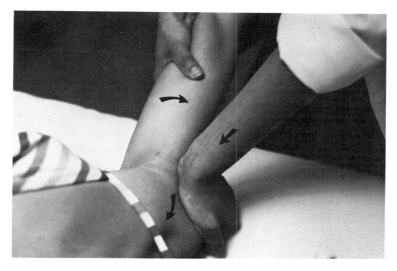

Fig. 11-11.

humerus; the heel of the left hand is placed over the lateral aspect of the head of the humerus. The force is applied through both hands. The right externally rotates the humerus. The left pushes on the most lateral aspect of the humeral head in a posterior direction, promoting external rotation of the humerus. A long-axis distractive force is applied during this technique. Graded oscillations or a thrust technique can be used.

Figure 11-11: External Rotation/Abduction/Inferior Glide of the Humerus

Patient position: supine, with the involved extremity supported by the table. The arm is abducted in the plane of the scapula.

Therapist position: facing laterally, with the right hand holding the distal humerus and the heel of the left hand over the head of the humerus. The forces are applied simultaneously. The right hand abducts the arm and externally rotates the humerus while maintaining the plane of the scapula position. The left hand simultaneously pushes the head of the humerus into external rotation and an inferior glide. The force applied can be a thrust or a prolonged stretch, both occurring at the end of the available range.

SCAPULOTHORACIC TECHNIQUES

A prolonged stretch is used with all the scapulothoracic techniques.

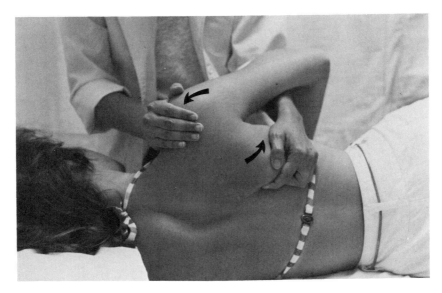

Fig. 11-12.

Figure 11-12: Scapula External Rotation

Patient position: side-lying, with the involved extremity accessible to the therapist.

Therapist position: facing the patient, with the left arm under the involved extremity through the axillary area. This allows the left hand to grasp the inferior angle of the scapula. The right hand holds the superior aspect of the scapula. The force is applied simultaneously, producing an external rotation of the scapula.

Figure 11-13: Scapula Distraction

Patient position: same as in Figure 11-12.

Therapist position: facing the patient, with the left hand grasping the inferior angle of the scapula and the right hand grasping the vertebral border of the scapula. Both hands pull the scapula up and away from the thoracic wall.

Figure 11-14: Inferior Glide of the Scapula

Patient position: same as Figure 11-12.

Therapist position: facing the patient, with the left web space surrounding the inferior angle of the scapula. The right hand holds the superior aspect of

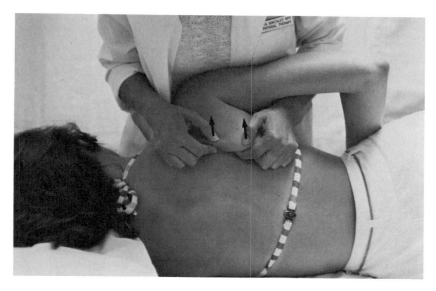

Fig. 11-13.

the scapula with a lumbrical grip. The right hand pushes in a caudal direction while the left hand moves under the inferior angle of the scapula.

Figure 11-15: Scapula Distraction, Prone

Patient position: prone, with the involved extremity supported by the table.

Therapist position: facing cranially, with the left hand under the head of

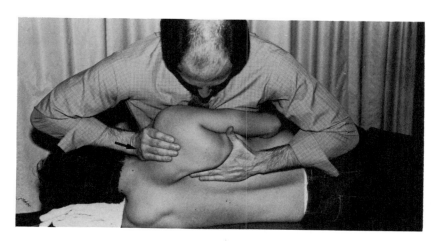

Fig. 11-14.

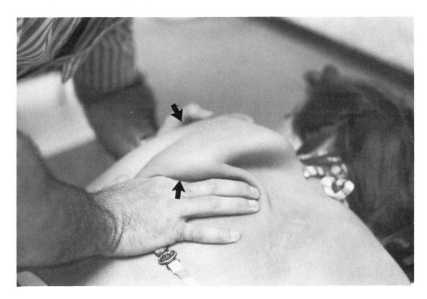

Fig. 11-15.

the humerus and the right web space under the inferior angle of the scapula. The forces are applied simultaneously. The left hand lifts the humerus while the right web space moves the inferior angle of the scapula.

STERNOCLAVICULAR AND ACROMIOCLAVICULAR TECHNIQUES

Figure 11-16: Superior Glide of the Sternoclavicular Joint

Patient position: supine, with the involved extremity close to the edge of the table.

Therapist position: facing cranially. The volar surface of the left thumb pad is placed over the inferior surface of the most medial aspect of the clavicle. The right thumb reinforces the dorsal aspect of the left thumb. Both thumbs push the clavicle superiorly. The graded oscillations are most successful with this technique.

Figure 11-17: Anterior Glide of the Acromioclavicular Joint

Patient position: supine and at a diagonal to allow the involved acromioclavicular joint to be over the edge of the table.

Therapist position: with the dorsal surface of the thumbs together, the

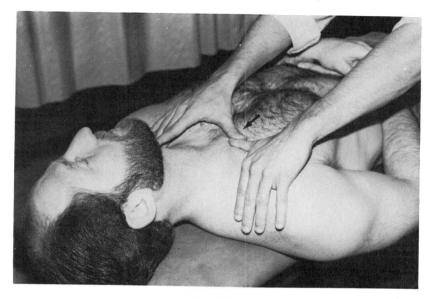

Fig. 11-16.

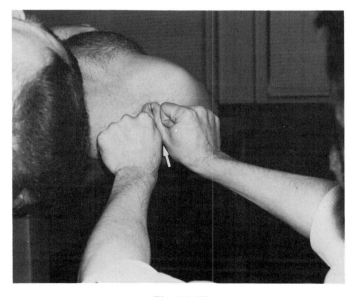

Fig. 11-17.

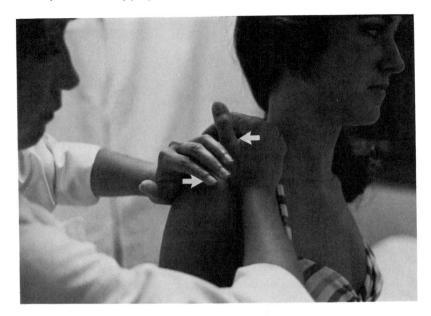

Fig. 11-18.

therapist places the distal tips of the thumbs posteriorly to the most lateral edge of the clavicle. Both thumbs push the clavicle anteriorly. The graded oscillations are mainly used with this technique.

Figure 11-18: Gapping of the Acromioclavicular Joint

Patient position: sitting close to the edge of the table.

Therapist position: facing laterally, with the heel of the left hand over the spine of the scapula and the thenar eminence of the right hand over the distal clavicle. The force is applied simultaneously. Both hands push the bones in opposite directions, obtaining a general stretch to the capsular structures of the acromioclavicular joint. Oscillations or a prolonged stretch are used with this technique.

The duration and amplitude of force suggested with each technique is based on my clinical experience.

SUMMARY

This chapter has reviewed several important mechanical, histologic, and neurophysiologic effects of mobilization. The shoulder joint is a complex organ. Mobilization is one aspect of treatment. The application of the mobilization techniques for the shoulder are dependent on the evaluation and assessment of the therapist. The indications and contraindications must be based on an understanding of the histology of immobilized and traumatized connective tissue. Remodeling of scar tissue is far more difficult than reversing the effects of short periods of immobilization. The most recent research indicates that early passive movement is important in the rehabilitation of joint restrictions. However, the velocity, amplitude, duration, and direction of force needed to produce a therapeutic effect requires further investigation. The role of mobilization in the future will be determined by the clinical research performed over the next decade.

ACKNOWLEDGMENTS

I would like to thank William Boissonnault, M.S., R.P.T., Steve Janos, R.P.T., Zita Gonzalez, R.P.T., and Amy Sowinski for their assistance with the technique pictures, and extend special thanks to Christy Moran and Helen Owens-Burkhart for their assistance with this chapter.

REFERENCES

1. Franks C, Akeson WH, Woo S, et al: Physiology and therapeutic value of passive joint motion. Clin Orthop 185:113, 1984
2. Stoddard A: Manual of Osteopathic Technique. Hutchinson, London, 1959
3. Maitland GD: Peripheral Manipulation. Butterworth, London, 1970
4. Clayton L (ed): Taber's Cyclopedic Medical Dictionary. FA Davis, Philadelphia, 1977
5. Friel J (ed): Dorland's Illustrated Medical Dictionary. 25th Ed. WB Saunders, Philadelphia, 1974
6. Warwick R, Williams P (eds): Gray's Anatomy. 35th British Ed. WB Saunders, Philadelphia, 1973
7. Wyke BD: The neurology of joints. Ann R Coll Surg Engl 41:25, 1966
8. Wyke BD: Neurological aspects of pain therapy: a review of some current concepts. p. 1. In Swerdlow M (ed): The Therapy of Pain. MTP Press Ltd., Lancaster, England, 1981
9. Akeson WH, Amiel D, Woo SL-Y: Immobility effects on synovial joints. The pathomechanics of joint contracture. Biorheology 17:95, 1980
10. Kelly M, Madden JW: Hand surgery and wound healing. p. 49. In Wolfort FG (ed): Acute Hand Injuries: A Multispeciality Approach. Little, Brown, Boston, 1980
11. Peacock EE, Jr: Wound Repair. 3rd Ed. WB Saunders, Philadelphia, 1984
12. Cohen KI, McCoy BJ, Diegelmann RF: An update on wound healing. Ann Plast Surg 3:264, 1979
13. Arem AJ, Madden JW: Effects of stress on healing wounds: intermittent noncyclical tension. J Surg Res 20:93, 1976
14. Woo S, Matthews JV, Akeson WH, et al: Connective tissue response to immobility: correlative study of biomechanical and biochemical measurements of normal and immobilized rabbit knees. Arthritis Rheum 18;257, 1975

15. Enneking W, Horowitz M: The inter-articular effects of immobilization on the human knee. J Bone Joint Surg 54-A:973, 1972
16. Evans E, Eggers G, Butler J, Blumel J: Immobilization and remobilization of rats' knee joints. J Bone Joint Surg 42-A:737, 1960
17. Haldeman S: Modern Developments in the Principles and Practice of Chiropractic. Appleton-Century-Crofts, East Norwalk, CT, 1980
18. Frank C, Woo SL-Y, Amiel D, et al: Medial collateral ligament healing: a multidisciplinary assessment in rabbits. Am J Sports Med 11:379, 1983
19. Tipton CM, James SL, Mergner W, Tcheng T: Influence of exercise on strength of medial collateral knee ligament of dogs. Am J Physiol 218:814, 1970
20. Kummel BM: Spectrum of lesion of the anterior capsule mechanism of the shoulder. Am J Sports Med 7:111, 1979
21. Poppen NK, Walker PS: Normal and abnormal motion of the shoulder. J Bone Joint Surg 58A:195, 1976
22. Saha AK: Theory of Shoulder Mechanism: Descriptive and Applied. Charles C Thomas, Springfield, IL, 1961
23. Light LE, Nuzik S, Personius W, Barstrom A: Low-load prolonged stretch vs. high-load brief stretch in treating knee contractures. Phys Ther 64:330, 1984
24. Warren CG, Lehman JF, Koblanski NJ: Elongation of rat tail tendon: effects of load and temperature. Arch Phys Med Rehabil 52:465, 1971
25. Warren CG, Lehman JF, Koblanski JN: Heat and stretch tech-procedure: an evaluation using rat tail tendon. Arch Phys Med Rehabil 57:122, 1976
26. Lehman JF, Masock AJ, Warren CG, Koblanski JN: Effects of therapeutic temperatures on tendon extensibility. Arch Phys Med Rehabil 51:481, 1970

12 | Management of Myofascial Dysfunction of the Shoulder

Patricia Scagnelli Hartman

MYOFASCIAL TRIGGER POINTS

Myofascial trigger points are often overlooked as a source of musculo-skeletal dysfunction. Trigger points occur frequently in the shoulder girdle musculature secondary to the many mechanical stresses directed to this region of the body. When a patient's complaint is of pain in the region of the shoulder, with or without restricted motion, the muscles of the shoulder girdle may be the origin of that pain.

Kellgren[1] concluded that pain referred from skeletal muscle usually followed spinal segmental patterns that were not dermatomal, but he noted many exceptions. Travell and Rinzler[2] showed that muscles referred pain extrasegmentally in characteristic patterns specific to each muscle. Travell and Simons[3] have done further work, and produced detailed documentation on myofascial pain and dysfunction.

This chapter focuses on trigger points and myofascial pain as a primary source of dysfunction. Clinically, the patient may have several factors causing dysfunction, only one of which is myofascial pain. Each patient should be given a thorough musculoskeletal evaluation, and the appropriate treatments should be rendered.

A generalized discussion of myofascial pain syndrome and its character-istics follows. Treatment is discussed in terms of techniques and modalities that have been most effective. The musculature of the shoulder girdle and their referred pain patterns is then reviewed.

Nature and Mechanism

A myofascial trigger point is a hyperirritable focus within a taut band of skeletal muscle located in the muscular tissue and/or its associated fascia. The point is painful on compression and can evoke characteristic referred pain and autonomic phenomena. The pain referred from the trigger point does not follow a simple segmental pattern, but is characteristic for each specific muscle.[2,3]

The literature on myofascial pain is confusing, and contains a profusion of terms, all attempting to describe muscle pain syndromes. Many of the terms have multiple meanings, depending on the author. The following terms are sometimes synonymous with myofascial pain and trigger points: myalgia,[4,5] myositis,[4,5] fibrositis,[4–6] fibromyositis,[4,5] myofibrositis,[4] fascitis,[4,5] myofasci-tis,[4,5,7] muscular rheumatism,[4,5] muscular strain,[4] nonarticular rheumatism,[6] myogelosis,[8] and interstitial myofibrositis.[9,10]

There is little information on the trigger point's exact histologic makeup and neurophysiologic mechanism. In a review of the literature, the term *fibro-sitis* is initially used at the turn of the century to explain tender muscles. In-flammatory changes in the fibrous structures of the muscles, nerves, and fascia were believed to be the cause of the pain.[6] Histologic investigation has failed to confirm this theory. The term *fibrositis* then became associated with non-specific muscle pain that lacked abnormal x-ray and laboratory findings[6] and that had no implication of pathogenesis.[5]

Other investigators continued to attempt to define the mechanism of the trigger point. In 1927, Albee[7] introduced the term *myofascitis*. He described a toxic condition of the blood caused by the colon with local manifestations in the muscle and fascia. Copeman and Ackerman[11] identified herniations of fatty tissue through their fibrous fascial compartments, which caused painful tension. They postulated that the production of pain at the trigger point took place in the fibrofatty tissue and not in the muscle.

Localized muscle spasm[12–14] was believed to be the cause of the palpable band or trigger point until the 1960s. Electromyographic (EMG) studies per-formed by Kraft et al.[6] in 1968 demonstrated that the area of "muscle spasm" was electrically silent. The concept of "spasm-pain-spasm" and the use of ethyl chloride spray or heat to "relax the spasm" was deemed not credible. Kraft et al.[6] proposed that altered kinin production in the skin could explain the palpable changes seen in the fibrositic muscles, the associated dermatographia, and the marked response to painful stimuli. Kinins are a group of polypeptides capable of inciting pain, causing vasodilation, and increasing capillary perme-ability.[6]

As EMG study done in 1985 by Friction et al.[15] confirmed that the local twitch response is specific to the fibers of the palpable taut band associated with the trigger point. The taut band of the trigger point at rest has no electric activity and is assumed to be composed of shortened fibers.

The term *interstitial myofibrositis*[9,10] gained popularity with several researchers who believed that the disorder was inflammatory and involved the interstitial connective tissue elements of the muscle. The findings of Ibrahim et al.[10] suggested that the patterns of serum and muscle isoenzymes in patients with myofibrositis are similar to those in patients with some connective tissue diseases. Brendstrup et al.[16] in 1957 and Awad[9] in 1973 took biopsies of fibrositic nodules and found local edema and interfascicular deposition of acid mucopolysaccharides in connective tissue of the muscle. Brendstrup et al.[16] proposed that the pain from the fibrositic muscles might be secondary to the resultant distention of the connective tissue of the muscle caused by interstitial edema.

A few investigators have demonstrated that the histologic findings of the muscle fibers are unspecific, but indicate that the muscle fibers are abnormal. Miehlke and Schuke and associates[17–19] found histologic changes, including fatty infiltration, increased number of fibrocytic and sarcolemmal nuclei, and loss of cross-striations of the muscle fibers. Henriksson et al.[20] and Yunus et al.[21] found a moth-eaten appearance of fibers evenly distributed over the whole cross-section and affecting only type I fibers. Also noted were mitochondrial abnormalities, and an abnormal relationship that existed between the mitochondria and the myofibrils. Energy metabolites and glycogen were also decreased significantly in these patients. Henriksson et al.[20] postulated that a primary metabolic disturbance or an overload myopathy was secondary to a more or less continuous increase in muscle tension. A recent study by Hagberg and Kvarnstrom[22] demonstrated that the EMG endurance time was short for muscles affected with myofascial syndrome, but normal in relation to EMG fatigue changes. Hagberg and Kvarnstrom[22] believed that the increased localized muscle fatigue possibly was caused by the decrease in mitochondria reported by Henriksson et al.[20]

Simons and Stolov[23] believed that the band-like induration could be caused by circumscribed transient muscle contraction rather than histologically demonstrable structural changes. Travell and Simons[3] have further developed this theory, proposing that the palpable band can probably be explained as a physiologic contracture of muscle fibers (a contraction without action potentials[3]). A contracture of muscle fibers in the band would make it feel hard and tense as compared with the surrounding fibers in the muscle. They propose that the initial activation of the trigger point starts with trauma that damages the sarcoplasmic reticulum. The sarcomeres are exposed to calcium, which initiates contractile activity. The sarcomeres that are exposed to calcium for an extended period would then maintain contractile activity as long as their ATP energy supply lasted. A sustained contractile force creates tension, and the contraction of these fibers results in a palpable band. The contractile force stops if the muscle is stretched and the sarcomere is elongated enough to separate the myosin heads from the reactive portion of the actin filaments. A reverberatory neural circuit may be established between nociceptors, the central nervous system, and motor units, resulting in chronic muscle band shortening, increased irritability, and motor unit firing on palpation.[15,24] This reverberatory neural circuit may be partially responsible for the local twitch response and its corresponding EMG changes.[15]

Hyperirritability of the trigger point may be explained by the sensitization of the muscle afferent nerve endings.[3,9] Awad[9] found nerve-sensitizing substances released from platelets (serotonin) and degranulating cells (histamine) in the area of the trigger point. The kinins reported by Kraft et al.[6] could also act as sensitizing agents.[3]

It is apparent that many discrepancies exist regarding the nature of trigger points. Some investigators reported normal histologic findings, whereas others reported unspecific abnormal findings in the muscle fibers. Travell and Simons[3] postulated that this could be a result of an acute versus chronic or dystrophic phase in the trigger point. In the acute phase, there would be no demonstrable histologic findings, whereas, in the dystrophic phase, abnormal histologic findings would be present in the muscle fibers.

Melzack et al.[24] believe that trigger points and acupuncture points represent the same phenomena. Pressure at certain points is associated with particular pain patterns, and brief intense stimulation of these points sometimes produces prolonged relief of pain.[24] In a study correlating spatial distribution and associated pain patterns, Melzack et al.[24] found 71 percent correspondence between trigger points and acupuncture points. The referred pain from both the trigger point and the acupuncture point can be explained as the result of mechanisms understood in terms of the "gate control theory" described by Melzack et al.[24] Further discussion of this topic is beyond the scope of this chapter, but may be found in Melzack et al.'s work.[24]

Clinical Characteristics

There are different classifications of trigger points. An active trigger point causes pain and decreased extensibility of a muscle. A latent trigger point is clinically silent with respect to pain, but may cause decreased extensibility and weakness of that muscle. The patient may not be aware of the latent trigger point until the clinician compresses it and the patient experiences the local and/or referred pain. Satellite trigger points may form in the referred pain region, whereas secondary trigger points may form in adjacent muscles owing to increased stresses placed on them from the primary muscle's hypersensitivity, shortened position, and weakness.[3]

Trigger points can be activated directly or indirectly. Direct activation occurs by acute overload, sustained muscle contraction, direct trauma, and chilling.[3] Indirect activation can result from other trigger points, visceral disease, arthritic joints, and emotional distress.[3]

Any sex or age group can develop trigger points, but the sedentary middle-aged woman is the most vulnerable.[3,6] The likelihood of developing active trigger points increases with age through the middle active years.[3] In the later years, when there is less strenuous activity, the trigger points may become latent and be exhibited primarily as stiffness and restricted motion.[3]

The patient's complaints are usually of stiffness at rest and a deep aching pain if allowed to stay in a prolonged position. Some relief is felt after the patient first changes position or moves. The patient usually reports that a moderate amount of activity causes increased aching as well as fatigue. Cold, damp weather as well as emotional stress or tension aggravate the symptoms. Complaints of weakness and stiffness in the involved muscle are common. Muscular strength can become unreliable, and the patient with shoulder girdle trigger points may report unexpected dropping of objects.

Symptoms and complaints relate to the most active trigger point. When treatment has begun and this trigger point has been eliminated, the pain pattern may shift to that of an earlier or less active trigger point.[3] This explains why many patients may report pain/symptoms shifting in location or from one side to the other.

The more hypersensitive the trigger point, the more intense and constant the referred pain and the more extensive its distribution.[1,3] The size of the muscle is not important.[1,3]

Phenomena other than pain are often caused by the trigger points.[3] Many autonomic symptoms, such as localized vasoconstriction, sweating, lacrimation, coryza, salivation, and pilomotor activity, can occur in the referred pain region. Proprioceptive disturbances such as imbalance, dizziness, and tinnitus also occur.

Travell and Simons[3] formulated a list of the general clinical characteristics of trigger points:

1.   When an active trigger point is present, passive or active stretching of the affected muscle increases the pain.

2.   The stretch range of motion (ROM) of the particular muscle is restricted.

3.   The pain is increased when the affected muscle is strongly contracted against resistance.

4.   The maximum contractile force of the affected muscle is weakened and is not associated with atrophy or pain unless the patient uses significant effort.

5.   Deep tenderness and dysesthesia are referred by active trigger points to the referred pain region.

6.   Autonomic disturbances sometimes occur in the referred pain region.

7.   Muscles in the vicinity of the trigger point feel tense to palpation.

8.   The trigger point is found in a palpable band as a sharply circumscribed spot of exquisite tenderness.

9.   Digital pressure applied to an active trigger point causes the patient to jump and cry out.

10.   Snapping palpation of the trigger point frequently evokes a local twitch response.

11.   Moderately sustained pressure on an irritable trigger point causes or intensifies pain in the referred pain pattern of that trigger point.

12.   The skin of some patients displays dermatographia (whealing) and panniculosis ("orange-peel" effect).

A myofascial pain syndrome due to active trigger points can be identified by history and physical examination.[25,26] Laboratory and imaging studies are useful only to rule out other disease processes, to identify perpetuating factors, and to substantiate diagnosis.[25] Myofascial pain syndromes are essentially single muscle syndromes with trigger points that may combine to form complex patterns involving many muscles in many regions of the body.[21,25]

The history of a patient with shoulder pain due to myofascial trigger point has certain characteristic features[26]: progressive spread of the pain from one site of the injury to adjacent areas, exacerbations and remissions of pain that may be related to physical activity, and a failure of customary therapy to provide relief.

Specific to the shoulder, Reynolds[26] characterizes the clinical diagnosis. There is an absence of articular signs, such as pain related to specific movement of the joint, a marked decrease in ROM, swelling, or crepitus. Active and passive ROM at the glenohumeral joint is normal or slightly decreased. Movement may be restricted in some directions and not others, signifying that the problem may be muscular. The pain is not neuralgic in character. Weakness may be present, but is not prominent. There is no atrophy. Spurling's test for cervical nerve root irritation is negative.

The key to diagnosis is palpation of the entire shoulder and adjacent area, with special attention to the muscles to discover trigger points.[26] Two findings are necessary for diagnosis[25]: exquisite spot tenderness at the trigger point and a palpable band of taut muscle fibers running through the trigger point. The muscle lacks full strength and ROM. Muscles on the side opposite the injury and in the neck also frequently become involved.[26]

Perpetuating Factors

Management of the many perpetuating factors of myofascial pain syndrome is necessary for the patient to get optimum relief. The shoulder girdle is especially vulnerable because its anatomic relationships make it susceptible to fatigue. There are three kinds of mechanical stresses that can cause or perpetuate a trigger point within the shoulder girdle[3]: postural stresses, constriction of muscles, and structural inadequacies.

The postural stresses refer to poor body mechanics, immobility, and poor posture. In the shoulder girdle, poor posture has been clinically referred to as the forward head posture, with resultant scapular elevation, abduction, and shoulder protraction. The ways in which this altered head, neck, and shoulder girdle relationship can cause or perpetuate dysfunction are described in Chapter 4.

Posture can also encompass sitting and sleeping positions. Prolonged sitting in a chair that does not offer adequate lumbar support[3] therefore allows an increased thoracic kyphosis, forward head, and protracted shoulders and can have the same effect as poor postural alignment in standing. Positioning of work materials while at a desk to avoid excessive reaching and twisting can also lessen the stress on the shoulder girdle muscles. Prolonged talking on the telephone using the shoulder and neck to hold the telephone can stress the shoulder girdle and cause dysfunction. Evaluation of patient's sleeping posture may also be enlightening as to the placement of stress on particular muscles.

Poor body mechanics can be stressful to the shoulder girdle by actions such as repetitive reaching, especially overhead.[3]

Prolonged immobility, such as bed rest, without using good positioning may affect the shoulder girdle by causing shortening of muscles or prolonged stretch or strain of a muscle. Immobilization after a fracture or dislocation of the humerus also has the potential to activate trigger points for the same reasons.[3]

Prolonged pressure on a muscle or constriction of a portion of a muscle can occur often in the shoulder girdle. Tight upper body clothing, such as a tight bra strap, can create enough constriction to perpetuate dysfunction. The strap of a heavy purse hung on the shoulder may also cause constriction.[3]

Structural inadequacies refer to body asymmetries.[3] The asymmetry must be compensated for, resulting in altered movement patterns. The change in normal function results in continual stress to the musculoskeletal system; and this abnormal stress can cause or perpetuate trigger points. An asymmetry as distal as a short leg can, through the kinetic chain, alter the position of not only the spine but also the shoulder girdle and head.

Fibrositis/Fibromyalgia

Over the last several years, there has been the emergence of what many[21,25,27,28] feel are two diagnostic categories: fibrositis (fibromyalgia) and myofascial pain syndrome. In the past, these two categories were not specifically described as separate entities. Although muscle stress, including mechanical trauma, plays a primary role in myofascial pain syndrome, trauma is not the primary causative factor in fibrositis/fibromyalgia.[27] The pain of fibrositis/fibromyalgia is chronic with systemic symptomatology.[27] Chronicity and widespread location is not a necessary condition in myofascial pain syndrome.[27]

In fibrositis/fibromyalgia, there are tender points present, not trigger points. A tender point is a localized area of tenderness found in muscle and other numerous nonmuscular structures that may or may not cause referred pain.[21,25] Myofascial trigger points are self-sustaining hyperirritable foci located in the skeletal muscle or its associated fascia.[25] Two hallmark findings of trigger points are the local twitch response elicited by snapping palpation of the trigger point and reproduction of the patient's pain by sustained pressure applied to the trigger point.[25] All trigger points are tender points.[25] Some tender points may be trigger points; some may be tender points in areas of referred pain by the active trigger point.[25]

Although a few investigators[25,27,28] refer to fibrositis/fibromyalgia as a separate entity, Yunus et al.[21] advocate using the term *primary fibromyalgia syndrome*. This syndrome is characterized by tender points in seven of 14 specified locations[27] or five of 40 locations[21] in muscular or nonmuscular tissue.

Yunus et al.[21] further classify the primary fibromyalgia syndrome as being rheumatologic in nature and having generalized aches and pains at three or more anatomic sites for more than 3 months with no underlying cause. There is modulation of symptoms by weather, physical activity, anxiety, stress, poor sleep, and general fatigue.[21,27] Chronic headaches, irritable bowel syndromes, and subjective swelling and numbness may also be present.[21,27] Such systemic features are not usually present in myofascial pain syndrome but may develop in those patients who have become chronic.[27]

Treatment of fibrositis/fibromyalgia is supportive and nonspecific.[28,29] Treatment of myofascial pain syndrome is directed specifically to the muscles involved with physical modalities[3,25,28] (see section on treatment).

The question posed is whether a patient with fibrositis/fibromyalgia has only extensive myofascial trigger points aggravated by severe perpetuating factors, or a separate systemic disorder, or some combination of fibrositis/fibromyalgia and myofascial pain syndrome.[25,28]

Physical Therapy Treatment

The treatments discussed here pertain only to trigger points. The clinician should be aware that myofascial pain is often only a part of the patient's dysfunction and other treatments are warranted as well.

Around a trigger point, the subcutaneous tissues are thickened and congested.[3] The skin becomes adherent to the underlying superficial fascia and loses its movement and elasticity. This is called panniculosis. The skin and superficial fascia should be checked for mobility in all directions. If an area of restriction is found, stroking techniques into the area of restriction should be used on the skin and superficial fascia.

Skin Rolling

Skin rolling is a technique frequently used when panniculosis is evident.[30] The skin and superficial fascia are picked up between the thumb and fingers, and are rolled backward over the advancing thumbs, which keep up the pressure behind the roll all the time. No lubricant is used and, when the area of the trigger point is reached, there is an "orange-peel" effect as well as an increase in pain.

Pressure

Sustained pressure or ischemic compression over a trigger point appears to block noxious impulses from the muscles and produces relief of pain as well as relaxation.[3,30] The relaxed muscle is stretched to the verge of discomfort, and a thumb or strong finger is pressed directly on the trigger point to create a painful sustained pressure. The pressure should be tolerable. This pressure is gradually increased and continued for approximately 1 minute.[3,30]

Massage

Massage techniques are used often in the treatment of myofascial pain. Massage has a mechanical effect of helping return venous blood, lymph, and catabolites into the mainstream of the circulation.[30] It aids the absorption of substances within the tissues.[3] Perhaps it produces an effect by washing out the sensitizing substances that are reported in the literature to accumulate around trigger points.[3] Williams and Elkins[31] advocate a firm, heavy friction type of massage rather than a kneading or stroking type in the treatment of their patients. Friction massage, which rubs the most superficial tissues over underlying structures, is often used to the tolerance of the patient. Travell and Simons[3] feel that a vigorous massage of hyperirritable trigger points can cause an adverse reaction with a marked increase in pain. Zohn and Mennell[30] advocate a firm kneading (length or across) or stretching massage.

In general, many clinicians find success by starting the treatment with the superficial fascial techniques and then progressing to light stroking techniques, adding more pressure gradually. The friction massage and deep, firm techniques are much more tolerable to the patient if the tissues are gradually prepared. In acute stages, firm massages cannot be used in many cases.

Stretching

Stretching techniques are the hallmark of the treatment program in a patient with myofascial pain dysfunction. The reasoning behind this lies in the theory mentioned earlier about the sarcomere's exposure to calcium, which produces a contractile force. The contractile force stops if the muscle is stretched and the sarcomere is elongated enough to separate the myosin heads from the reactive portion of the actin filaments. To inactivate the trigger point fully, the muscle must be extended to its full normal length.[3] The stretching should be on the verge of causing pain, but should evoke only local discomfort and not referred pain.[3] Optimal tension is about two-thirds of the muscle's normal stretch ROM.[3]

Stretching in itself may cause pain and a reflex spasm to develop in a muscle with a very irritable trigger point. When this occurs, a vapocoolant spray can be used. Flouri-methane spray (Gebauer Chemical Co, Cleveland,

OH) is the vapocoolant frequently used. In the spray and stretch method, the jet stream of the vapocoolant is applied once to cover the length of the muscle before the stretch is applied. The muscle is slowly stretched with a steady increase in force, as described previously, and the spray is directed in parallel lines from the trigger point over the muscle and through the area of referred pain. After a full stretch is completed, the return must be smooth and gradual.

The vapocoolant acts as a counterirritant.[12] Intense stimulation on the skin by the cold is transmitted by larger afferents faster than the noxious pain impulses from the muscle,[30] creating a refractory period during which reception of the noxious impulses is blocked. During this period, the muscle can be relaxed and stretched to a normal resting length.[30] When the normal resting length is obtained, the normal tonic reflexes are restored and the muscle is capable of normal, pain-free function.[30] There is also some degree of direct depression of cutaneous receptors by cooling.[12] The vapocoolant spray also has effects similar to those of a light stroking massage.[12]

Recently activated, acute, single muscle trigger point syndromes may respond to passive stretch and hot packs without vapocooling, whereas more chronic cases require both stretch and spray.[3] If the condition becomes chronic, the vapocoolant's effect may be significantly diminished.[12] As pain decreases, stiffness with a decrease in ROM is the chief complaint. The muscles during this stage are less responsive to stretch and spray.[3]

The Lewit and Simons[3,32] technique places the muscle to be stretched on a manually resisted isometric contraction followed by relaxation. The clinician passively stretches the involved muscle to a point just short of pain or onset of resistance to further movement. The patient exerts a prolonged, gentle isometric contraction against minimal resistance for approximately 10 seconds, then relaxes. When there is full relaxation, the clinician instructs the patient to take a deep breath and exhale completely. During exhalation, the muscle is stretched further, but only as far as muscle relaxation allows (slight resistance from the new position). The procedure is repeated. A set of three to five repetitions usually provides as much progress as could be obtained in one session.[32] If increased stretch ROM is not obtained after isometric contraction, the contraction time is increased to 30 seconds.[32] The technique itself can be taught to the patient and can be used as a home stretching exercise.

The Lewit and Simons technique is successful because the stretch equalizes the lengths of the sarcomeres throughout each involved muscle fiber and thereby normalizes the function of the contractile elements of the muscle.[32] Therefore, the most important factor in the success of this technique is precision in aligning the stretch to the involved muscle fibers.

Zohn and Mennell[30] advocate that ice massage be used if vapocoolant is not available. The ice cube is held by the edge of a small towel, which is also used to wipe up the water from the melted ice, keeping the skin dry. The ice is applied out from the trigger point and over its referred pain pattern in parallel lines. Once the skin gets cold and red in a histamine-like response, the patient becomes conscious of a tender mass over the site of maximum pain.[30] When this sensation disappears, the pain is usually relieved and the treated part is cold and numb. Stretching is then begun.

Stretching immediately after trigger point injection has been shown to be beneficial.[3,26,28] For a discussion on trigger point injections, the reader is referred to Chapter 13 or to the work of Travell and Simons.[3]

Ultrasound

Ultrasound has been used with some success as an adjunct to the therapy. One technique starts with a setting of 0.5 W/cm^2 with a circular motion that completes one circle in 2 to 3 seconds.[33] The circle is tight enough to overlap the trigger point. Many other clinicians use ultrasound at a setting of 1.0 to 2.0 W/cm^2 in a circular motion as described above.

The literature on the effects of ultrasound on muscle reports an alteration of cell permeability, producing changes in isometric tension, decreased membrane potentials, and retardation of the deterioration of specific muscle proteins.[33,34] Because the nature of trigger points remains in dispute, it is difficult to draw conclusions as to specific benefits of ultrasound. If the trigger point does indeed have a dystrophic phase, as suggested previously by Travell and Simons,[3] ultrasound effects would appear to be beneficial in reversing or retarding the process. The mechanical action of the sound waves may help to prevent or reverse symptoms arising from adhesions within the interstitial tissue.[30] A recent study by Klemp et al.[35] reported that ultrasound decreased the muscle blood flow in muscles with trigger points. It was generally believed that treatment of trigger points with ultrasound increased the muscle blood flow.

Ultrasound in combination with electric stimulation has also demonstrated some therapeutic results.[3,30,36] The mechanical pumping by the electric stimulation probably dissipates the products of increased metabolism or edema away from the muscle being treated and restores its physiologic state to near normal.[30]

Heat

Heat in the form of hot packs is effective as an adjunct to therapy. Dry heat is not as effective as wet heat. Application of a hot pack after stretching helps reduce post-treatment muscle soreness.[3] The wet heat promotes further reduction of muscle tension.[3]

Transcutaneous Electric Nerve Stimulation

Some clinicians[37,38] advocate the use of transcutaneous electric nerve stimulation in the treatment of myofascial pain syndrome. Phero et al.[38] reported that electrodes may be placed directly over the area of pain, on the trigger point, within the dermatome where the pain is located, over myotomes, or over superficial peripheral nerves. Acupuncture and motor points have also been used.[38] Optimal stimulation will occur with at least two of these entities existing at the same location.[38]

Pressure Algometry

A hand-held pressure algometer has been recently used to determine a psychophysiologic index of trigger and tender points. It consists of a plunger mounted on a calibrated spring. Several studies[29,39-41] have been done to show that the pressure algometer is reliable to tender and trigger point sensitivity, especially when the sensitivity is defined as the amount of pressure needed to elicit a threshold response.[40]

Many investigators[25,28,29,39-41] advocate the use of the pressure algometer to quantify the clinical outcome of treatment. In myofascial pain syndrome, trigger point sensitivity has been reported to be associated with decreased subjective reports of referred pain intensity.[39]

Summary

Trigger points occur frequently in the shoulder girdle musculature due to the many mechanical stresses directed to this region of the body. A trigger point is a hyperirritable focus within a taut band of skeletal muscle located in the muscular tissue and/or its associated fascia. The trigger point is painful on compression and can evoke characteristic referred pain specific to each muscle as well as autonomic phenomena. A tender point is not a trigger point, whereas a trigger point is always a tender point.

More research is needed to determine the nature and mechanism of the trigger point. Some researchers report normal histologic findings, whereas others report unspecific abnormal findings of the muscle fibers. This may be a result of an acute versus chronic phase in the trigger point. A recent explanation for the taut band or trigger point is that it is a physiologic contracture of muscle fibers.

Because of the uncertain nature and mechanism of the trigger point, speculation exists as to why some treatments are beneficial in the treatment of myofascial pain dysfunction. The most important aspect of treatment centers around proper stretching of the involved muscle. Stretching may elongate the sarcomere enough to separate the myosin heads from the reactive portion of the actin filaments and interrupt the physiologic contracture. Vapocoolant spray and icing coupled with stretching give additional benefits. Massage, ultrasound, transcutaneous electric nerve stimulation, and heat have also been beneficial. Pressure algometry may be useful in quantifying the clinical outcome of treatment.

SHOULDER GIRDLE MUSCLES

The following is an overview of some of the shoulder girdle musculature that refers pain to the region of the shoulder. A brief discussion on referred pain, common patient complaints, findings on evaluation, trigger point locations, and stretch techniques for each particular muscle will be provided. The reader is referred to the bibliography for more detailed information on each particular muscle.

Subscapularis

The subscapularis muscle refers pain mainly to the posterior aspect of the shoulder and posterior arm down to the elbow.[2,3] There is also a strap-like area of referred pain and tenderness around the wrist, with the dorsum of the wrist usually more painful and tender than the volar[2,3] (see Fig. 2-4).

The patient usually presents with restriction of movement in shoulder abduction and external rotation. Resisted shoulder adduction and internal rotation may be weak and painful. Pain is present at rest and with motion.

Many times, the patient has been diagnosed as having adhesive capsulitis or frozen shoulder when Travell and Simons[3] believe that the trigger points in the subscapularis may be the original culprit. They feel that the subscapularis trigger points may sensitize the other shoulder girdle musculature into developing secondary and satellite trigger points. This could lead to a full-blown restriction in glenohumeral motion.

Trigger points are in the scapular fossa along the axillary border of the scapula[2,3] and occasionally more medially toward the superior angle of the scapula.[3]

For stretch position, see Figure 12-1.

Supraspinatus

The supraspinatus muscle's referred pain causes a deep ache around the shoulder,[42] especially in the middle deltoid region. It extends down the arm and forearm, sometimes focusing at the lateral epicondyle of the elbow.[2,3]

The patient's chief complaint is pain, especially during abduction of the shoulder, and a dull ache at rest. Snapping and clicking sounds occur around the shoulder due to the tautness of the supraspinatus fibers interfering with the normal glide of the humeral head.[3] Resisted abduction and sometimes resisted external rotation of the shoulder are weak and painful. The patient may be unable to abduct the arm fully.

Two trigger points lie in the supraspinatus fossa of the scapula.[2,3]

For stretch position, see Figure 12-2.

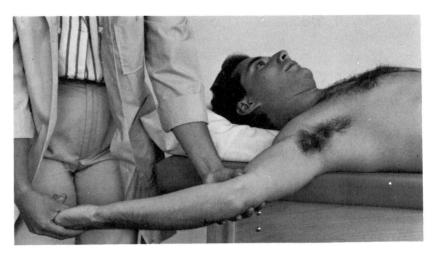

Fig. 12-1.   Stretch for subscapularis.

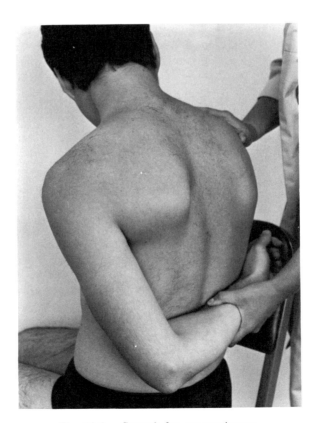

Fig. 12-2.   Stretch for supraspinatus.

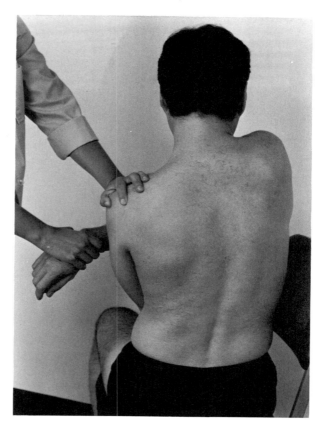

Fig. 12-3. Stretch for infraspinatus.

Infraspinatus

The infraspinatus muscle refers pain to the anterior shoulder/deltoid region,[1-3,13,14,43,44] down the anterolateral aspect of the arm to the lateral forearm,[1-3,13,14,43] the radial aspect of the hand,[1-3,43,44] and, occasionally, the fingers[2,3,13] (see Fig. 2-5).

The patient may complain of shoulder girdle fatigue, weakness of grip, and loss of mobility at the shoulder.[43] A restriction in simultaneous internal rotation and adduction of the shoulder is often present.[3] Difficulty in lying on the same side or supine at night can occur due to the compression and stimulation of the trigger point by the weight of the thorax.[3] Resisted external rotation and adduction may be painful and weak, while passive abduction and internal rotation may be painful and restricted.

There are three trigger points, all located in the infraspinatus fossa of the scapula.[2,3]

For stretch position, see Figure 12-3.

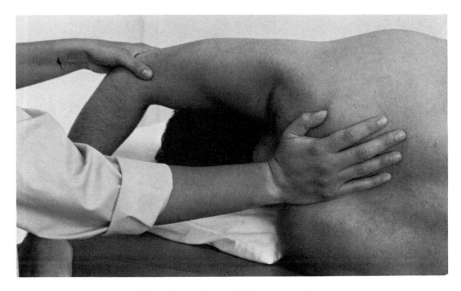

Fig. 12-4.   Stretch for teres minor.

Teres Minor

The teres minor muscle refers pain in the posterior deltoid muscle region[3] (see Fig. 2-6).

The patient's complaint is more of pain than of restricted motion of the shoulder with internal rotation. Resisted external rotation of the shoulder may be painful and weak. Resisted adduction of the shoulder is occasionally painful.

The trigger point is found on the lateral edge of the scapula between the infraspinatus above and the teres minor below.[3]

For stretch position, see Figure 12-4.

Teres Major

The teres major muscle refers pain to the posterior deltoid region and over the long head of the triceps brachii.[3,42] It may refer pain into the shoulder joint posteriorly and occasionally to the dorsal forearm, but rarely to the scapula or elbow.[3]

The patient complains of pain on motion or reaching overhead. Rest pain is mild.[3] Resisted internal rotation, resisted extension, and resisted adduction of the shoulder all may be painful and weak. Passive abduction and external rotation of the shoulder may be restricted.

The trigger points are located medially overlying the posterior surface of the scapula and laterally in the posterior axillary fold.[3]

For stretch position, see Figure 12-5.

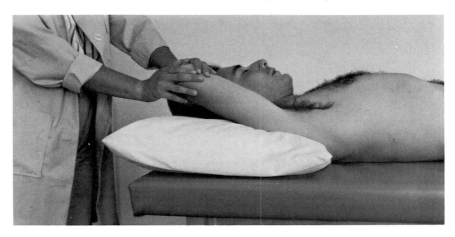

Fig. 12-5. Stretch for teres major.

Deltoid

The deltoid has no distal projection of referred pain. The anterior deltoid refers pain to the anterior middle deltoid region.[2,3,30] The posterior deltoid refers pain to the middle and posterior deltoid region.[2,3,30]

The patient will report experiencing pain deep in the deltoid region with motion of the shoulder, especially with abduction and extension movements of the shoulder combined. Resisted abduction and flexion of the shoulder are painful and weak, with involvement of the anterior deltoid; resisted abduction and extension are painful and weak, with involvement of the posterior deltoid.

Trigger points are located in the anterior portion of the shoulder for the anterior deltoid[3] and more distally along the posterior margin of the muscle for the posterior deltoid.[3]

For stretch position, see Figures 12-6 and 12-7.

Latissimus Dorsi

The latissimus dorsi muscle refers pain to the inferior angle of the scapula and mid-thoracic region.[1,3] It may also extend to the back of the shoulder, down the medial aspect of the arm, forearm, and hand, including the ring and little fingers.[3]

The patient will complain that reaching forward and upward with the arm causes pain. Resisted shoulder internal rotation and extension are painful and sometimes weak. Passive shoulder flexion with external rotation may be painful and restricted.

The trigger points are located in the axillary portion of the muscles.[3]

For stretch position, see Figure 12-8.

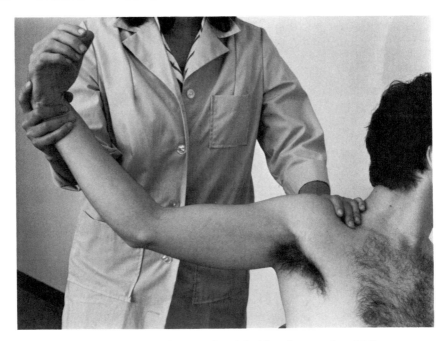

Fig. 12-6.   Stretch for anterior deltoid and coracobrachialis.

Levator Scapula

The levator scapula muscle refers pain to the neck and back of the head,[2,3,43] the vertebral border of the scapula,[2,3] and the posterior shoulder[2,3,43] (see Fig. 7-10).

The patient will report stiffness at the base of the neck.[3,43] There will be some restriction in cervical rotation to the same side as the involved muscle. There may also be an elevated scapula or shoulder shrug on the involved side.

Trigger points are located at the angle of the neck[3] and at the superior angle of the scapula.[2,3]

For stretch position, see Figure 12-9.

Rhomboid Major and Minor

The rhomboid major and minor muscles refer pain to the vertebral border of the scapula[3] and may spread up over the supraspinatus portion of the scapula.[1,3]

Snapping and crunching noises during movement of the scapula may be due to trigger points in the rhomboid muscles.[3] Motion of the glenohumeral joint does not aggravate the symptoms.

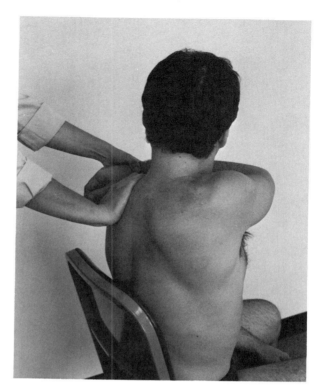

Fig. 12-7.   Stretch for posterior deltoid.

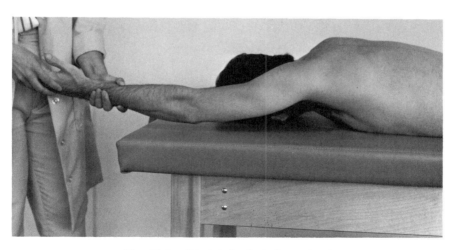

Fig. 12-8.   Stretch for latissimus dorsi.

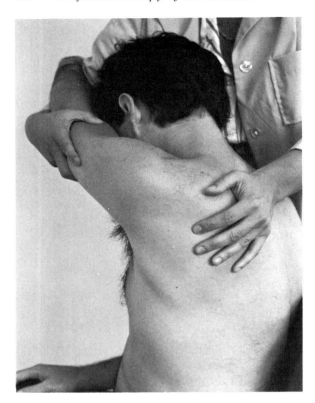

Fig. 12-9. Stretch for levator scapula.

Trigger points are located along the scapular vertebral border.[3,44]
For stretch position, see Figure 12-10.

Pectoralis Major

The pectoralis major muscle refers pain substernally,[3] to the anterior chest and breast,[2,3] the anterior shoulder,[2,3] and the ulnar aspect of the arm to the fourth and fifth fingers.[2,3]

Generally, a patient will complain of pain in the anterior shoulder and subclavicular region.[3] Breast pain and diffuse soreness may also be a complaint.[3] Symptoms similar to cardiac pain may also be present.[3]

Examination of the patient reveals a protracted shoulder on the involved side. Resisted horizontal adduction and internal rotation of the shoulder may be painful and weak. Passive stretch of the shoulder into horizontal abduction with external rotation is restricted and painful.

Trigger points are found throughout all portions of the muscle.[3]

For stretch position, see Figure 12-11.

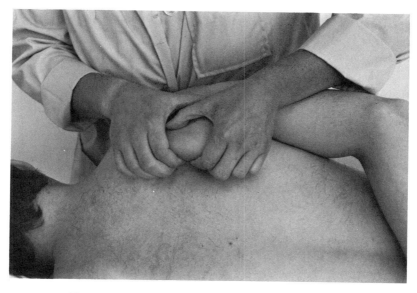

Fig. 12-10. Stretch for rhomboid major and minor.

Pectoralis Minor

The pectoralis minor muscle refers pain primarily to the anterior shoulder,[2,3] but also to the anterior chest[2,3] and sometimes down the ulnar side of the arm, forearm, and last three fingers.[2,3] Its pattern of referral is similar to that of the pectoralis major muscle (see Fig. 7-11).

The patient's complaints of pain are similar to the pain experienced from a pectoralis major trigger point, cardiac pain included. The shortened pectoralis minor may entrap the brachial plexus and cause a distribution of symptoms similar to thoracic outlet syndrome.

Examination of the patient usually reveals an increase in protraction of the shoulder girdle complex on the involved side. Passive movement of the shoulder into horizontal abduction and external rotation will be restricted and painful, and may cause neurovascular symptoms into the upper extremity. Scapulothoracic mobility may also be restricted.

Trigger points are located near the muscle's attachment to the coracoid process and in the belly of the muscle.[3]

For stretch position, see Figure 12-11.

Coracobrachialis

The coracobrachialis muscle refers pain to the anterior deltoid region, the posterior aspect of the arm over the triceps, the dorsum of the forearm, and down to the dorsum of the hand.[3] The pain skips the elbow and wrist.

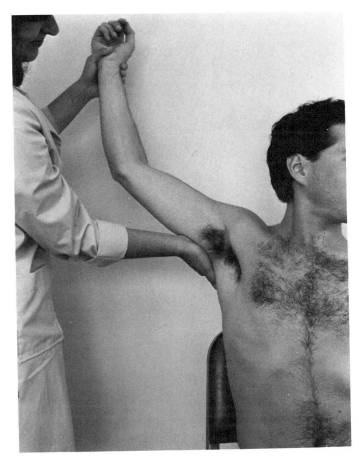

Fig. 12-11. Stretch for pectoralis major and minor.

The patient complains of upper extremity pain, especially in the anterior shoulder and posterior arm. Reaching behind the body across the low back is painful and limited.[3] Reaching up in abduction and flexion at the shoulder may be painful.[3] Resistive shoulder flexion can be painful and weak, whereas passive extension of the shoulder may be painful and restricted.

The trigger point is located in the superior part of the muscle near its attachment to the coracoid process.[3]

For stretch position, see Figure 12-6.

Biceps Brachii

The biceps brachii muscle refers pain up over the muscle belly and into the anterior deltoid region of the shoulder.[3] The patient may also experience milder pain downward in the antecubital space[3] and volar forearm and hand.[45]

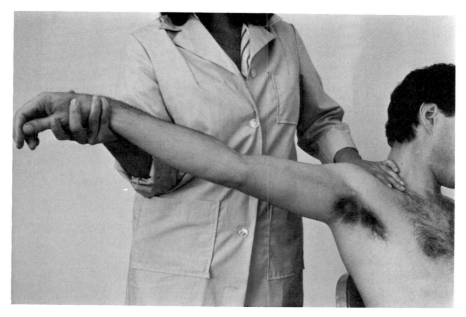

Fig. 12-12.   Stretch for biceps brachii.

The chief complaint is that of superficial anterior shoulder pain.[3] Weakness and pain may be present when the patient attempts to raise the hand above the head. Resisted elbow flexion with the wrist supinated will be painful and weak. Combined passive elbow and shoulder extension may be painful and restricted.

The trigger points are located in the distal one-third of the muscle.[3]

For stretch position, see Figure 12-12.

Triceps Brachii

The triceps brachii muscle has several variations of its referred pain pattern due to its three heads and subsequent trigger points. Areas of referred pain are as follows[3]: upward over the posterior arm to the back of the shoulder; the base of the neck in the upper trapezius region and sometimes down the dorsal forearm, skipping the elbow; the lateral epicondyle; the medial epicondyle; and the fourth and fifth digits.

With all of the possibilities of referred pain, the patient's complaint will be that of a hard-to-localize pain in the posterior shoulder region.[3] Extension of the elbow may be painful. Passive elbow flexion may be painful. Resisted elbow extension may be painful and weak.

Trigger points are located in each of the three heads, and the referred pain pattern depends on the location.[3]

For stretch position, see Figure 12-13.

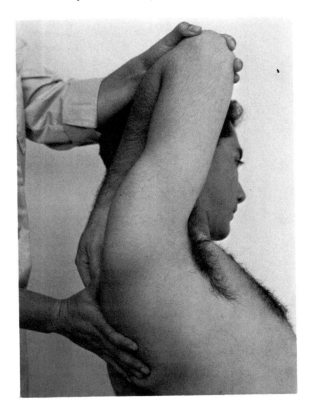

Fig. 12-13. Stretch for triceps brachii.

ACKNOWLEDGMENTS

I would like to thank Joyce Klien, R.N., C.A.N.P., for her assistance with the photography.

REFERENCES

1. Kellgren JH: Observations on referred pain arising from muscle. Clin Sci 3:175, 1938
2. Travell J, Rinzler SH: The myofascial genesis of pain. Postgrad Med 11:425, 1952
3. Travell J, Simons DG: Myofascial Pain and Dysfunction. The Trigger Point Manual. Williams & Wilkins, Baltimore, 1983
4. Berges PU: Myofascial pain syndromes. Postgrad Med 53:161, 1973
5. Bennett RM: Fibrositis: misnomer for a common rheumatic disorder. West J Med 134:405, 1981
6. Kraft GH, Johnson EW, LeBan MM: The fibrositis syndrome. Arch Phys Med Rehabil 49:155, 1968
7. Albee FH: Myofascitis. A possible explanation of many apparently dissimilar conditions. Am J Surg 3:523, 1927

8. Jordan HH: Myogelosis: the significance of pathologic conditions of the musculature in disorders of posture and locomotion. Arch Phys Ther 23:36, 1942
9. Awad EA: Interstitial myofibrositis: hypothesis of the mechanism. Arch Phys Med Rehabil 54:449, 1973
10. Ibrahim GA, Awad EA, Koltke FJ: Interstitial myofibrositis: serum and muscle enzymes and lactate dehydrogenase-isoenzymes. Arch Phys Med Rehabil 55:23, 1974
11. Copeman WSC, Ackerman WL: Edema or herniations of fat lobules as a cause of lumbar and gluteal "fibrositis." Arch Intern Med 79:22, 1947
12. Travell J: Ethyl chloride spray for painful muscle spasm. Arch Phys Med 33:291, 1952
13. Long C: Myofascial pain syndromes: part II—syndromes of the head, neck, and shoulder-girdle. Henry Ford Hosp Med Bull 4:22, 1956
14. Travell J, Rinzler S, Herman M: Pain and disability of the shoulder and arm: treatment by intramuscular infiltration with procaine hydrochloride. JAMA 120;417, 1942
15. Friction JR, Auvinen MD, Dystra D, Schiffman E: Myofascial pain syndrome: electromyographic changes associated with local twitch response. Arch Phys Med Rehabil 66:314, 1985
16. Brendstrup P, Jesperson K, Asboe-Hansen G: Morphological and chemical connective tissue changes in fibrositic muscles. Ann Rheum Dis 16:428, 1957
17. Miehlke K, Schuke G, Eger W: Clinical and experimental studies on the fibrositis syndrome. Rheumaforsch 19:310, 1960 (Ger)
18. Miehlke K, Schuke G: So-called muscular rheumatism. Internist 2:447, 1961 (Ger)
19. Schoen R, Miehlke K: Fibrositis or so-called muscle rheumatism. Med Klin 57:708, 1962 (Ger)
20. Henriksson KG, Bengtsson A, Larsson J, et al: Muscle biopsy findings of possible diagnostic importance in primary fibromyalgia (fibrositis, myofascial syndrome). Lancet 1395, Dec 1982
21. Yunus MB, Kalyan-Raman UP, Kalyan-Raman K: Primary fibromyalgia syndrome and myofascial pain: clinical features and muscle pathology. Arch Phys Med Rehabil 69:451, 1988
22. Hagberg M, Kvarnström S: Muscular endurance and electromyographic fatigue in myofascial shoulder pain. Arch Phys Med Rehabil 65:522, 1984
23. Simons DG, Stolov WC: Microscopic features and transient constriction of palpable bands in canine muscle. Am J Phys Med 55:65, 1966
24. Melzack R, Stillwell DM, Fox EJ: Trigger points and acupuncture points for pain: correlations and implications. Pain 3:3, 1977
25. Simons DG: Myofascial pain syndromes: where are we? where are we going? Arch Phys Med Rehabil 69:207, 1988
26. Reynolds MD: Myofascial trigger points in persistent posttraumatic shoulder pain. South Med J 77:1277, 1984
27. Wolfe F: Fibrositis, fibromyalgia, and musculoskeletal disease: the current status of the fibrositis syndrome. Arch Phys Med Rehabil 69:527, 1988
28. Simons DG: Fibrositis/fibromyalgia: a form of myofascial trigger points? Am J Med 81:93, 1986
29. Tunks E, Crook J, Norman G, Kalaber S: Tender points in fibromyalgia. Pain 34:11, 1988
30. Zohn DA, Mennell JM: Musculoskeletal Pain: Diagnosis and Physical Treatment. Little, Brown, Boston, 1976

31. Williams HL, Elkins ED: Myalgia of the head. Arch Phys Ther 23:14, 1942
32. Lewit K, Simons DG: Myofascial pain: relief by postisometric relaxation. Arch Phys Med Rehabil 65:452, 1984
33. Gersten JW: Nonthermal neuromuscular effects of ultrasound. Am J Phys Med 37:235, 1958
34. Fischer E, White EA, Hendricks SL, et al: Effect of moderate and weak ultrasound exposures upon normal and denervated mammalian muscle. Am J Phys Med 37:284, 1958
35. Klemp P, Staberg B, Korsgrd J, et al: Reduced blood flow in fibromyotic muscles during ultrasound therapy. Scand J Rehabil Med 15:21, 1982
36. Bonica JJ: Management of myofascial pain syndromes in general practice. JAMA 164:732, 1957
37. Grosshandler SL, et al: Chronic neck and shoulder pain. Focusing on myofascial origins. Postgrad Med 77:149, 1985
38. Phero JC, et al: Transcutaneous electrical nerve stimulation and myoneural injection therapy for management of chronic myofascial pain. Dent Clin North Am 31:703, 1987
39. Jaeger B, Reeves JL: Quantification of changes in myofascial trigger point sensitivity with the pressure algometer following passive stretch. Pain 27:203, 1986
40. Reeves JL, Jaeger B, Graff-Radford SB: Reliability of the pressure algometer as a measure of myofascial trigger point sensitivity. Pain 24:313, 1986
41. Fischer AA: Reliability of the pressure algometer as a measure of myofascial trigger point sensitivity. Pain 28:411, 1987 (letter)
42. Kelly M: New light on the painful shoulder. Med J Aust 1:488, 1942
43. Sola AE, Williams RL: Myofascial pain syndromes. Neurol 6:91, 1956
44. Pace JB: Commonly overlooked pain syndromes responsive to simple therapy. Postgrad Med 58:107, 1975
45. Steinbrocker O, Isenberg SA, Silver M, et al: Observations on pain produced by injection of hypertonic saline into muscles and other supportive tissues. J Clin Invest 32:1045, 1953

13 | Medical Management of Myofascial Pain Dysfunction

Sanford E. Gruskin

Myofascial pain, as most pain dysfunction syndromes, has received myriad classifications. When connected with the head, neck, and shoulder girdle, it is most commonly referred to as tension, psychogenic, or nervous headache. Recently, these headaches have been classified under the heading of muscle contraction headaches and included with those of vascular origin.[1-6] Although Shaber refers to these as acute and chronic, he asks whether the disease process is genetic (intrinsic), acquired (extrinsic), or both.[7] Rather than further confuse the picture by interjecting new classifications, two states affecting myofascial pain are defined that directly relate to the mode of medical management of this malady. It will be unnecessary to go through a muscle-by-muscle diagnostic examination or to define the general characteristics of myofascial pain, as this has been covered elsewhere. The physical therapy aspects will also be referred to only in the most general terms since this too has been thoroughly covered.

The purpose of this chapter is to classify only when it has bearing on the specific medical management of these patients. In this regard, reference is made to only two general classes, those of extrinsic and intrinsic etiology. Extrinsic etiology implies that the specific traumatic force is extrinsic to the patient, namely, an outside force directly traumatizing specific muscles. A psychogenic or tension-related muscle contraction is considered to be of intrinsic etiology. These terms are not to be confused with those of Shaber[7] (genetic [intrinsic] and acquired [extrinsic]), but are related to the mitigating circumstances that precipitate the myofascial pain episode involving the neck and shoulder girdle. A diagnostic protocol will be developed whereby patients can be classified as primarily those with extrinsic or intrinsic etiologic factors that precipitate pain dysfunction. Once the patient is properly classified, proper medical management can be determined.

Extrinsic patients are those who have an active external force that directly precipitates their pain dysfunction. Among this group is the athlete who is constantly irritating the neck or shoulder girdle during physical workouts, the laborer who carries heavy loads and strains or injures specific muscle groups, and the secretary who cradles a phone on the shoulder, directly traumatizing the muscles. During the past few years, we have been able to identify a new group of patients that fall into the extrinsic classification. We are seeing an increasing number of patients with pain localized primarily to the suboccipital muscles and secondarily to the upper trapezius muscles. It seems that these patients are secretaries who, until recently, used the typewriter and have now converted to word processing computers. The computer screens are positioned at a greater distance from their heads than were the typewriters, and we find that they assume a significant forward head position to maintain the same eye distance to the screen as they did from the typewriter paper. It may seem that the extrinsic patients would be relatively easy to diagnose. As compared with those of intrinsic etiology, they are, if not easier to diagnose, considerably easier from a management standpoint. These patients readily identify the active trigger point and admit to the episodes that precipitate pain. This group consists predominantly of men (in a ratio of 2:1). As obvious as the findings seem, it is still important to proceed with a thorough history and data base examination and to analyze the material in a logical, sequential manner to allow detection of a more serious problem that can otherwise be overlooked.

The second classification for myofascial pain is intrinsic, distinct from the previously mentioned extrinsic myofascial pain that "intrinsic" is related to direct muscle contraction from tension. These patients are far more difficult to manage, as there is a tendency to treat the pain as a symptom and not as a total disease state. The intrinsic patients are usually middle-aged and may be defensive in nature. Headache is often the focus of pain that brings them in for examination.

It is important to question these patients thoroughly relative to their social and psychological profile. A specific data base is used for the history and examination, with questions designed to cover all aspects of social, occupational, and physical history as well as guide the practitioner through a complete examination. Use of a specific data base serves several functions. Patients do not feel that they are being singled out for the psychological profile. The data base allows easy access into the psychological aspects of the disease and gives patients the impression that they are not alone with their problem. This group consists predominantly of women (in a ratio of 3:1) in their middle years. Usually, they have seen a multitude of practitioners, generally leaving with no specific diagnosis and the impression that the doctor thinks their pain is functional. To a practitioner taking a history, it is apparent that many of these patients have a round-shouldered posture with a forward head position. They often actively contract their musculature during the history, most notably the masseter muscles in clenching their teeth.

On direct questioning, patients often deny having a psychological or tension problem. However, when specifically asked about their sleeping habits, they admit to having difficulty maintaining sleep and awaken after only a short period, remaining restless throughout the night. Previous investigators have discussed in detail the emotional state of these patients and agree that they exhibit a tense personality, having difficulty coping with daily activities and handling stress.[2,6,8,9] They may be emotionally unstable, with a dependence on others. The patients often use the myofascial pain to their benefit, allowing them to cope with the stresses and escape the responsibilities that they are unable to handle. The relationship between chronic pain and depression has been approached by several researchers.[1,9,10] France et al. discuss the possibility of two relationships existing between chronic pain and depression. They believe that one group of patients reacts to the chronic pain disorder by becoming depressed, whereas a second group develops chronic pain as a symptom of the depression.[9] The relationship may be somewhat more complicated than these investigators suggest. Others have found that the chronic intrinsic patient can be effectively managed with smaller doses of antidepressants than can the classic depressed patient.[1] As a first step in the medical management of myofascial pain, our patients were sent for a Minnesota multiphasic personality inventory (MMPI). However, this immediately built a barrier between patients and doctors because patients felt that we were implying that their problem was functional and not organic. The use of the MMPI has since been abandoned in favor of a psychological profile developed through careful questioning of the patient over several visits. Observance of posture and movements of a significant number of patients during the history taking has shown that they will elicit trigger point tenderness involving the upper trapezius muscle. A patient's confidence can be enhanced by predicting these trigger points at the initial examination. Before the specific trigger point is palpated, the patient is told that this will elicit referred pain to the area of their initial concern. In medical management of pain, it is important to gain the patient's confidence and trust. Patients who are antagonistic, challenging all aspects of the treatment, will remain an enigma. In summary, profiles have been developed of patients who experience pain dysfunction from an extrinsic versus an intrinsic factor (Table 13-1). The extrinsic patients are usually somewhat younger in age, predominantly male, and can usually point to a specific occurrence that causes their pain dysfunction. Their pain tends to be unilateral in distribution. They rarely admit to associated headaches. The psychological profile does not contribute anything of significance. In contrast, the intrinsic patients are somewhat older and are predominantly women. They usually cannot identify any specific factor that causes their dysfunction. The pain assumes a bilateral distribution with sides not necessarily equal in intensity. These patients usually have associated headaches. Thorough questioning may elicit emotional instability. They may admit to difficulty maintaining sleep. This, they may feel, causes not only the muscle pain, but precipitates many of the family emotional disorders. They

Table 13-1. Profile of Patients Experiencing Pain Dysfunction from an
Extrinsic versus an Intrinsic Factor

	Extrinsic	Intrinsic
Identifiable etiologic factor	Yes	No
Sex predilection	2 : 1 M	3 : 1 F
Age (yr)	20–39	30–59
Visible muscle contractions	No	Yes
Distribution	Unilateral	Bilateral
Sleep disorder	Falling asleep	Maintaining sleep
Associated headaches	No	Yes
Previous treatment	No	Yes
Emotional instability	No	Yes

may admit to a lack of ability to perform various obligations due to their pain
dysfunction.

THE EXTRINSIC PATIENT

Patients with myofascial pain dysfunction of extrinsic etiology, if treated
properly, will experience results that are complete and rapid. These patients
should be approached with the full scope of treatment at onset to alleviate their
pain dysfunction and return them to muscular harmony. After patients are
classified into the extrinsic grouping, the mechanism of their pain is discussed.
The specific etiologic factor is detailed to the patient. Usually in consultation
with the physical therapist, a modified work pattern is suggested. Recommen-
dations for change in lifting patterns are discussed when this is felt to be the
etiologic factor. We have found striking improvement when we have advised
patients to modify their eye screen position on a word processor whereby they
can place their head in an erect position. This is done either by modifying the
focal distance on their glasses or repositioning the screen closer to their heads.
They are then placed on one of the nonsteroidal anti-inflammatory agents.
These drugs provide significant analgesic as well as appropriate anti-inflammatory action. Patients must be placed on a sufficient dose of this medication.
Our primary preference is flurbiprofen (Ansaid) at a dose of 100 mg three times
a day, tapering to twice a day after 2 weeks. Our experience is that this is well
tolerated by the patient with minimal side effects. Other nonsteroidal anti-
inflammatory drugs we use are ibuprofen (Motrin) at a dose of 600 mg three
times a day, diflunisal (Dolobid) at a dose of 500 mg twice a day, or naproxen
(Naprosyn) at a dose of 500 mg twice a day. These are highly effective medications, and the choice depends on convenience of administration and previous
drug therapy. A patient may have previously been given one of these drugs,
but on an as-needed basis, which does not provide a sufficient constant blood
level to obtain the appropriate anti-inflammatory effects. In such cases, that
drug is avoided and another is used in its place. Patients then do not feel that
they are being treated as they have previously been treated. The new medication, if it does not have any pharmacologic advantages, at least possesses

certain psychological advantages. The nonsteroidal anti-inflammatory agents are contraindicated in patients with a sensitivity to salicylates. These agents cause gastric irritation and are not to be used in patients with peptic ulcers or a history of gastrointestinal bleeding. They are also to be avoided in patients with impaired renal function. Platelet function is altered with these drugs, and anticoagulant therapy should be adjusted accordingly. The most common side effect from these agents is gastric irritation and nausea, which can be diminished to a large extent if patients take them with meals. If this is ineffective, switching from one nonsteroidal anti-inflammatory agent to another often alleviates the problem. Less frequent side effects include dizziness, headaches, nervousness, tinnitus, depression, insomnia, urticaria, neutropenia, agranulocytosis, aplastic anemia, thrombocytopenia, and acute renal failure. Aspirin should not be used in conjunction with the nonsteroidal anti-inflammatory agents as it has a tendency to increase the incidence of gastrointestinal problems and to diminish the anti-inflammatory activity.[11,12]

For those patients who have difficulty getting to sleep due to their extrinsic pain dysfunction, one of the benzodiazepines is prescribed. In this class, the choices are triazolam (Halcion) in a dose of 0.25 mg or temazepam (Restoril) in a dose of 15 mg, 30 minutes prior to bedtime. These specific benzodiazepines are selected because of their short half-life ($+\frac{1}{2}$). Restoril has a $+\frac{1}{2}$ of 9 to 12 hours and Halcion has a $+\frac{1}{2}$ of 3 to 5 hours. These drugs allow the patients to reach a restful level of sleep rapidly, preventing further traumatization of the musculature and allowing them to awaken without the hangover of many hypnotic agents. These medications are prescribed for a short period of time for those patients whose pain dysfunction limits their sleeping. As with other benzodiazepines, they should be avoided in patients who are pregnant. In addition to the obvious effects of drowsiness, dizziness, and lethargy, these drugs produce nausea in a small percentage of patients. They can also contribute to mental confusion and memory impairment. A limited number of patients will complain of constipation, diarrhea, xerostomia, and altered taste. These drugs are not addictive; however, the patients may have some minor withdrawal symptoms and difficulty sleeping after prolonged use followed by discontinuation of the drug.[11,12] In 1989, the amnesic effects of Halcion were successfully used by an attorney in the defense of his client. The Food and Drug Administration (FDA) investigated this matter and recommended a labeling change to the package insert for Halcion to reflect amnesic symptoms. In my clinical practice, I have experienced no incidence of amnesia in patients being treated with Halcion. Following appropriate medication with the nonsteroidal anti-inflammatory drugs and the benzodiazepines, patients are instructed to undergo physical therapy. They are seen approximately 2 weeks later. If a patient's symptoms have improved, the benzodiazepines can be discontinued and the dosage of the nonsteroidal anti-inflammatory agent can be decreased. A patient who has shown no improvement during the 2-week period is maintained at the same level of medication and is scheduled for appropriate trigger point injections.

THE INTRINSIC PATIENT

Patients with intrinsic myofascial pain dysfunction cannot be approached as having a symptom-based problem. They have had their symptoms over a period of years and at times have used the dysfunction to manipulate those around them and, at best, have integrated the pain into their life-style. To approach this as a symptom-oriented disease state will lead to failure. The patients cannot expect, nor can the practitioners anticipate, a rapid improvement of their symptomatology. It must be realized that certain patients cannot successfully be managed. However, with a systematic, logical approach, many patients will return to normal function. Within this group, however, some patients will need the adjunctive care of a psychotherapist. At times, it is apparent that the patients are asking for psychological supportive care, although it is the rare patient who feels comfortable enough to voice these problems. More often, after a number of visits and as patients develop more trust in the pain management, they can appropriately be led into psychotherapy.

These patients, having seen multiple practitioners before their visit, will list a number of drugs they have previously taken and are presently taking. It is often difficult to convince the patients that they are on the appropriate drugs, but that they need more than the agents alone. They need a combination of medication, aggressive physical therapy, and the understanding of those who treat them.

As with the extrinsic patients, the pain and inflammatory aspects of the myofascial dysfunction of these patients are treated with nonsteroidal anti-inflammatory agents in the same dosage previously described. It is necessary to explain to these patients in considerable detail the mechanism of action of these agents and the need to take them as directed without expecting immediate relief. Throughout the regimen, these patients should be constantly reminded to expect very gradual improvement of their symptoms.

The intrinsic patients with long-term tension-based pain dysfunction are approached as depressive patients. They frequently change their personalities to suit the circumstance. These individuals do not necessarily have difficulty getting to sleep, but have difficulty in maintaining their level of sleep. The first line of medication is one of the benzodiazepines; however, rather than Restoril or Halcion, an agent with a longer $+ \frac{1}{2}$ that is more of a sedative antidepressant than a hypnotic is prescribed. Alprazolam (Xanax) 0.5 mg three times a day is used initially, with the dosage adjusted as needed. If patients become drowsy and have difficulty functioning, the dosage is decreased to 0.25 mg in the morning, at noon, in early evening, and 0.5 mg at bedtime. Those with mild anxiety and depression problems seem to respond very well to the use of Xanax. The contraindications and side effects from Xanax are similar to those previously described with the other benzodiazepines. After the above medications are prescribed, an aggressive physical therapy program is maintained. Patients are seen for follow-up evaluation in approximately 2 weeks. After the 2-week interval, the patients are rarely symptom-free. If they report that they are symptom-free and able to function fully in their environment, it is doubtful they were placed in the appropriate category. Those that seem to be functioning better and have some diminution of their pain will be maintained on the same regimen and continued physical therapy.

Approximately 50 percent of these patients will have trigger point areas that are resistant to the usual physical therapy modalities and will require trigger point injections. The muscles that generally require trigger point injections are the upper trapezius, suboccipital, levator scapuli, and sternocleidomastoid muscles. Those patients who seem to make little or no progress with the Xanax and trigger-point therapy are withdrawn from Xanax and placed on cyclobenzaprine (Flexeril) at a dose of 10 mg three times a day. They are maintained on their nonsteroidal anti-inflammatory agents. Flexeril, like Xanax, is a benzodiazepine; however, it is closely related to the tricyclic antidepressants, both from a structural and pharmacologic standpoint. Like the tricyclic drugs, many of the side effects include anticholinergic manifestations, namely, drowsiness, xerostomia, tachycardia, and blurred vision. This drug should be avoided in patients with cardiac arrhythmias or heart block.[11,12] Patients should be maintained on Flexeril for 4 to 5 weeks. If there is no improvement with the combination of the nonsteroidal anti-inflammatory agents, Flexeril, physical therapy, appropriate trigger point injections, and psychotherapy, tricyclic antidepressants are considered.

Although many investigators[1,2,6,9,13] discuss the use of the tricyclic antidepressant agents at an earlier stage of treatment, these drugs should not be prescribed until the other chemotherapeutics have been tried and the patients have received a psychiatric consultation. The tricyclics used are imipramine, a dibenzazepine derivative, and amitriptyline, a dibenzocycloheptadiene derivative. These drugs have a high incidence of side effects, most notably involving the antimuscarinic effects of the drugs. There is also the risk of cerebral toxicity. As noted with Flexeril, these medications may cause cardiac toxicity that can result in hypotensive episodes and arrhythmias; they should be used with care in patients with cardiac disease. The tricyclics interact with numerous other medications; therefore, appropriate caution must be exercised. Side effects may include xerostomia, metallic taste, constipation, epigastric pain, dizziness, tachycardia, palpatation, blurred vision, and urinary retention.[11] The dosage should be 100 to 200 mg/d. Several investigators refer to their use in a somewhat less than antidepressive dosage.[1,2,9] It is best to prescribe larger doses for short periods of time (3 to 5 weeks) and then decrease the dosage accordingly.

In a new approach recently tried with younger patients in good health who seem to have anxiety episodes related to the home or work environment, patients are placed on an exercise program involving daily runs, bicycling, or aerobic classes, starting at 20 minutes per day and working up to 1 hour per day, 6 days per week. The patients are placed on a diet consisting of 80 percent carbohydrates, 10 percent protein, and 10 percent fat, supplemented with L-tryptophan twice a day, which promotes the release of beta-endorphin and helps nullify pain. The L-tryptophan also allows them increased relaxation and sleep. At this juncture, we are not certain that the exercise program itself is not causing a sufficient distraction for those patients in that their stress and tension are directed toward athletic endeavors and away from the muscle contraction associated with myofascial pain dysfunction. In November 1989, the FDA had reports of around 250 cases of a blood disorder known as eosinophilia myalgia syndrome. All the patients who developed this syndrome had been taking L-tryptophan. It was felt that there were two possibilities linking L-tryptophan to eosinophilia myalgia syndrome: that this syndrome has been present for quite some time and the causal relationship not recognized or, more likely, that certain batches of L-tryptophan were contaminated and it is the contaminant causing the disorder. Until the matter is clarified, we are no longer recommending the use of L-tryptophan.

TRIGGER POINT INJECTIONS

Credit must be given to Travell when we discuss trigger points and their treatment. She was years ahead of the rest of the profession in recognizing the role and treatment of trigger points.[6] Trigger point injection is now a recognized approach to myofascial pain dysfunction.[3,6,14] There is little question of the need for trigger point injections. The discussion centers on the subtleties of the technique and the agents used for the injection.

Agents or techniques advocated consist of dry needling, gammaglobulin, and sarapin, as well as the local anesthetics bupivacaine (Marcaine), procaine (Novacaine), lidocaine (Xylocaine), and mepivacaine (Carbocaine).[3,6,14] Some researchers advocate the addition of cortical steroids to the local anesthesia, whereas others use only isotonic saline solution.[6] Local anesthesia provides several immediate benefits. It provides a less painful injection procedure and allows for pain-free stretching of the patient by the physical therapist immediately after the injection. Furthermore, the patient's confidence is gained because of the immediate reversal of the positive trigger point findings. The stretching no longer produces pain, the range of motion is increased, palpation is pain free, there is a decrease in the tenseness of the musculature, and muscle strength is increased.[6] Vasopressor agents are contraindicated not only because of the increased hazard of accidental intravenous injection and myotoxicity, but also because the local anesthetic together with the vasopressor may increase muscle necrosis, compounding the problem.[6,15] Three percent Carbocaine supplied in 1.8-ml carpules is an effective and convenient agent for trigger point injections. The Carbocaine is prepackaged in carpules; the sterility chain is maintained because multiple entries into a vial are not necessary. Carbocaine is available without the addition of a vasopressor agent and conveniently fits in the syringe used in most dental and many medical facilities. A 27-gauge stainless steel needle (length 1½ in) is used. This length is sufficient to reach the designated trigger point and allows the tactile sense to determine when the trigger point is penetrated.

The injection procedure is considered a sterile procedure. The patient removes all binding clothes from the area of the injection and sterile drapes are provided. The operator wears sterile gloves and all materials are autoclaved or otherwise sterilized before use. The skin is prepared with a betadine solution covering the area of penetration and a sufficient adjacent area so that the operator on palpating the trigger point will not cross-contaminate the site of injection. The area of the trigger point is palpated and is identified by the operator both by feeling the tautness of the region and by precipitating the referred pain. The skin overlying this area is stretched by the practitioner, who places the index finger and middle finger on either side of the skin overlying the trigger point, spreading these fingers to stretch the skin; with a sharp motion, the needle is inserted. A small amount of local anesthetic is injected as the trigger point is approached. Aspiration is always accomplished prior to any injections. As the operator contacts the trigger point, resistance can be felt and the local anesthetic is injected into the region. The injection technique requires a keen tactile sense to determine the exact moment at which the trigger point is penetrated. With an increasing number of injections, this becomes easier. Following the initial injection, the needle is withdrawn slightly and multiple injections are made in a circumferential pattern around the trigger point. The needle is then withdrawn, the area is gently massaged, and the additional trigger points are approached in a similar manner.

The most common trigger point injections of the neck and shoulder are the upper trapezius, suboccipital, levator scapuli, and sternocleidomastoid muscles. The upper trapezius muscle is approached with the patient in a sitting position with the head tilted toward the affected side. The trigger point is identified on bimanual palpation; the overlying skin is stretched with the middle and index fingers, with penetration between these fingers.

The suboccipital muscles, consisting of the recti capitis posteriores major and minor and the obliqui inferior and superior, are approached with the patient lying face down with the head extended over the edge of the table. These injections often involve the hairline, which, during the period of preparation, is thoroughly soaked in the betadine solution. The trigger points are identified on palpation, and the needle is inserted in a superior direction toward the base of the skull. Aspiration is accomplished before any anesthetic is administered because of the proximity of the vertebral artery.

The levator scapulae is approached from behind with the patient lying with the affected side upward. The trigger point is identified on manual palpation, and the index and middle finger are spread to stretch the skin as the needle is inserted. The needle should not penetrate deeply to assure that the thoracic cavity will not be entered.

The sternocleidomastoid muscle is approached with the patient in a sitting position with the operator above and behind the patient. The head is flexed toward the affected side and the operator grabs the muscle between the thumb and index finger, identifying the trigger points. Extreme care is necessary with this injection owing to the vital structures adjacent to muscle. The external jugular vein courses along the outer aspects of the sternocleidomastoid muscle. Aspiration during the injection is mandatory. Following the trigger point injections, the patients are immediately sent for physical therapy. They undergo active stretching after the trigger point injections, followed by moist heat application. After discharge from the physical therapist, the patients are instructed to maintain moist heat on the area for several hours.

CONCLUSIONS

It is imperative that a logical, sequential procedure be followed in medical management of myofascial pain dysfunction to the neck and shoulder. It cannot be overemphasized that these patients must be properly classified and then treated in a progressive manner. A haphazard approach to medical management of these patients will be frustrating at best. At times, these patients have seemed to be an integrated part of the practice; however, when their treatment can be brought to a successful conclusion, it is most gratifying.

REFERENCES

1. Peter K: Headache—diagnosis and effective management. West J Med 140:157, 1984
2. Martin M: Muscle-contraction (tension) headache. Psychosomatics 24:319, 1983
3. Rubin D: Myofascial trigger point syndromes: an approach to management. Arch Phys Med Rehabil 62:107, 1981
4. Nuechterlein K, Holroyd J: Biofeedback in the treatment of tension headache. Arch Gen Psychol 37:866, 1980
5. Ahles T, King A, Martin J: EMG biofeedback during dynamic movement as a treatment for tension headache. Headache 24:41, 1984
6. Travell J, Simons D: Myofascial Pain and Dysfunction. The Trigger Point Manual. Williams & Wilkins, Baltimore, 1983
7. Shaber P: Skeletal muscle: anatomy, physiology, and pathophysiology. Dent Clin North Am 27:435, 1983
8. Bell N, Abramowitz S, Folkins C, et al: Biofeedback, brief psychotherapy and tension headache. Headache 23:162, 1983
9. France R, Houpt J, Ellinwood E: Therapeutic effects of antidepressants in chronic pain. Gen Hosp Psychiatry 6:55, 1984
10. Carron H: Control of pain in the head and neck. Orolaryngol Clin North Am 14:631, 1981
11. Gilman A, Goodman L, Gilman A: The Pharmacological Basis of Therapeutics. 6th Ed. Macmillan, New York, 1983
12. Angel J: Physicians' Desk Reference. 38th Ed. Medical Economics, Oradell, NJ, 1984
13. Lance J: Headache. Ann Neurol 10:1, 1981
14. Rask M: The omohyoideus myofascial pain syndrome: report of four patients. J Craniomandibular Pract 2:256, 1984
15. Benoit P: Reversible skeletal muscle damage after administration of local anesthetics with and without epinephrine. J Oral Surg 36:198, 1978

14 | Shoulder Girdle Fractures

Michael J. Wooden
David J. Conaway

Shoulder pain, stiffness, and weakness after fracture are common problems presented to the orthopaedic physical therapist. Fractures are always accompanied to some degree by soft tissue injury, leaving serious implications for rehabilitation well after the fracture has healed. Even if the fracture itself heals solidly, it is the soft tissue recovery that will determine the ultimate outcome of function.[1]

This chapter presents a brief overview of some of the more common shoulder girdle fractures. For each, general rehabilitation guidelines are offered. The effects of trauma and immobilization are also summarized.

STAGES OF FRACTURE HEALING

As in any other body region, displaced fractures of the shoulder girdle must be immobilized to allow the fracture to progress through the stages of healing. Immediately following the fracture is the *acute, inflammatory stage*[2] of hematoma formation. In this stage of vasodilation and serous exudation, inflammatory cells are brought to the area to remove necrotic soft tissue and bone from the ends of the fragments. As the hematoma becomes more organized at the start of the *reparative stage*,[2] a "fibrin scaffold" is provided for the reparative cells, which differentiate and begin to produce collagen, cartilage, and bone. These cells, primarily osteoblasts, invade the hematoma through capillary formation to form a callous of immature bone. Meanwhile, osteoclast cells resorb necrotic bone from the ends of the fragments. In the *remodeling*

329

stage,[2] resorption and new bone formation continue as trabecular bone patterns are laid down in response to the stress applied. By this time, the immobilization period should be ending so that the necessary "stress" is provided by remobilization of the limb.

The length of time required for each healing stage is influenced by many factors.[2] Some of these include the severity of the trauma, how much bone is lost, the presence of infection, which bone is fractured, how effective the immobilization is, and the patient's age, general health, and level of activity.

EFFECTS OF IMMOBILIZATION ON SOFT TISSUES

The combination of trauma to soft tissues and subsequent immobilization needed for bone healing contributes to stiffness of periarticular connective tissue structures and weakness of the surrounding musculature.[3] Much has been researched and written about changes in histologic, biochemical, and mechanical properties. To summarize, the most significant motion-limiting effects are as follows:

1. Loss of extensibility of capsule, ligaments, tendons, and fascia. Immobilization results in a decrease in water and glycosaminoglycan content. This contributes to an increase in aberrant cross-linking and a loss of movement between fibers.[4-6]
2. Deposition of fibrofatty infiltrates between joint structures acting as intra-articular "glue."[7]
3. Breakdown of hyaline articular cartilage.[8]
4. Atrophy and adaptive length changes in muscle.[9,10]

Conversely, it has been shown that movement tends to prevent or reduce these changes in connective tissue[4,11] and muscle.[9,10] The problem for us, as clinicians, is knowing when to begin active motion and when to progress to passive exercise. This requires close communication with the physician and an understanding of the stages of soft tissue healing. Evaluation of the direction of restriction, pain, and reactivity is essential in determining the readiness of movement.[12]

CLAVICLE FRACTURES

Clavicle fractures (Fig. 14-1) most commonly occur from a fall on the lateral aspect of the shoulder or, less commonly, onto the outstretched arm.[13] The clavicle typically fractures at the juncture of the middle one-third and distal one-third (Fig. 14-2) and often in the middle one-third (Fig. 14-3).

The shoulder is immobilized for 14 to 21 days, either in a clavicle (or figure eight) brace or a sling. Badly comminuted, delayed union, or surgically repaired fractures will require more immobilization.

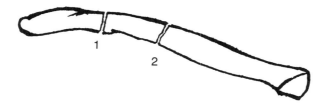

Fig. 14-1. Clavicle fractures at the (**1**) juncture of the middle and distal thirds and the (**2**) middle one-third.

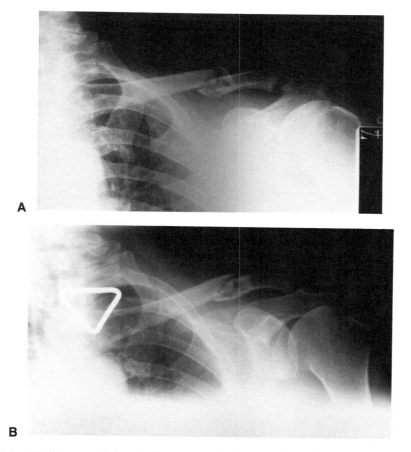

Fig. 14-2. Radiograph of clavicle fracture at the juncture of the middle and distal thirds (**A**) before reduction and (**B**) after reduction.

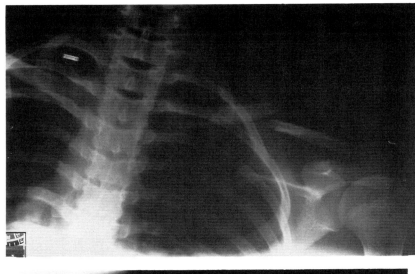

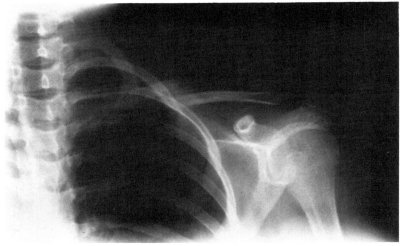

Fig. 14-3. Radiograph of clavicle fracture in the middle one-third (**A**) before reduction and (**B**) after reduction.

Rehabilitation

Active range of motion (ROM) exercises should begin within 14 to 21 days. Exercises should involve the shoulder girdle (elevation, depression, protraction, and retraction) and the shoulder joint (pendulum and wand exercises). In most cases, a home program is sufficient. In unusual cases of prolonged immobilization and excessive stiffness, passive mobilization may be necessary. Evaluation and treatment should include accessory and physiologic movements of the sternoclavicular, acromioclavicular, glenohumeral, and scapulothoracic joints. The latter is often overlooked, but may be particularly important because of immobilization in a retracted position.

Prolonged immobilization can also result in muscle weakness and even in visible atrophy. Resistive exercises can begin when the fracture appears solidly healed and when pain with movement is reduced.

SCAPULA FRACTURES

Scapula fractures are usually the result of a direct blow.[13] Most are non-displaced; therefore, little or no immobilization is required.

Neck of the Scapula

The fracture line extends from the suprascapular notch to the lateral border (Fig. 14-4, no. 1). Downward displacement of the glenoid fragment is not usually severe.

Body of the Scapula

Fragments are well protected by layers of muscle, even if comminuted (Fig. 14-4, no. 2).

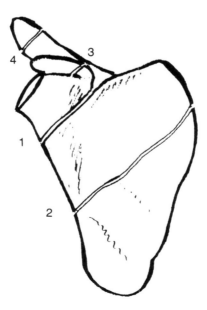

Fig. 14-4. Scapular fractures of the (**1**) neck, (**2**) body, (**3**) coracoid process, and (**4**) acromion process.

Coracoid Process

The fracture is usually not displaced, but occasionally is displaced downward (Fig. 14-4, no. 3).

Acromion Process

Again, this is not often displaced. If the fracture is communited or badly displaced, fragments can be removed surgically (Fig. 14-4, no. 4).

Rehabilitation

In most cases, active ROM exercises can begin within the first few days, and a home program will suffice. However, occasional prolonged immobilization because of severe displacement or surgical treatment may necessitate passive mobilization and muscle strengthening. All joints in the shoulder girdle complex should be evaluated, with particular emphasis on the scapulothoracic and its related musculature. If a direct blow to the scapula was the cause of injury, thoracic spine and rib mechanics should also be evaluated.

FRACTURES OF THE HUMERUS

Fractures of the upper humerus can involve the greater tuberosity, neck, or shaft (Fig. 14-5). Mechanisms of injury are varied, as are the needs for immobilization and surgery. The effects of trauma and immobilization on glenohumeral joint soft tissues have especially significant implications for rehabilitation.

Greater Tuberosity

Fractures of the greater tuberosity are usually the result of a fall on the shoulder, most commonly in elderly individuals.[13] In nondisplaced fractures (Fig. 14-6) splinting should be avoided so that active exercise can begin soon. An avulsed and displaced fragment must be reduced to avoid impingement with the acromion or coracoacromial ligament, which will result in painful, limited abduction.[13,14] These are often treated surgically with a fixation screw. Additional clearance acromioplasty or removal of the acromion may be necessary. Postoperative immobilization is from 14 to 21 days.

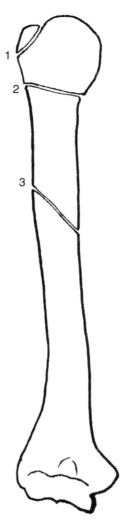

Fig. 14-5. Fractures of the upper humerus in the (**1**) greater tuberosity, (**2**) neck, and (**3**) shaft.

Neck of the Humerus

Humeral neck fractures are caused by a fall on the outstretched arm or the elbow, often in elderly, osteoporotic women.

Since shoulder joint stiffness is a common complication of humeral neck fractures, early movement is desirable. The immobilization required depends on the severity of the displacement. In impacted and nondisplaced fractures

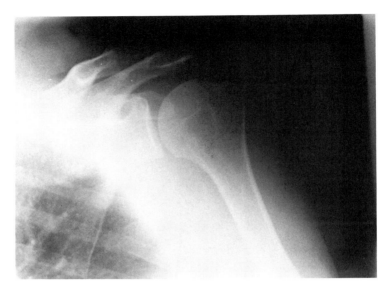

Fig. 14-6. Radiograph of nondisplaced greater tuberosity fracture.

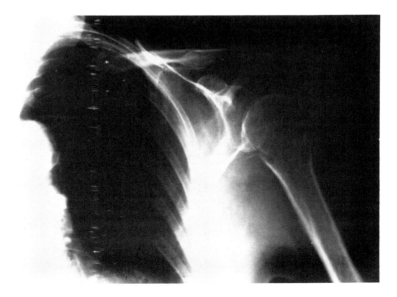

Fig. 14-7. Radiograph of impacted humeral neck fracture.

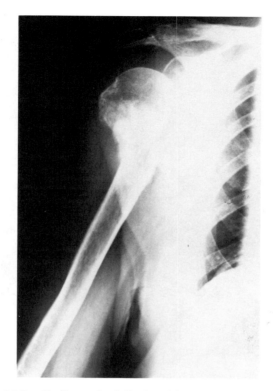

Fig. 14-8.   Radiograph of displaced humeral neck fracture.

(Fig. 14-7), the arm can come out of the sling frequently for exercise. If the fragments are displaced (Fig. 14-8), the arm may need to be immobilized in a sling held tightly to the chest for 14 to 21 days. Occasionally, an abduction splint is needed for as much as 4 weeks. Immobilization will be variable in cases of open reduction, internal fixation with plates or intramedullary rods.

Shaft of the Humerus

Humeral shaft fractures usually involve the middle one-third, resulting from a direct blow or a twisting force that causes a spiral fracture (Fig. 14-9).

As in other upper humerus fractures, early joint motion is desirable. However, immobilization is greatly variable, depending on the stability and whether casting or surgical fixation is used.

Rehabilitation

Because the glenohumeral joint is particularly susceptible to stiffness, early remobilization, when safe, is essential. Even while the arm is in a sling or cast, the patient should be taught careful active exercises or be seen frequently for

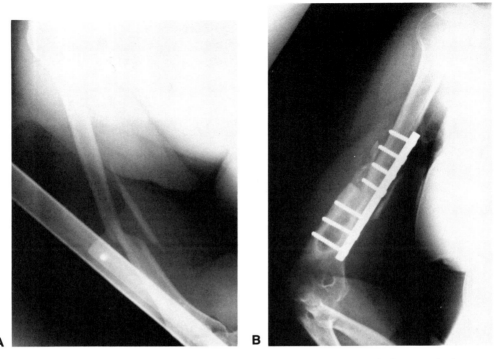

Fig. 14-9. Radiographs of spiral/oblique humeral shaft fracture (**A**) before surgical reduction and (**B**) after open reduction, internal fixation.

active assistance-providing exercises. As the immobilization period ends, the exercises should be increased gradually in range and vigor.

Once the fracture is stable and reactivity is reduced at least to moderate (i.e., pain and end-range resistance are simultaneous[12,15]), careful passive mobilization can begin. Each movement should be tested for reactivity prior to mobilizing, since some structures may be more inflamed and painful than others. For example, immobilizing the arm in a sling or in a position of adduction and internal rotation can result in a "capsular pattern" limitation.[16] In this capsular pattern, all movements at the glenohumeral joint, especially external rotation and abduction, will be restricted.[17] Therefore, mobilization should emphasize stretching the anterior and inferior portions of the capsule. During mobilization, pain should always be respected. When reactivity is moderate to high, grades I and II accessory mobilizations are used to reduce pain and promote relaxation. When reactivity is low to moderate, grades III and IV accessory and physiologic mobilizations are used to increase ROM.[18] While most effort will be concentrated at the glenohumeral joint, other joints in the shoulder girdle should be assessed after prolonged immobilization. The reader is referred to Chapter 11 for a detailed summary of shoulder joint and girdle mobilization techniques.

Immobilizing the shoulder girdle can result in significant muscle weakness. Muscles commonly involved are the upper and middle trapezius, the pectorals, and all muscles of the rotator cuff. To minimize weakness and atrophy, specific isometric exercises should be instructed early. After immobilization, if the fracture is stable, reactivity is not high, and ROM is at least 50 percent, submaximal effort progressive resistive exercises can begin, with progression to maximal effort as tolerated. Isokinetic devices are preferred because "stops" can be used to protect the joint and because resistance can be applied to all planes of movement, including functional diagonals. Chapter 3 outlines the use of shoulder isokinetics.

SUMMARY

Fractures of the shoulder girdle are common and, because of soft tissue trauma and immobilization, often result in stiffness, especially at the glenohumeral joint. When possible, early movement is essential. After a period of immobilization, all joints of the shoulder complex should be assessed, regardless of the location of the fracture.

REFERENCES

1. Gradisar IA: Fracture stabilization and healing. p. 118. In Davies G, Gould J (eds): Orthopaedic and Sports Physical Therapy. CV Mosby, St. Louis, 1985
2. Cruess RL: Healing of bone, tendon and ligament. p. 147. In Rockwood CA, Green DP (eds): Fractures in Adults. JB Lippincott, Philadelphia, 1984
3. Engles M: Tissue response. p. 3. In Donatelli R, Wooden MJ (eds): Orthopaedic Physical Therapy. Churchill Livingstone, New York, 1989
4. Akeson WH, Amiel D, Woo S: Immobility effects on synovial joints: the pathomechanics of joint contractures. Biorheology 17:95, 1980
5. Woo S, Matthews JV, Akeson WH, et al: Connective tissue response to immobility: an accelerated aging response. Exp Gerontol 3:289, 1968
6. LaVigne A, Watkins R: Preliminary results on immobilization: induced stiffness of monkey knee joints and posterior capsules. Proceedings of a Symposium of the Biological Engineering Society, University of Strathclyde. University Park Press, Baltimore, 1973
7. Enneking W, Horowitz M: The intra-articular effects of immobilization on the human knee. J Bone Joint Surg 54A:973, 1972
8. Ham A, Cormack D: Histology. 8th Ed. JB Lippincott, Philadelphia, 1979
9. Tabary JC, Tabary C, Tardieu S, et al: Physiological and structural changes in cat soleus muscle due to immobilization at different lengths in plaster casts. J Physiol (Lond) 224:221, 1972
10. Cooper R: Alterations during immobilization and regeneration of skeletal muscle in cats. J Bone Joint Surg 54A:919, 1972
11. Akeson WH, Amiel D, Mechanic GL, et al: Collagen crosslinking alteration in joint contractures: changes in reducible crosslinks in periarticular connective tissue collagen after 9 weeks of immobilization. Connect Tissue Res 5:5, 1977

12. Wooden MJ: Mobilization of the upper extremity. p. 239. In Donatelli R, Wooden MJ (eds): Orthopaedic Physial Therapy. Churchill Livingstone, New York, 1989
13. Adams JC: Outline of Fractures, Including Joint Injuries. 9th Ed. Churchill Livingstone, London, 1987
14. Turek SL: Orthopaedics: Principles and Their Applications. Vol. 2. 4th Ed. JB Lippincott, Philadelphia, 1980, p. 938
15. Paris SV: Extremity Dysfunction and Mobilization. Institute Press, Atlanta, 1980
16. Moran CA, Saunders SR: Evaluation of the shoulder: a sequential approach. p. 17. In Donatelli R (ed): Physical Therapy of the Shoulder. 1st Ed. Churchill Livingstone, New York, 1987
17. Cyriax J: Textbook of Orthopaedic Medicine. Vol. 1. Diagnosis of Soft Tissue Lesions. Ballierre Tindall, London, 1978
18. Maitland GD: Peripheral Manipulation. 2nd Ed. Butterworth, London, 1978

SUGGESTED READINGS

Chapman MW (ed): Operative Orthopaedics. JB Lippincott, Philadelphia, 1988
Crenshaw AH (ed): Campbell's Operative Orthopaedics. Vol. 3. WB Saunders, Philadelphia, 1970
Cruess R: Adult Orthopaedics. Churchill Livingstone, New York, 1984
DePalma AF: The Management of Fractures and Dislocations. WB Saunders, Philadelphia, 1970
Park WH, Hughes SPF (eds): Orthopaedic Radiology. Blackwell Scientific Publications, London, 1987
Rodgers LF: Radiology of Skeletal Trauma. Churchill Livingstone, New York, 1982

15 Total Shoulder Replacement

Larry F. Andrews
Carol Ann Gunnels

Although several prosthetic replacements for the upper part of the humerus were introduced in the 1950s, reports of artificial shoulder joints appeared as early as 1894. The first artificial shoulder joint consisted of a constrained prosthesis that had a humeral component composed of an iridescent platinum. The humeral head was made of a hard rubber ball, crossed by two deep grooves placed at right angles to each other. Each groove contained two separate loops of metal, one joining the rubber ball to the platinum stem and the other holding the glenoid by screws. This was the first reported constrained or fixed fulcrum prosthesis; it lasted approximately 2 years.

Most of our present-day prostheses are really an extension of work previously done in the area of the hip. Prosthetic development in the shoulder occurred because less radical procedures, such as resectional arthroplasties and arthrodesis, had failed to produce satisfactory results. Although worthwhile, standard operations such as humeral head resection, reattachment of rotator cuffs to the proximal humerus, glenohumeral arthrodesis, and autogenous fibular graft replacements to the upper humerus had serious drawbacks. Humeral head resection and arthrodesis greatly limited glenohumeral motion and may not have totally eliminated shoulder discomfort. Similarly, autogenous fibular grafts decreased shoulder motion and were also subject to fracture. Therefore, to provide more motion and greater relief of pain, surgeons began to perform other arthroplastic procedures.

Hemi-replacements affecting the humeral head resulted in satisfactory outcomes for patients with uninvolved glenoids and shoulder muscles of good to normal strength. Materials such as acrylic and cobalt chrome were used to replace the proximal humerus. Some even combined fenestrations (as did the Austin-Moore prosthesis for the hip) within the prosthesis to allow for attachment of tendons and muscles surrounding the shoulder.

The problem, however, was often not confined to the humeral head alone. As the disease process advanced, it became necessary for replacement considerations of the glenoid as well as the humerus. Glenoid liners of metal or plastic were used initially. These early designs depended on strong shoulder muscles, especially the deltoid and rotator cuff.

Because of inadequate musculature surrounding the glenohumeral joint, surgeons turned toward fixed fulcrums. It was thought that these constrained prostheses could be used for irrevocably damaged glenohumeral joints with the added loss of stabilization resulting from a weakened rotator cuff. In a constrained prosthetic design, the main considerations were durability of parts and attachment of the prosthesis to the scapula (glenoid) without subsequent loosening.

To enhance the longevity of the fulcrum (or articulation process) in the constrained prosthesis, designs included two balls in opposition, as in universal joints or reversed configurations, using thin-walled, large cups with interarticulating large spheres extending from metal glenoids. To provide better deltoid leverage of the humerus, larger spheres were used in the fulcrum. It was thought that the larger radius enhanced not only strength but also degrees of motion (Fig. 15-1).

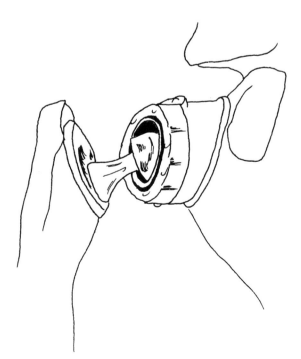

Fig. 15-1. The constrained prosthesis was designed to eliminate the need for rotator cuff muscles.

Post et al. felt that success with constrained prostheses depended more on protection of the scapular vault (bony configuration behind the glenoid) than on any ingenious design. Anything that destroys the thin cortical vault of the glenoid, its subcondylar plate, or cancellous bone mass increases the chances of loosening. Other complications have included dislocations and glenoid and prosthetic neck fractures.[1]

Neer et al. found the active motion following the constrained prosthetic procedures disappointing. The fixed fulcrums failed to provide the power necessary for external rotation so essential for good function. They also felt that these prostheses invited mechanical failure.[2]

Cofield agreed, and studied the unconstrained designs of Neer et al. "Unconstrained" implies that only the cartilage will be replaced. All other structures will be repaired. The major argument for an unconstrained over a constrained total shoulder replacement as presented by Cofield is that the failure rate of the unconstrained implants is less than that of the constrained. If the additional constraint can be offered by repair rather than arthroplasty, long-term results would be much more consistent and complications fewer.[3]

The early designs of prostheses were offered to treat simultaneous loss of articular cartilage and instability engendered by rotator cuff disease. However, as it became apparent that rotator cuff disease was not always present in these conditions, the trend toward the unconstrained prosthesis evolved. Together with this evolution, there was a trend toward better repair of surrounding soft tissues, such as the rotator cuff. Partial anterior acromioectomies were performed to prevent impingement of soft tissue and overlying bone. Often, with rotator cuff injuries, all that was necessary was suture of torn edges to cancellous bone of the upper humerus; at times, transposition of subscapularis was used as an adjacent cuff closure. Thus, a larger percentage of rotator cuff tears were treated without resorting to unduly complex or uncertain surgical techniques.

The unconstrained replacement is not effective if there is a deficient deltoid muscle and if there is poor closure of the rotator cuff in the face of a non-functioning cuff mechanism (Fig. 15-2).[4]

DIAGNOSTIC CATEGORIES REQUIRING TOTAL SHOULDER REPLACEMENT

Regardless of the diagnosis necessitating total shoulder replacement (TSR), one common feature was prevalent: cartilaginous erosion. Studies by Poppen et al. offered one explanation for this destructive process. The excursion of the humeral head on its glenoid surface in the superior inferior plane was less than 1.5 mm in normal subjects. This occurred during each 30° of motion with a normal compressive force on the glenoid. These studies demonstrated how increased excursion along varying centers of rotation resulted if the shear force directed upward or downward was excessive. This increase in excursion occurred when there was a muscle imbalance secondary to pain or a tear or functional loss of the rotator cuff. As the deltoid muscle pulled

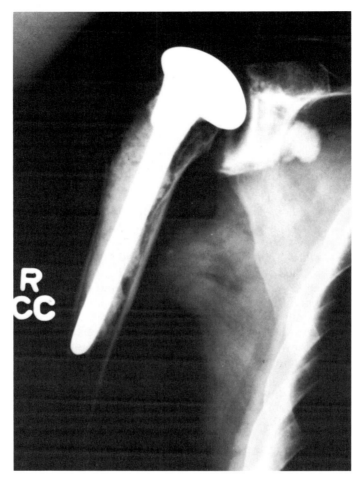

Fig. 15-2. The unconstrained prosthesis consists of a metal humeral component and a plastic glenoid, as demonstrated by the metal clip.

upward (shear) without the compressive counterforce provided by the rotator cuff, destruction of the cartilage resulted.[5] Each of the following diagnostic categories provides variations from the normal biomechanical function of the shoulder that lead to cartilaginous erosion and, thus, the need for TSR.

Osteoarthritis

"The lesion of primary glenohumeral osteoarthritis is remarkably constant and consistent." The areas of wear and sclerosis develop at the maximum point of joint reaction force: 90° of abduction.

> The head becomes surrounded by marginal osteophytes which are more prominent inferiorly and posteriorly. In advanced cases, the glenoid becomes flattened and eroded posteriorly, as also occurs in the arthritis of recurrent dislocation and in the rheumatoid patient. The sloping glenoid may result in a posterior subluxation of the humeral head which in extreme cases resembles an old posterior dislocation.[2]

The forces necessary to generate this type of wear require the rotator cuff to be intact, as was found to be the case in shoulders of patients who were treated surgically (Fig. 15-3).

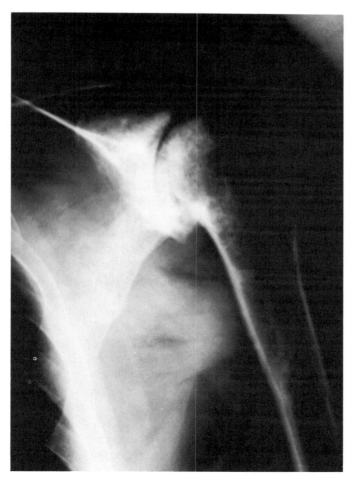

Fig. 15-3. Shoulder x-ray film depicting osteoarthritis.

Chronic Dislocation

A second classification of TSR candidates includes those with histories of chronic dislocation. Years of recurrent dislocation and, in many cases, previous surgeries cause tightening of the joint capsule and produce a fixed subluxation in the opposite direction from the dislocation, which leads to severe degenerative arthritis.

> Glenoid involvement was more severe than is usual in the shoulder with osteoarthritis. Some degree of erosion of the posterior part of the glenoid is characteristically present, making it necessary to lower the high side or elevate the low side when inserting the glenoid component.[2]

Bone grafts under the glenoid are required in some shoulders.[2]

Rheumatoid Arthritis

A large percentage of female TSR candidates have rheumatoid arthritis. Bilateral shoulder disability along with elbow disability is much more common in these patients than in other diagnostic categories. The presence of attenuated rotator cuffs, adherence of the long head of the biceps within the synovial sheath, and arthritis of the acromioclavicular joint has often been noted. There are, however, significant differences in the severity of the disease. Middle-aged women may have a mild form of rheumatoid arthritis. Although moderate to severe cases reveal a thinning of the rotator cuff, tears of complete thickness of the rotator cuff are often small and readily repaired. With the most severe degree of arthritis, massive disintegration of the rotator cuff is common, resulting in a softened rotator cuff that does not hold sutures and does not function. The exposed humeral head in these patients erodes deeply into the acromion, the outer aspect of the clavicle, and the coracoid.

To enhance the results of TSR in the rheumatoid patient, excision of the acromioclavicular joint is done at the time of surgery. The prevention of shoulder stiffness and support of surrounding surgically repaired structures necessitates the need for an abduction splint.

Most of the rheumatoid patients with both elbow and shoulder complaints are first treated by TSR, as the relief usually has a beneficial effect on the elbow (Fig. 15-4).[2] A reduction in pain, with a possible increase in motion of the shoulder, relieves some of the burden placed on the elbow during functional activities. Soft tissue and multiple joint involvement of the glenohumeral, acromioclavicular, and thoracoscapular joints often prohibits the patient from gaining overhead use of the arm. For the patient with rheumatoid arthritis, pain relief is the primary benefit of TSR.

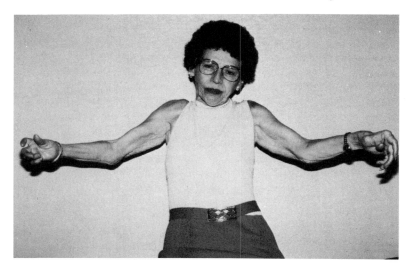

Fig. 15-4. Patient with rheumatoid arthritis demonstrating upper extremity involvement of shoulders, elbows, and hands.

Trauma

Patients with trauma-induced total shoulders usually have had previous surgical procedures. They include those with displaced fractures and fracture–dislocations of the proximal end of the humerus of more than 6 month's duration. Muscle contracture and scarring, difficulty with bony union of the tuberosities, associated nerve injuries, and shortening of the humeral shaft make treatment difficult; thus, the rehabilitation program proceeds at a slower rate. Neer found that the interval from injury to operation ranged from 7 months to 15 years and averaged more than 2 years.[2]

Revision

The most difficult operative procedure is the prosthetic revision. Many prostheses had previously been inserted for fractures and were often anchored with acrylic cement. Other difficulties include massive rotator cuff defects, previously weakened deltoids, and more than 2 cm of bone loss at the proximal head of the humerus and glenoid. Finally, weakened deltoids often result from radical acromionectomies.

Miscellaneous

Other less frequently seen diagnoses necessitate TSR. Shoulders with longstanding massive tears of the rotator cuff are characterized by attrition of the articular cartilage with thinning and a bumpy, so-called pebblestone appearance with decalcification and eventual collapse of the subchondral bone. With time, the humeral head becomes irregular. Without its smooth cartilaginous covering, it erodes into the acromion, clavicle, and coracoid process. Thus, surgical reconstruction is especially difficult in these shoulders. Some diagnoses, such as chondrosarcoma, may require long humeral components and grafts to maintain humeral length. To preserve this normal length, it is often important to fix the humeral component with methylmethacrylate. This is significant for assuring glenohumeral stability and preservation of length of the deltoid muscle for possible humeral elevation. It serves to remove strain from the bone graft shaft junction. However, it must be remembered that some patients with glenohumeral fusion who complain of loss of motion and generalized shoulder pain are treated by TSR on a limited basis—to regain rotation and reduce discomfort.[2]

PATIENT PROFILE

Patient selection depends on several factors, but pain is the primary factor that is considered when the decision regarding TSR is made. Patients being considered for TSR usually have such severe pain that their sleep is disturbed. Their pain has continued despite conservative treatment such as medications, physical therapy, and steroid injections. Many patients have undergone previous surgical procedures aimed at alleviating their pain.

Loss of motion and strength varies among patients presenting for TSR. The stage of their disease process and their presenting diagnosis seem to influence these two factors. Patients can often initially compensate for decreased glenohumeral motion by scapulothoracic motion. However, with progression of the disease, especially rheumatoid arthritis, the patient can no longer compensate in this manner and a significant loss of motion is noted. The increased incidence of rotator cuff tears in patients with rheumatoid arthritis influences the loss of strength with which the patient is initially seen.

As a result of an increase in pain and a decrease in range of motion (ROM) and strength, the patient notes limitations in functional activities. Combing hair, washing the opposite axilla, using a back pocket, and dressing often become difficult, if not impossible. Many patients compensate by changing hand dominance or, in the case of bilateral involvement, must seek assistance (Fig. 15-5).

Infection and extensive paralysis are contraindications to surgery. Patients who have weakness of the shoulder musculature can be considered candidates with the knowledge that their rehabilitation will be limited. All patients must be motivated and must cooperate fully in their postoperative rehabilitation if satisfactory results are to be achieved.

SURGICAL CONSIDERATIONS

A competent surgeon, skilled in all aspects of shoulder surgery, is the prime consideration in surgery. Preoperative consideration must be taken into account. A good physical therapy evaluation should be performed to determine

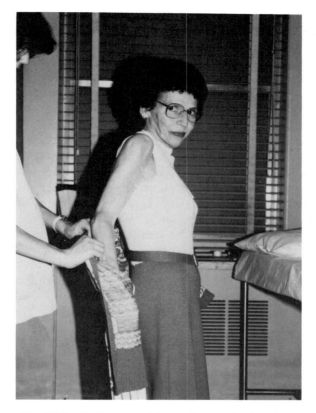

Fig. 15-5.   Patient requiring assistance in dressing.

the patient's loss of motion and strength. This evaluation may help the surgeon determine the need for a constrained or unconstrained prosthesis. A good medical consultation can help determine if there are any contraindications to the surgery.

Constrained TSRs are indicated in those patients who have constant pain or inaccurate rotator cuff function and in those who would not do as well with other standard operations. The surgeon must take into account the bone stock available in the scapula and the availability of shoulder girdle musculature. If there is severe osteoporosis from various causes, such as tumor or surgical excavation of the glenoid vault, it would be prudent for the surgeon to avoid a constrained replacement since loosening may be the side effect. Post et al. believed that there should also be a strong serratus anterior and trapezius to stabilize the scapula for a constrained prosthesis to be considered. A strong deltoid is also advisable, except in cases in which passive motion is acceptable. In reality, patients, according to Post et al., do well with constrained prostheses even in the face of an inefficient deltoid if they understand the limitations of motion.[1]

The unconstrained total shoulder prosthesis probably is the more popular since the use of components (with satisfactory results) designed by Neer have been reported more in the literature. Fleming, Chairman of the Orthopedic Department of Emory Clinic, Atlanta, GA, uses the Neer unconstrained shoulder prosthesis and feels that it can be used very well with an intact rotator cuff. He states that it is necessary to have the rotator cuff repaired with some type of graft material or to have the subscapularis transferred to the greater tuberosity. Fleming also states that the superior and inferior glenohumeral ligament complexes should be reattached very well, as they are as important as the rotator cuff because they provide anterior stability. In making an approach to the shoulder initially, it is now thought to be very important not to take down any aspect of the deltoid, but to make a deltoid pectoral approach. This makes rehabilitation much easier on the patient and provides for a greater possibility for elevation of more than 90°. Fleming also discourages total acromionectomies, as do others, because of the effect they have on the function of the deltoid. If there is a total acromionectomy, the humeral head may ride superiorly, thus defeating the force couple provided by the rotator cuff musculature and the deltoid. Therefore, in most cases, partial acromionectomy is performed, especially if impingement is found. This helps reduce pain in the arthritic acromioclavicular joint of the rheumatoid patient. The difficulty with the unconstrained prosthesis can occur if the anterior tissues are destroyed to such an extent that they cannot be closed over the prosthesis. This is often the case with radiation necessary for treatment of cancer and with trauma of the shoulder.

The importance of evaluating the postoperative results of various types of prostheses before attempting to use these designs is stressed. The wide use of the Neer total shoulder prosthesis can probably be attributed to the in-depth studies available on the results of the shoulder surgery.

Early mobilization has been shown to decrease early postoperative pain. Use of continuous passive motion devices has been beneficial in cases in which the anterior aspect of the shoulder remains intact. Any repairs are protected for approximately 3 months before resistance is added to the exercise routine.

Complications may involve nerve paralysis, infections, and prosthetic loosening. Of particular note, most surgeons report radiolucent lines that, in the weight-bearing extremities, are thought to be related to prosthetic loosening. There is no general concensus on what the radiolucent line is, but it is agreed that the area is not filled with bone. With a non–weight-bearing prosthesis, such as a total shoulder, the prosthesis is thought to hold up much longer. Possibly, designs such as a porous coat will be used in the future and will discontinue the need for methylmethacrylate or other cements within the humerus, thus making revisions easier when necessary.

In final analysis, the surgical considerations depend on the patient's profile (i.e., their involvement of soft tissue extrinsic to the underlying bony defects), with the main goals of surgery for the patient being the loss of pain and an increase in daily functions.

POSTOPERATIVE MANAGEMENT

Following good surgical technique, the most important aspect for the total shoulder patient is postoperative management. The results of surgery would be unacceptable without maximum mobility of the joint provided by early and continued passive movement. Strengthening of the musculature around the shoulder, with emphasis on the rotator cuff and deltoid, must be continued throughout the life of the patient.

Post et al.[1] described an exercise program of passive and active assistive ROM exercises for patients following a constrained TSR. They emphasized that motion, especially external rotation, should never be forced beyond the limits found at the time of surgery. The pendulum exercise was not recommended, nor was vigorous and heavy use of the shoulder (as in push-ups). These exercises could cause loosening of the prosthesis. These investigators found that the severity of the disease process in most patients receiving TSR made active overhead motions impossible.

Neer has provided guidelines for postoperative management of the patient with an unconstrained shoulder.[6] Depending on the involvement of the patient's surrounding support structures, modifications for the rehabilitation process can be determined. During the first 4 or 5 days, the patient is typically placed in a shoulder immobilizer. Recently, continuous passive motion machines have been used to provide earlier mobilization. Abduction braces are sometimes provided for patients with repairs of the rotator cuff. The healing of certain structures, such as a repaired rotator cuff, may require 6 to 12 weeks of protection from active motion. Pendulum exercises followed by over-the-door pulley exercises are then important for patient independence in passive mobility of the joint. Passive stretching should be included in the exercise program indefinitely to maintain motion (Fig. 15-6).

Mobilization of the joint in the trained hands of a therapist is often beneficial, especially for the severely involved shoulder. Isometrics may be initiated early, as long as they are performed correctly. Slow tension is important to minimize tissue stress and joint movement when performing the isometric exercises (Fig. 15-7).

The main emphasis is on protection of the surgical repair. With initiation of resistive exercises, the elbow should remain flexed and by the side of the trunk. Rubber tubing is helpful to start early isometric exercises and for progression of the program to active resistive exercises (Fig. 15-8).

Following unconstrained TSR, Clayton et al. reported improvement in shoulder function of greater than 100 percent over preoperative ratings, while the ROM increased relatively little.[7] In his studies, Cofield[3,4] found that patients typically regained approximately two-thirds of normal active motion, the best results being seen in patients with osteoarthritis.

Each patient's program of rehabilitation should be individually designed, with goals modified according to the soft tissue constraints of both the involved shoulder and other joints, such as the elbow and hands. Patients should un-

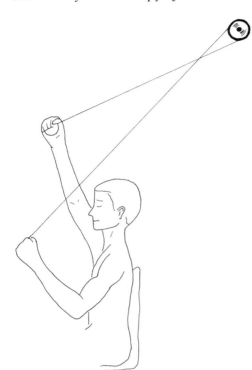

Fig. 15-6.   Patient demonstrating the use of an over-the-door shoulder pulley for elevation of more than 90°.

derstand that once the early phases of rehabilitation have been completed, a maintenance program is to be followed. This allows for small gains in mobility and strength once progress has plateaued.

Short-term complications, which include excessive pain and swelling, require modifications of exercise schedules and external treatments of ice and heat. Long-term complications, such as infection or prosthetic loosening, can be addressed by the surgeon as they occur.

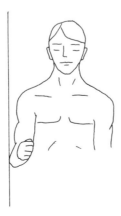

Fig. 15-7.   Middle deltoid strengthening with isometric exercise.

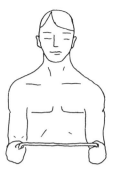

Fig. 15-8. Isolation of external rotators with use of rubber tubing.

Total shoulder replacement is considered a success when the goals for relief of pain and increase in function are achieved. Expectations of a return to normal strength and motion may not be realistic. Finally, functional activities and life-styles must be modified to the patient's benefit following surgery (Fig. 15-9).

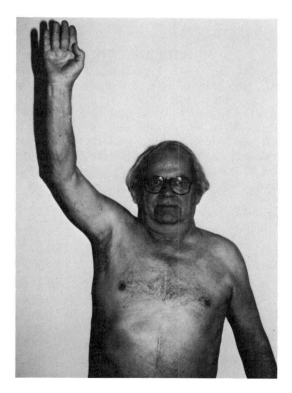

Fig. 15-9. Successfully rehabilitated patient following total shoulder replacement with unconstrained prosthesis.

SUMMARY

The two types of TSR prostheses currently in use are the constrained and unconstrained; the one predominantly used is the unconstrained prosthesis. Thorough evaluation of arm strength, functional needs, and patient expectations must be made prior to determination of prosthetic type for the patient's surgery. With the constrained prosthesis, preoperative muscle loss of the shoulder is usually more severe. Relief of pain and increases in function following surgery are gratifying for the patient. However, because of the increase in muscle involvement, active overhead motion is often not possible. Patients with constrained prostheses should avoid repeated stress of the shoulder to prevent loosening.

With the unconstrained prosthesis, a return to near-normal motion and function can be expected following stretching and strengthening exercises. With this type of prosthesis, the reconstruction and rehabilitation of the muscle is of utmost importance. Relief of pain and improvement of functional activities have been consistently achieved. Because the anatomy remains near normal with the unconstrained prosthesis, it is felt that motion, function, and prosthetic endurance will be superior to the constrained prosthetic device. This is probably the reason for the wider use of the unconstrained total shoulder prosthesis.

REFERENCES

1. Post M, Jablon M, Miller H, Singh M: Constrained total shoulder joint replacement: a critical review. Clin Orthop 144:135, 1979
2. Neer CS, Watson LD, Stanton FJ: Recent experience in total shoulder replacement. J Bone Joint Surg 64-A:319, 1982
3. Cofield RH: Total joint arthroplasty: the shoulder. Mayo Clin Proc 54:500, 1979
4. Cofield RH: Unconstrained total shoulder prostheses. Clin Orthop 173:97, 1983
5. Poppen K, Walker N, Peter S: Normal and abnormal motion of the shoulder. J Bone Joint Surg 58-A:195, 1976
6. Neer CS: Arthroplasty of the shoulder: Neer technique. 3M, St. Paul
7. Clayton ML, Ferlic DC, Jeffers PD: Prosthetic arthroplasties of the shoulder. Clin Orthop 164:184, 1982

16 | Arthroscopic Surgery of the Shoulder

Joseph S. Wilkes

Arthroscopy of the shoulder and adjacent subacromial bursa is proving to be as valuable as arthroscopic surgery of the knee. The practical application of shoulder arthroscopy is only a recent development, even though the first shoulder arthroscopy was performed approximately 50 years ago on cadavers.[1] The development of shoulder arthroscopy has been a natural consequence from arthroscopy of the knee and the greater ease of taking care of some intra-articular pathology by arthroscopic methods. Arthroscopy of the shoulder was developed out of the need for more specific documentation of diagnoses in an otherwise imperfect labeling of painful syndromes of the shoulder despite adequate physical and radiographic examinations. Naturally, operative procedures have developed for simplification of shoulder surgery. The more extensive arthroscopic procedures, specifically rotator cuff repairs and stabilizations, have yet to pass the test of time for satisfactory results, although the initial results from the more recent procedures are certainly promising.[2,3]

INDICATIONS

The most frequent indication for arthroscopic surgery of the shoulder is diagnostic examination. Etiologies for unexplained pain or disability of the shoulder can be elucidated through diagnostic examination of the shoulder with the arthroscope. Also useful is the confirmation of clinically suspected lesions. Even though these lesions are unable to be corrected arthroscopically, they can be definitely identified and a clinical course of treatment can be planned. Some problems that can be evaluated by diagnostic arthroscopy are capsulitis, tendonitis, degenerative changes and/or chondromalacia, and impingement. Also, postsurgical problems with the shoulder sometimes can be brought to light through arthroscopic examination.[4]

The other major indication for shoulder arthroscopy is operative arthroscopy; there are presently many problems that can be solved or minimized through operative arthroscopy of the shoulder. One of the more beneficial indications with very good results is removal of loose bodies, whether from synovial chondromatosis or traumatic or degenerative lesions.[3,4]

Synovectomy of the glenohumeral joint for chronic or acute synovitis can be well accomplished with shoulder arthroscopy. This can be important in reducing pain and dysfunction in patients with rheumatoid, traumatic, or degenerative arthritis and also in patients with inflammatory synovitis. The procedure performed through the arthroscope allows access to all compartments of the glenohumeral joint without extensive surgical exposure, as would be necessary through an open approach. This allows for early motion and less time to return to full function.

A symptomatic torn glenoid labrum has become a more common indication for shoulder surgery because of its ease of access through arthroscopic surgery.[3–5] Previously, only severely debilitating tears of the anterior labrum or symptomatic labral tears in high-level throwing or racquet-using atheletes were considered for surgery.[6] This is a common lesion in athletes involved in all throwing and racquet sports as well as in some occupations, especially with overhead activities. The anterior labrum is the most common area to be torn, and tears of the anterior superior labrum can be addressed by debridement. Tears of the anterior inferior labrum may represent an instability pattern, and attention should be addressed to this area rather than addressing only the labral tear.[4]

The determination of instability can be elusive no matter what the method of evaluation, but there are some typical pathologic findings with arthroscopic evaluation. In anterior instability, the inferior one-half of the anterior labrum is separated from the glenoid margin, thereby allowing the inferior and, occasionally, the middle glenohumeral ligaments to be lax. Also, a frank stretching of the capsule can be identified, allowing subluxation and/or dislocation of the humeral head. Diagnostic evaluation in these instances confirms evidence of subluxation or dislocation and also identifies the instability pattern and the type of repair that may be most effective.[3,4] Bankert lesions can readily be identified by arthroscopy. There are several types of capsulorrhaphy being performed in an arthroscopically assisted method. All of these are being currently evaluated for effectiveness as opposed to open procedures.[2,7]

Until recently, arthroscopic evaluation of rotator cuff tears had been a diagnostic procedure for confirmation of pathology. The gentle debridement of rotator cuff tears can bring about a lessening of discomfort and, thereby, sometimes allows increasing function. Also, techniques for arthroscopically assisted repairs of relatively small rotator cuff tears have seen some success.

Impingement syndrome, which is an irritation of the supraspinatus tendon and/or subacromial bursa from various causes, can be an indication for shoulder arthroscopy. Investigation of the subacromial bursa by arthroscopy can confirm subacromial bursitis and rotator cuff irritation, and can frequently help in the determination of the grade of tendonitis in the supraspinatus tendon. If there appears to be abrasion of the supraspinatus tendon from the subacromial bursal surface, coracoacromial decompression with release of the coracoacromial ligament and partial debridement of the undersurface of the acromion can relieve symptoms in this area.[3,4,8]

Some less common indications for shoulder arthroscopy might be in adhesive capsulitis, with evaluation of the glenohumeral joint and capsular distention before manipulation. Also, evaluation and sometimes debridement of unresponsive bicipital tendonitis can be helpful. The debridement of chondromalacia of the glenoid or humeral surface can be helpful in relieving symptoms. The evaluation of postoperative persistent problems can be valuable because the diagnostic tests are frequently less accurate after surgical intervention and are hard to interpret; therefore, diagnostic arthroscopy and, sometimes, corrective arthroscopy can be performed for postoperative pain problems.[3,4,5] Although rare, osteochondritis dissecans of the humeral head can be evaluated by arthroscopy, and debridement of the lesion can frequently relieve the pain it causes.[4,9] It may also be possible that early stages of osteochondritis dissecans could be percutaneously drilled and pinned by arthroscopically assisted methods.

SURGICAL TECHNIQUE

Shoulder arthroscopy is performed under general anesthesia with the patient in the lateral decubitus position (Fig. 16-1) or occasionally in the supine, semisitting position. When in the lateral position, the shoulder to be operated on is placed in the abducted, slightly flexed position, with the arm in a gently distracting apparatus. After preparing and draping the patient, the bony landmarks are palpated about the shoulder, identifying the coracoid process, the acromioclavicular joint, the lateral tip of the acromion, and the posterior lip of the acromion (Fig. 16-2A). With a finger on the coracoid process, a posterior portal is identified in line with the glenohumeral joint approximately 1.5 cm inferior to the acromion and medial to the tip. An 18-gauge needle is then inserted through this site to ensure good alignment with the glenohumeral joint and to inflate the glenohumeral joint with saline (Fig. 16-2B). The arthroscope is then introduced through this portal after a small stab wound incision is made. Through this portal, the glenohumeral joint usually can be inspected in its entirety.

Accessory portals are frequently needed for inflow and working instruments. For the glenohumeral joint, the most common accessory portals are one or more anterior portals between the subscapularis and supraspinatus medial or lateral to the biceps tendon. Another accessory portal is identified coming through the supraspinatus muscle mass medial to the acromion, between the acromion and the clavicle.

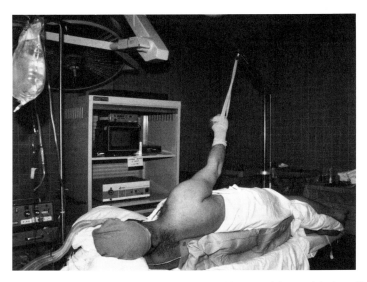

Fig. 16-1. The patient is placed in the lateral decubitus position, with the affected arm abducted between 45° and 60° and flexed anteriorly 15° to 20°. The arthroscopic cabinet for the instruments and the viewing screen are placed on the anterior aspect of the patient, with the surgeon generally standing in the posterior aspect.

For visualization of the subacromial bursa and the coracoacromial ligament, the posterior portal for the arthroscope usually can be used with reinsertion into the subacromial bursa. Likewise, the anterior portal is usually just lateral to the coracoacromial ligament and can be used from an anterior approach. If a third portal is needed, a puncture just lateral to the tip of the acromion through the deltoid muscle provides good access to the subacromial space. Because of the deltoid muscle, the portals for shoulder arthroscopy are not as readily reentered as the arthroscopic knee portals. To avoid problems with reinsertion, cannulas used with instruments are placed in the shoulder spaces and, when moving from one portal to another, switching sticks, which are rods placed from one portal to another through the cannulas, can be used to maintain these portals.

ARTHROSCOPIC ANATOMY

From the posterior portal in the glenohumeral joint, the biceps tendon is readily visualized and is used as an orientation landmark during the arthroscopy. The tendon can be visualized from its entrance at the bicipital groove to its insertion on the glenoid tubercle. The anterior labrum courses from the glenoid tubercle anteriorly and inferiorly on the anterior rim of the glenoid (Fig. 16-3A). The glenoid surface can be visualized at this time, determining the

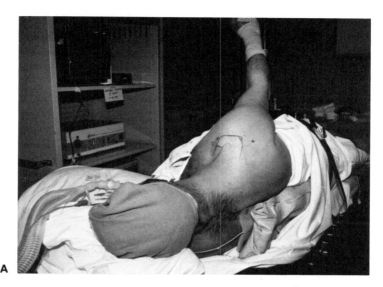

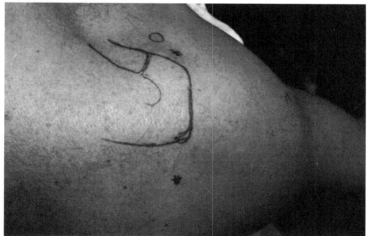

Fig. 16-2. (A) The landmarks for entering the shoulder arthroscopically are the acromioclavicular joint and the coracoid process, seen outlined here. The anterior and posterior portals are drawn as black dots. (**B**) A closer view of the anatomic landmarks for the anterior and posterior portal. The posterior portal orientation is to enter posteriorly and aim anteriorly and medially approximately 25° toward the coracoid process. The anterior portal is just lateral to the line between the coracoid process and the acromion. Both of these portals can be used secondarily for arthroscopic approaches to the subacromial bursa.

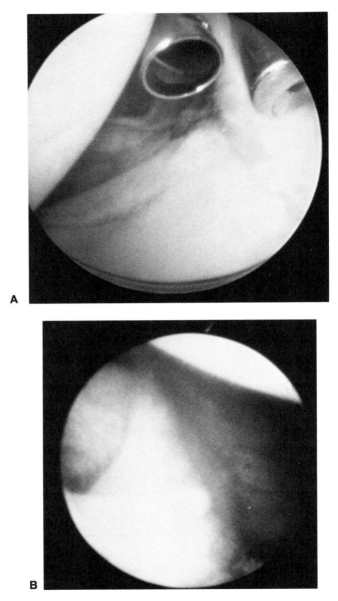

Fig. 16-3. **(A)** To the upper left is the humeral head. Between the two metallic instruments is the biceps tendon; the anterior labrum is seen coursing from the attachment of the biceps tendon along the anterior glenoid, and the surface of the glenoid is shown toward the bottom of the figure. **(B)** Anteriorly and inferiorly is the inferior glenohumeral ligament coursing away from the anterior glenoid labrum. The humeral head is at the upper right. (*Figure continues.*)

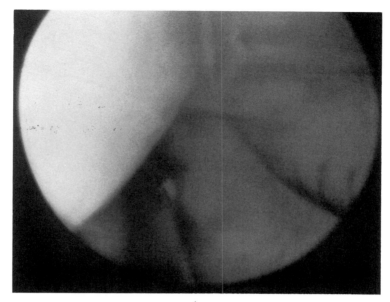

C

Fig. 16-3 *(Continued).* **(C)** The rotator cuff attaches to a ridge along the humeral head at the greater tuberosity, seen here at approximately the 12-o'clock position with the rotator cuff coursing to the right and the humeral head seen at the upper left.

integrity of the cartilage surface. The anterior labrum can be probed and its integrity established. Just superior to the biceps tendon is the superior glenohumeral ligament, which is frequently difficult to visualize. Inferiorly on the anterior surface of the capsule, the subscapularis bursa is identified and the subscapularis tendon can be seen crossing the front of the capsule. The middle glenohumeral ligament courses obliquely across the subscapularis tendon and inserts in the capsule at the glenoid neck in a variable position. Moving further inferiorly, the inferior glenohumeral ligament can be seen arising from the dimple in the anterior glenoid surface, which is approximately one-half of the distance from the glenoid tubercle to the inferior lip, and it courses inferiorly and anteriorly around the humeral head (Fig. 16-3B). Inferior to this is the inferior recess, which can be identified by the large, spacious area inferior to the humeral head; frequently, a posterior–inferior glenohumeral ligament can be identified that mirrors the position of the anterior–inferior glenohumeral ligament posteriorly. The inferior and posterior glenoid labrum can be seen and probed. Coursing back superiorly, the undersurface of the rotator cuff, specifically the supraspinatus, can be identified as it sweeps over the superior humeral head and inserts into the greater tuberosity (Fig. 16-3C). The humeral surface can be identified and, with rotation of the arm, the entire humeral surface generally can be seen.[4,5,10]

In visualizing the subacromial bursa from the posterior aspect, the coracoacromial ligament can generally be seen coursing from superior to anterior

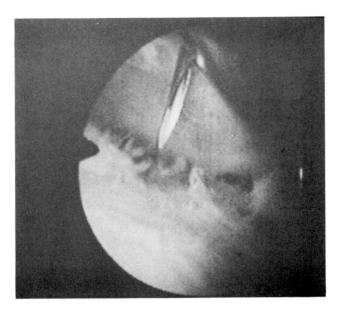

Fig. 16-4.   The needle has been placed into the subacromial bursa just anterior to the acromial clavicular joint. Just inferior to the needle, the superior surface of the rotator cuff can be seen.

away from the arthroscope. If this is not readily available as a landmark, a needle passed through or just anterior to the acromioclavicular joint allows for orientation. The coracoacromial ligament can be seen underneath the acromion as it attaches. The inferior capsule of the acromioclavicular joint can be identified. The superior surface of the rotator cuff can be seen and probed and its attachment to the greater tuberosity inspected. At this point, surgical arthroscopy can be performed to correct identified problems (Fig. 16-4).

SURGICAL PROCEDURE

Synovectomy

Inpatients with rheumatoid arthritis, severe synovitis, degenerative changes, and inflammatory arthropathy can be significantly helped by synovectomy. Previously, synovectomy of the shoulder was performed through an open procedure and was a major operation for the patient and surgeon. Through the arthroscope, synovectomy can be performed with relative ease. A small amount of epinephrine and anesthetic can control postoperative pain and bleeding fairly well. This allows for early postoperative range of motion and an overall decrease in recovery time.

Loose Bodies

The arthroscopic removal of loose bodies in shoulders with locking- or catching-type symptoms from mobile loose bodies has been extremely helpful. There is a minimum of time away from normal activities. This, as well as the majority of arthroscopic shoulder procedures, is done on an outpatient basis.

Chondroplasty

With loose bodies, chondral lesions frequently will be found in the glenohumeral joint. Also, with degenerative changes of the joint, chondral lesions can be identified. If these lesions are thought to represent significant pathology associated with pain or dysfunction or would contribute to significant future dysfunction, a chondral shaving or abrasion type chondroplasty can be performed. Again, this is fairly straightforward in the shoulder joint and is performed on an outpatient basis.

Labral Lesions

Labral tears are very common.[11] A current indication for operative shoulder arthroscopy is a symptomatic labral tear (Fig. 16-5). These tears are easily identified during diagnostic shoulder arthroscopy and, with intra-articular knives and motorized instruments, the labral lesions not representing instability patterns can be easily debrided. This allows for a reduction in the symptoms and an increase in function.

Bicipital Tendonitis Rupture

In bicipital tendonitis of a chronic nature, arthroscopic debridement of the involved portion of the tendon can be helpful in allowing symptoms to subside. If the biceps tendon has ruptured, there is frequently a stump remaining in the intrascapular area that causes popping and painful catching symptoms. This can be debrided through arthroscopic methods.

Rotator Cuff Lesions

The rotator cuff and, specifically, the supraspinatus tendon can be visualized adequately on the undersurface through arthroscopy of the glenohumeral joint or on the superior surface through arthroscopy of the subacromial bursa (Fig. 16-6). For partial tears or incomplete tears of the rotator cuff, the lesions can be identified, and it has been found that debridement of the margins of the partial tear can be helpful in stimulating more effective healing response and

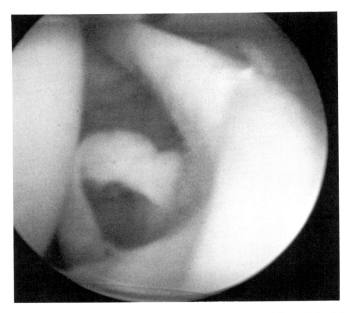

Fig. 16-5. Torn anterior labrum: the humeral head is to the left and the biceps tendon is to the upper right; between them is the loop of torn anterior labrum.

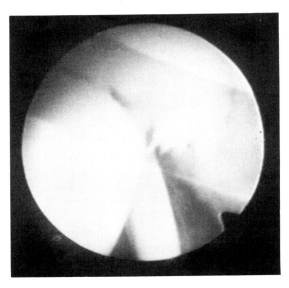

Fig. 16-6. The tear in the rotator cuff is seen as the fraying, just as the rotator cuff attaches to the humeral head.

allows for reduction in symptoms. In situations in which there is a large, irreparable tear of the rotator cuff, painful use of the shoulder is frequently incapacitating. Debridement of the margins of the torn rotator cuff has been found to relieve the pain, at least in some cases, but does not allow for increase in function. The smaller, complete tears of the rotator cuff are more difficult to deal with arthroscopically, and methods are currently being developed and undergoing trials that involve an arthroscopically assisted rotator cuff repair.

Calcific tendonitis of the rotator cuff is not an infrequent finding. For resistant calcific tendonitis, arthroscopic examination and debridement of the calcific deposit has been found to be extremely beneficial.

Instabilities

The most common type of instability in the shoulder is anterior–inferior, with incompetence of the anterior–inferior glenohumeral ligament. This is the type of instability that is most readily addressed by arthroscopically assisted methods. During arthroscopic examination of the shoulder, incompetence of the anterior–inferior glenohumeral ligaments can be identified.[4] Through arthroscopically assisted methods, a staple or suturing technique can be used to repair the ligament and capsule anteriorly.[4,7] These methods are being used on a widespread basis, but are still in a trial state. The long-term results are not yet available. Posterior, inferior, and global instabilities are more difficult to deal with adequately by arthroscopically assisted methods.

Subacromial Pathology

The subacromial space can be easily reached while doing shoulder arthroscopy from the same posterior portal with redirection. In cases of persistent or unrelieved subacromial bursitis, subacromial bursectomy can be helpful. In these cases, grade I or II impingement lesions can be frequently identified on the supraspinatus tendon. If impingement syndrome has been a prominent feature of the symptoms in these patients, coracoacromial decompression with resection of the coracoacromial ligament and debridement of the inferior portion of the acromion can be helpful in relieving these symptoms. In this procedure, the ligament is transected and debrided and the inferior acromion on the anterior aspect is resected approximately 3 mm anteriorly and is beveled posteriorly for approximately 1 cm. This procedure effectively accomplishes the same decompression as an open Neer acromioplasty,[8] allowing for decompression of the rotator cuff and, specifically, the supraspinatus tendon to give freer movement without pressure on the tendon, thereby relieving symptoms and abrasion of the tendon.

POSTSURGICAL TREATMENT

Postoperatively, the majority of arthroscopic shoulder procedures use rest and ice for the first 24 to 48 hours to allow for decrease in inflammation resulting from instrumentation of the joint. In procedures for diagnosis or debridement, motion and exercises may begin as soon as the patient can tolerate them and progress to normal function. At approximately 36 hours, the large bandage used to soak up early postoperative drainage is changed, bandages are applied to the wounds, and the patient is allowed to shower. Very vigorous and heavy activities are avoided for a minimum of 2 weeks. For procedures requiring repair, such as rotator cuff or stabilization procedures, 3 to 4 weeks of relative immobilization are necessary to allow for a biologic healing response to reduce the incidence of recurrent lesions. Subsequently, rehabilitation is undertaken for regaining motion, strength, and function.

Overall, the response to arthroscopic surgical procedures has shown a dramatic decrease in the amount of dysfunctional time for the majority of surgical procedures associated with arthroscopy as opposed to open procedures.[4] Although the final study results are not available on the arthroscopically assisted repairs of the rotator cuff and stabilization, it appears that these procedures are effective, with less postoperative pain, lessened hospitalization, and a shorter rehabilitation time due to the decreased amount of dysfunction in the muscles, as opposed to open procedures.

SUMMARY

Arthroscopic surgery of the shoulder has developed much like that of the knee and has resulted in the development of many surgical procedures that sometimes can be performed more effectively, or at least with less morbidity, than with open procedures. The return to function appears to be faster, and the visualization of the glenohumeral joint as well as the subacromial bursa is more complete and less traumatic than after an open arthrotomy.

One must always be cognizant of the possible problems and complications associated with any procedure. A general anesthetic can be associated with problems in any procedure. Infection also can be a problem, although due to the minimum exposure and operative time of this procedure, this has not been a major problem. The shoulder joint is not as anatomically well defined on the surface as the knee; therefore, one must be extremely careful in placing the portals to avoid damage to the neural and vascular structures. Overall, the complication rate in shoulder, arthroscopy is very low, and the benefits appear to be very promising.

Expectations for the future include more defined procedures for arthroscopically assisted rotator cuff repairs and stabilizations, for anterior instabilities as well as for posterior and inferior instabilities. The development of lasers for use in the shoulder is currently undergoing experimentation with the hope that they will prove to be beneficial in arthroscopic shoulder procedures.

REFERENCES

1. Burmon MS: Arthroscopy or direct visualization of joints: an experimental cadaver study. J Bone Joint Surg 13:669, 1931
2. Rockwood CA, Jr: Shoulder arthroscopy. J Bone Joint Surg 70-A:639, 1988
3. Sisk TD: Arthroscopy of shoulder and elbow in Campbell's operation. p. 2609. In Crenshaw AH (ed): Orthopedics. 7th Ed. CV Mosby, St. Louis, 1987
4. Johnson LL: Arthroscopic Surgery: Principles and Practice. 3rd Ed. CV Mosby, St. Louis, 1986
5. Wilkes JS, Andrews JR: Arthroscopic Surgery in Throwing Athletes. AOSSM Annual Meeting. Lake Tahoe, NV, 1981
6. McMaster WC: Anterior glenoid labrum damage: a painful lesion in swimmers. Am J Sports Med 14:383, 1986
7. Gross RM: Arthroscopic shoulder capsulorraphy: does it work? Am J Sports Med 17:495, 1989
8. Gartsman GM, Blair ME Jr, Noble PC, et al: Arthroscopic subacromial decompression: an anatomical study. Am J Sports Med 16:48, 1988
9. Ishihawe H, Ueba Y, Yonezawa T, et al: Osteochondritis dissecans of the shoulder in a tennis player. Am J Sports Med 16:547, 1988
10. Andrews JR, Carson WG, Ortega K: Arthroscopy of the shoulder: technique and normal anatomy. Am J Sports Med 12:1, 1984
11. DePalma AF: The unstable shoulder. p. 415. Surgery of the Shoulder. 2nd Ed. JB Lippincott, Philadelphia, 1973

APPENDIX

Biomechanical Factors in Overuse Dysfunction

Robert A. Donatelli

BIOMECHANICAL FACTORS

Impingement syndrome, rotator cuff tears, and frozen shoulder are three overuse injuries to the shoulder that can be related to abnormal biomechanical factors.

Predisposing Overuse Injury to the Shoulder

- Repetitive movement producing muscle fatigue of the rotator cuff muscles
- A single incident of overuse causing fatigue (e.g., unconditioned muscles are asked to perform several hours of a sporting event or a work-related activity)
- Fatigue of a muscle places increased stress on the musculotendinous junction, the weakest part of the muscle and the part most susceptible to injury
- Muscle strain to the rotator cuff muscles, causing a trigger point and weakness of the muscles and/or one of the rotators

- Weakness of the rotator cuff reduces the stabilizing and compressive forces to the glenohumeral joint
- Deltoid muscle group produces excessive shearing forces to the glenohumeral joint, causing instability

Precipitating Factors in Overuse to the Shoulder

- Increased shearing forces to the glenohumeral joint produce an *impingement of glenohumeral structures* under the acromial arch (e.g., bursitis-tendonitis)
- Patient reports pain with overhead activities; continued irritation of glenohumeral structures and inflammation

Perpetuating Factors in Overuse to the Shoulder

Patient will either
A. Immobilize the limb resulting in
    Connective tissue changes
    Reduced GAG
    Poor collagen fiber alignment
    Pain and immobilization continues; the end result will be *frozen shoulder*
OR
B. Continue to use the limb resulting in
    Continued pain and inflammation
    Compensatory movement patterns of the shoulder

Compensatory movement patterns of the shoulder
- Continued abnormal stress to the musculotendinous junction of the rotator cuff muscles
- Pain and weakness of the rotators causing greater impingement of glenohumeral structures, secondary to overpowering deltoid muscle

Possible pathologies secondary to abnormal mechanics as noted above.
- *Rotator cuff tear*
- Labrum tear
- Spur formation under the acromion process—mechanical irritation to the glenohumeral structures within the acromial arch
- Immobilization secondary to pain–connective tissue changes—*frozen shoulder*

ASSESSMENT OF BIOMECHANICAL DYSFUNCTION

Active Range of Motion

- Glenohumeral joint motion restricted in elevation and external rotation
- External rotation limited in the adduction position, indicating dysfunction of the subscapularis

- External rotation limited at 45° of abduction, indicating dysfunction of the glenohumeral ligament and capsule, in addition to subscapularis
- Scapula mobility excessive in elevation and abduction; a prominent lateral border of the scapula with elevation, just below the axilla area
- Scapula hypermobility secondary to muscle imbalance of the scapula force couple

Passive Range of Motion

- External rotation limited in the adducted position, in the 45° abduction position, and the 90° position, with an abnormal soft-tissue end feel
- Scapula distraction, limited, secondary to muscle tightness of the levator/upper trapezius muscles and subscapularis
- A/C and S/C joint mobility reduced secondary to limited clavicular elevation and rotation

Palpation

- Trigger points within the
    Subscapularis
    Latissimus
    Teres Major
    Clavicular portion of the pectoralis major
    Belly of the supraspinatus
    Levator scapularis and upper trapezius muscles
- Tendon damage of the supraspinatus

Muscle Strength Testing

- Isokinetic strength testing of the rotator cuff muscles
- Normal ratio of the rotators: External rotators are .6–.7 of the internal rotators when the test is performed at 45° of abduction or in the plane of the scapula.

TREATMENT OF BIOMECHANICAL DYSFUNCTION

- Continuous passive stretching of the tight internal rotators in the plane of the scapula
- Soft tissue mobilization of the restricted soft tissue structures and muscular trigger points
- Mobilization of the glenohumeral capsule, anterior and inferior techniques
    - Scapula distraction techniques to

1) Stretch subscapularis by distraction of the vertebral border of the scapula in the sidelying position
2) Promote clavicular elevation at the A/C joint and rotation at the S/C, by distraction and rotation of the inferior angle of the scapula in the sidelying position
3) Stretch the levator scapulae by a rotation distraction of the scapula in the sidelying position

- Muscle strengthening of the rotator cuff muscles
    - Strengthening of the rotators in the plane of the scapula using isokinetics
    - Diagonal patterns for strengthening functional movements of the shoulder on an isokinetic device
    - PNF patterns
    - Home programs

Index

Page numbers followed by f indicate figures; page numbers followed by t indicate tables.